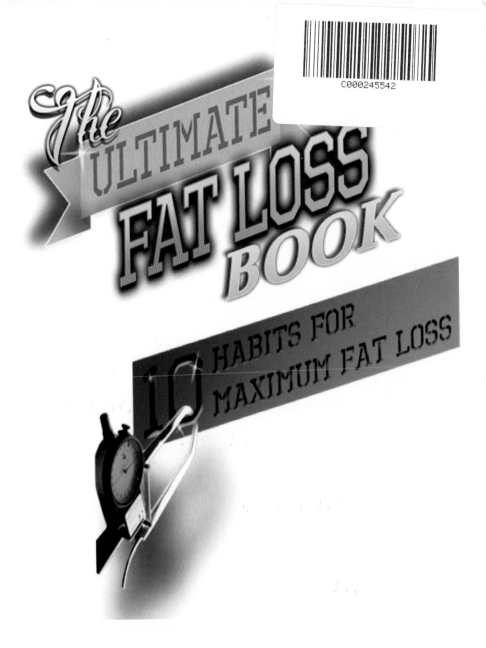

The **ULTIMATE FAT LOSS BOOK**

10 HABITS FOR MAXIMUM FAT LOSS

Phil Richards

Published by Phil Richards Performance

A catalogue record for this book is available from the British Library.

ISBN 978-0-9927227-0-8

Published by Phil Richards Performance

For more copies of this book, please email: enquiries@philrichardsperformance.co.uk Tel: 01639 861593

Designed and Set by SWATT Design Ltd
Eastleigh, SO50 4NP

Printed Tyson Press
Chester, CH4 9QR | London, W1d 2EU

THE ULTIMATE FAT LOSS MANUAL

10 HABITS FOR MAXIMUM FAT LOSS

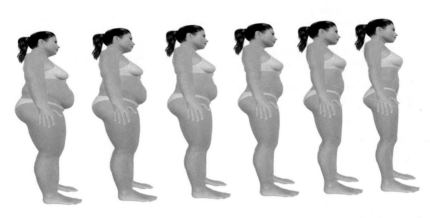

"Please let me take this opportunity to say thank you for purchasing "10 Habits for Maximum Fat Loss", which, in reality, is also 10 habits for maximum health. Remember, without health you simply won't have safe, effective and long term fat loss.

I was personally overweight for many years and feel that this has given me a much greater insight on the difficulties on losing weight. I have always been fanatical about fitness and nutrition but, after my research, I realised that what was making me fat was not a lack of exercise or what I ate. In my case, it was stress and toxicity.

I've had the privilege for the last several years of being able carry out full time research into nutrition and conditioning strategies for health, fat loss and performance. This is on the back of working as a head strength, nutrition & conditioning coach in professional rugby for 10 years where, in my last year in professional sport, I also worked as a consultant to three professional teams, at Premiership level, in three different sports, as a full time fat loss expert.

The information I gathered over a period of time whilst working in professional sport is quite literally astonishing. For example I saw professional players train up to 8-12 times per week, play Premiership rugby/soccer and still gain body fat as they didn't control the stress in their lives. This helped me learn that one of the most important things to enhance fat loss is emotional health. After emotional health you need a well functioning detoxification system. I don't care how much you train, you will usually get fatter in the long term without a detoxification plan and good emotional stability. These have a detrimental effect on our body's ability to lose fat as you will find out in the upcoming habits.

The way that most people today attack fat loss is a bit like pushing an elephant up a hill - it becomes very difficult to shift the fat. The information presented in this Ultimate Fat Loss Manual will hopefully give you the right information to lose fat safely, effectively and for the long-term. There are no gimmicks in this manual, it is based on my extensive experience and hardcore scientific facts. Trust

...ck-fix measures on how to lose fat - it simply boils down to the 10 habits presented

me, ion in the 10 habits is what I have found worked for me over many years as a professional in ...onditioning and nutrition coach, working with thousands of professional athletes. The 10 ...have arisen from giving countless lectures and seminars over the years to elite sports teams and ...e trainers. This is one of the reasons why it is written in the bullet point style which may appear ...en to some. The other reason why I chose to write the manual in this way, and why I have included so many pictures, is because I wanted to make this manual easy to read, simple to follow and appealing to the eye.

Everyone has strong opinions on nutrition, exercise and lifestyle and I can only share with you what I learnt on my journey as a coach and am still learning to this day.

In writing this manual I have taken a Bruce Lee approach; reading and drawing from the knowledge out there and then using what I feel works and then creating my own style. I have read many books, articles and journals over the years as part of the research from this manual and have drawn knowledge from some of the best minds in the field of health, fitness and fat loss. In this manual I have tried to give credit to all sources, where possible. However, due to the extent of the research that I have undertaken I am sure you can appreciate that it may not have always been possible to track down original sources, although I have strived to do so.

Please enjoy the manual. If you do, please share it with as many people who you think will benefit from the information it contains."

Phil Richards

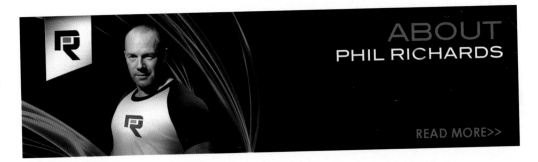

Amongst professional athletes, Phil Richards is regarded as one of the leading strength, conditioning and nutrition experts in the world. He has prepared professional boxers for title fights, led premiership rugby teams to league titles & cup finals and transformed the careers of professional athletes in many sports and disciplines.

Phil regularly lectures and consults for elite athletes and teams as well as running workshops and seminars based on the principles and knowledge he has gained over a 25 year career of working with some of the World's leading experts in his field. Having studied with figures such as Louie Simmons (Westside Barbell), Dr Eric Serrano (Leading Hormonal Expert) and the late great Charlie Francis (Speed Coach), Phil has probably interned with more experts in the field of strength, conditioning and nutrition than any other coach in the world. Phil also holds various qualifications in nutrition and is also an advanced cellular nutritional microscopist. Phil is also Europe's first Westside Barbell Certified Strength Coach which is like the Phd in the strength training world.

> "PHIL RICHARDS IS ONE OF SELECT FEW CHOSEN TO BE AN AMBASSADOR OF THE WESTSIDE BARBELL SYSTEM IN EUROPE. THROUGH HIS MULTIPLE INTERNSHIPS, SPORTING SUCCESS AND SEMINARS HE HAS CLEARLY SHOWN A HIGH LEVEL OF COMPETENCY IN TEACHING THE WESTSIDE METHODS. PHIL ALSO BRINGS A NEW DIMENSION TO THE INDUSTRY WITH HIS REVOLUTIONARY SUPPLEMENTS OF WHICH HAVE GREATLY IMPROVED MY OVERALL HEALTH IN A SHORT SPACE OF TIME. I AM PROUD TO HAVE PHIL RICHARDS TO BE AMONG THE HAND SELECTED WESTSIDE CERTIFIED GYMS AND AMBASSADORS."

LOUIE SIMMONS
WESTSIDE BARBELL

> "I HAVE KNOWN AND WORKED WITH PHIL RICHARDS FOR A NUMBER OF YEARS NOW. DURING THIS TIME I HAVE ALWAYS FOUND HIM TO BE EXTREMELY KNOWLEDGEABLE ON THE SUBJECTS OF TRAINING AND NUTRITION. THOSE FORTUNATE ENOUGH TO HAVE THE OPPORTUNITY TO WORK WITH HIM SHOULD TAKE ADVANTAGE OF IT."

CHARLIE FRANCIS
BEN JOHNSON'S SPRINT COACH

> "PHIL RICHARDS' KNOWLEDGE OF TRAINING AND NUTRITION IS ABOVE THE REST AND HE CAN CORRECT ANY ATHLETE'S WEAKNESS BY APPLYING HIS SUPERB LEVEL OF KNOWLEDGE AND EXPERTISE".

DR ERIC SERRANO
WORLDS LEADING HORMONAL EXPERT

Phil applies this wealth of learning to a no nonsense approach to build health, strength and performance. Throughout Phil's successful career he has worked with and consulted for the 'who's who' in world sport including; Amir Kahn (World Champion Boxer), Worcester Warriors (Professional Rugby), London Harlequins (Professional Rugby), Swansea RFC (Professional Rugby), Leicester Tigers, (Professional Rugby), Wigan Warriors (Rugby League), Hull FC (Rugby League), Bolton Wanderers

(Professional Football), Glenn Ross (World Masters Strongest Man), Nick Dunn (World Triathlon Champion), Stuart Stokes (Olympian Steeplechaser) and many, many more. Phil Richards has dedicated his life to finding out exactly what really works in the field of nutrition, strength and conditioning - and his track record is undeniable. Phil gets results!

In 2009, Phil began applying this experience and knowledge into developing a range of nutritional products that would deliver health and performance to athletes and members of the general public alike. Since then, the range has grown to some 20+ products and is now being shipped worldwide to athletes, teams and clients across the globe. These products have been developed for one thing, RE-SULTS. Phil has been meticulous in ensuring every single ingredient in every single product is well sourced and is there only to benefit the product, and therefore the athlete and the general public.

www.philrichardsperformance.co.uk

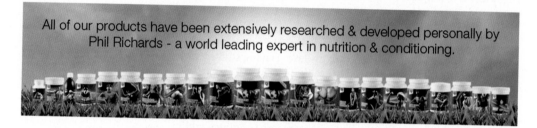

All of our products have been extensively researched & developed personally by Phil Richards - a world leading expert in nutrition & conditioning.

The information in this manual is not meant as medical advice. The training programs, nutrition plans and supplement plans were developed by the author as an adjunct to improved health and fitness. These programs may not be suitable for everyone. All individuals, especially those who suffer from any disease or are recovering from any injury or illness, should seek the advice from a qualified medical professional before making any lifestyle changes. The author has been thorough in his research. However, he is neither responsible nor liable for any harm, injury or illness resulting from any of the information provided in this manual. The views expressed in this manual are that of Phil Richards and not of Phil Richards Performance Ltd.

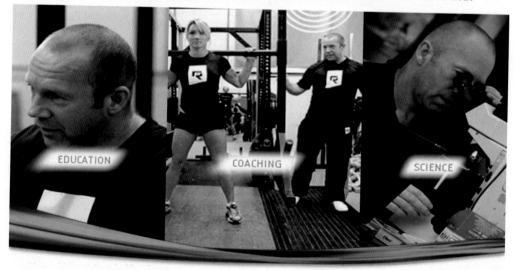

EDUCATION   COACHING   SCIENCE

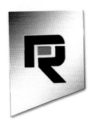

Contents

Contents

I dedicate this book to my best friend and son, Mansel, my beautiful princess, little Ava May, and, also, my Mother, for helping me during my darkest times.

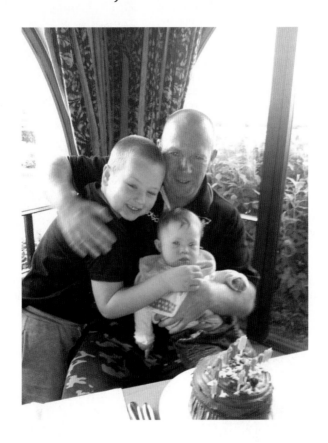

Special mention - this book would not have been written without the help of my research scientist, Jamie Pugh. He has been truly amazing and I am exceptionally grateful for his help in organising the most unorganised man in the world, me, and getting this book to print.

Introduction

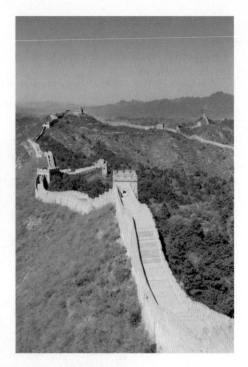

- Let's start this book off with one of my favourite analogies;

- When observing something of true greatness, like the Great Wall of China. Can you imagine the effort and the sacrifice that would have gone into this monumental structure? Imagine looking up at the Great Wall with a group of people. Everyone there is admiring its presence, except for one person who has spotted a damaged brick. They focus their whole attention on that one brick and miss the whole, incredible presence and magnificent architecture of this Great Wall. So, if you see a spellling mitsake, or incorrect gramma in this manual, don't focus on it. Move on and appreciate the content of the book. I want to inform you, that I left school with no formal qualifications.

- In the same way: don't focus on what is wrong in your life, focus on what is right in your life.

- Extract from this book what you need, ignore what you don't. If there is something that you disagree with, then move on. Remember, this book is my opinion and, hopefully, it will help many people, whatever their circumstances, live a happier and healthier life.

- As you read this book, begin to put the pieces of the 10 habits jigsaw in place. Put them in one piece at a time and eventually, when all of the pieces fit together, you will get a leaner, happier and healthier body.

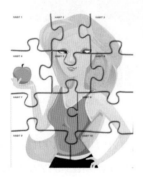
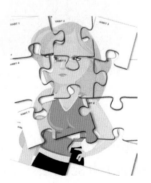

- When you read this book, you could easily become overwhelmed by the number of changes that you feel you may need to make in your life to become lean, happy and healthy. Let me give you another analogy which I have used for many years with my athletes and teams.

Chase one rabbit, and catch it.

Chase two, and you catch nothing!

- Focus in on what is the most important change that you need to make. When you achieve that, move on to the next. For example, after reading the book you might recognise that your breakfast is making you fat and that you need to do more exercise. Spend one week changing your breakfast so that it becomes a habit. Then, the following week, start introducing some exercise. This way you will make changes very gradually and you will get into the habit of living a healthier lifestyle.

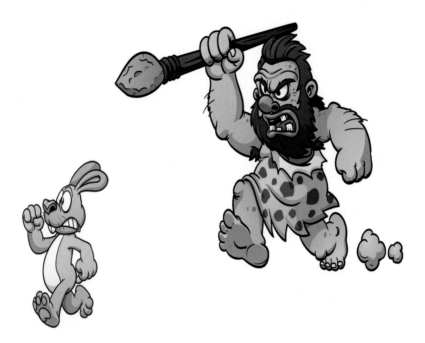

HABIT 1

THE FURTHER WE MOVE AWAY FROM THE NATURE, THE FATTER WE BECOME

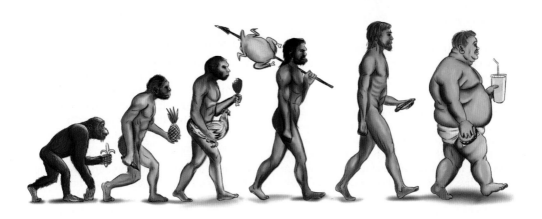

"Since applying everything that I have learnt from Phil during the multiple internships that I have attended with him, I have thrown my microwave out, had all of my amalgam fillings removed, replaced junk foods with organic foods, replaced tap water with filtered water and have benefited massively from Phil's supplements. Since then my health has sky-rocketed and can honestly say that I definitely would not have won UK's strongest man 2008 & 2010 as well as Worlds Masters Strongest Man without the help of Phil. What he has taught me after 20+ years in this business has totally transformed me."

Glenn Ross (UK & World's Masters Strongest Man)

- In this Habit let's look at the multiple ways in which our toxic world is making us sicker, fatter and exhausted.

- Today, in the UK it has been estimated that nearly 2/3s of adults and over 30% of children are over weight or obese.

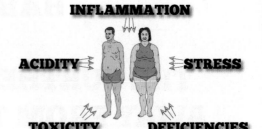

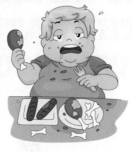

- If you are living in the Western World, look around you and try to spot the vibrantly healthy people who are lean and full of energy. If you see someone happy in our society today you would probably think there is something wrong with them, as we have created a society where smiling is almost frowned upon.

5 causes of us becoming sick and overweight

- We are always being told that we are living longer today than we have ever lived before. That is nonsense. Humans are genetically programmed to live for up to 120-140 years old depending on which research you read and have been for thousands of generations. On average we do live longer only because we don't have the dangers that our ancestors had. But are we healthier? I very much doubt it and the research clearly shows this.

- Ask yourself this question; if we are healthier now than at any other time in human history, why can't you get a car parking spot in any hospital in the UK during the day? Why are we dying on mass from cancer, heart disease & brain diseases in our millions? Remember, you don't catch these diseases, we build them from within when our internal environment becomes polluted from the army of toxins we are exposed to every day from our food, water and environment.

- You need to realise that there is no money in healthy people for the pharmaceutical industry and the junk shit food industry to make their trillions of pounds of profits. You are not supposed to be healthy, it is that simple. Let me spell this out crystal clear, the only cure to disease is prevention.

- Learn to detoxify, nourish yourself with clean water, good food, amazing thoughts and you have a very strong probability of becoming disease-proof. Remember, nature does not program you to become diseased; it wants healthy creatures. Yes of course there is a small exception that are born with genetic difficulties, like my beautiful daughter who has down syndrome. But 95% of us are born to be healthy.

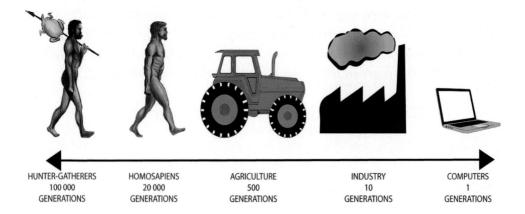

HUNTER-GATHERERS	HOMOSAPIENS	AGRICULTURE	INDUSTRY	COMPUTERS
100 000	20 000	500	10	1
GENERATIONS	GENERATIONS	GENERATIONS	GENERATIONS	GENERATIONS

Our genetic constitution has changed little in 10,000 years its make-up evolved from biological processes eons earlier. Proto-humans evolved about 5 million years ago, began using stone tools 2 million years ago, and ate meat. The staggering flow of time is apparent when we consider generations.

"The diet that made us human is the one that will keep us human. That diet is rich in fruits, vegetables, nuts, seeds, high quality animal protein, especially offal & fish. Our diet has the power to radically improve or impair our health and intelligence. It also has the power to create disease and reduce our IQ. This is known as dumbing down of society."

- There are 5 reasons why we become sick, tired and fat:

  1. TOXICITY
  2. ACIDITY
  3. DEFICIENCIES
  4. INFLAMMATION
  5. STRESS

- If all 5 of these are addressed then it is virtually impossible to be overweight or sick. You must also remember it is 100% impossible to be fat and healthy. Therefore, health should be your priority in losing body fat.

- There are races of people who are all slim, who are stronger and faster than us who have continued the diet of their ancestors. They all have straight teeth and perfect eyesight. Obesity is very rare amongst these people. From the research by Western-Price, it was confirmed that when people moved away from their natural diet, health deteriorated very quickly.

- Weston-Price was a dentist in the early 20th Century who published a book entitled "Nutrition and Physical Degeneration". In the book he described his global travels which he spent studying the diets and nutrition of various cultures. The book concluded that aspects of a modern Western diet (such as flour, sugar, and modern processed vegetable fats) cause nutritional deficiencies that are a cause of many dental issues and health problems.

- These people live by nature's rules and nourishes themselves with unadulterated foods and drinks clean water. They get natural sunlight, are grounded (have a close connection with the earth e.g. barefoot walking) and are not swimming in electro magnetic frequencies. They live as close knit communities who care for each other the strong help the weak. Children are allowed to be children and not manufactured in a system which moulds them how the system wants them to be which is basically to become a tired, overweight TAX payer as is usually the case in our Westernised culture.

- The impact of our environment has been illustrated by a study of Pima Indians. Those living in Arizona have among the highest prevalence of obesity. Despite the similar genetic predisposition, Pima Indians living a traditional lifestyle in a remote section of Mexico have significantly lower levels of body fat. These groups were only separated around 700 years ago.

- 99% of our genetic heritage dates back to before the appearance of humankind. Only 1% of our biological makeup has appeared since human and great ape lines separated some seven million years ago. The point is to reflect upon how little an opportunity there has been to for our body's to adapt to the age of agriculture and our present junk food diet.

- Looking at the scene of human nutrition from this perspective, it is obvious that throughout

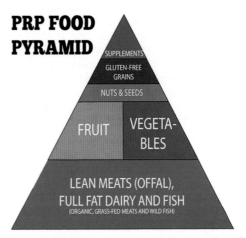

PRP FOOD PYRAMID

SUPPLEMENTS
GLUTEN-FREE GRAINS
NUTS & SEEDS
FRUIT | VEGETABLES
LEAN MEATS (OFFAL), FULL FAT DAIRY AND FISH
(ORGANIC, GRASS-FED MEATS AND WILD FISH)

The diet of our Paleolithic ancestors was one that was made up of fresh, in-season, organic foods. It did not come in a packet and it was not produced in a factory. You must find the right ratios of food from the pyramid to suit your metabolic type. Some get lean on higher carbs, some on higher amounts of protein.

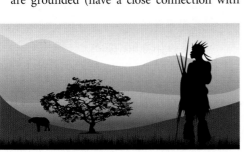

Our ancestors had to be exceptionally fit and healthy to simply survive

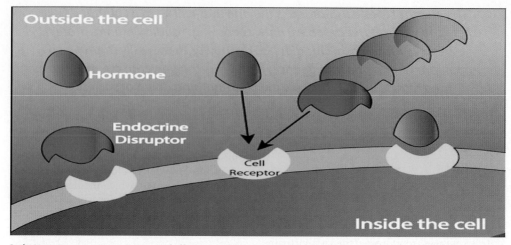

In the 21st century we are swimming in a pool of hormone and mitochondrial disruptors which are literally causing chaos with our ability to think clearly, lose fat efficiently and have plenty of energy for life.

human evolution man relied on wild foods with high nutrient ratio compared to today. Our physiology was initially adapted by, and is still adapted to, wild not modern foods. We spent 99.8% of our existence as a species as hunter-gatherers.

- The fact that our paleolithic diet is far healthier for us than our modern westernised diet comes from archaeological studies of ancient skeletons.

- Studies tell us that the Paleolithic humans were in remarkably good health. Paleolithic humans were tall and slender; cavities and signs of malnutrition or stress in bones were rare, muscle attachments were strong.

- Cambridge University experts say that humans are past their peak and that modern-day people are 10% smaller and shorter than their hunter-gatherer ancestors. And if that's not depressing enough, our brains are also 10% smaller. These findings reverse perceived wisdom that humans have grown taller and larger, a belief which has grown from data on more recent physical development. The decline has happened over the past 10,000 years.

- An average person 10,000 years ago weighed between 12st 8lb and 13st 6lb, with this being made up of much more lean body weight than our more modern, chubby man. Today, the average is between 11st and 12st 8lb. The timing points to the switch from a hunter-gatherer lifestyle to agriculture, which began 10,000 years ago. While farming would have made food plentiful, focussing on a smaller number

of foodstuffs could have caused vitamin and mineral deficiencies that stunted growth.

- The blame has been put on agriculture, with restricted diets and urbanisation compromising health and leading to the spread of disease. The theory has emerged from studies of fossilised human remains found in Africa, Europe and Asia.

Some experts have claimed that brain capacity is actually decreasing due to the reduction of omega 3 consumption, which has been estimated to be as much as 80%.

- In short, the evolution of the human brain is in reverse, our brains are now very slowly shrinking.

What Paleolithic People Did Not Eat
- Cow's milk, cereal grains (introduced after 10 000 BC)
- Table salt (NaCl)
- White sugar (after 1800)
- Potatoes (after 1750)
- Highly processed foods (mostly after 1800)
- Pesticide residues (after 1930), radioactive foods (after 1945)
- Artificial/synthetic additives (mostly after 1950)

- And this trend will continue unless we return to the omega 3 rich brain stimulating diets of our Palaeolithic ancestors.

Feed your genes

- You must remember that the ability to store fat has allowed the human race to survive for millions of years.

- No system is infallible though and unfortunately today we have an abundance of substances that have been artificially added to our water, food, environment and wash care products etc., which keeps us in fat storage mode. And, it doesn't matter how hard you hit the gym you will get fatter or at least the same unless you know how to play the fat loss game today, it is a completely different game to that even 50 years ago!

"The old idea that weight gain is simply a matter of calories in, calories out is falling apart. New evidence proves that weight gain can occur in the absence of excess calorie intake.

For example, in a recent study rats given toxic chemicals gained weight and increased their fat storage without increased caloric intake. In six months, these rats were 20 percent heavier and had 36 percent more body fat than rats unexposed to chemicals."

- It has been estimated that about 80% of the food on the shelves of supermarkets today didn't exist a 100 years ago! If you look at most supermarkets, 80% of the produce in there is

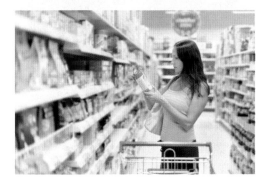

packaged for long life storage. If there is one thing I have learnt as a nutritionist, the quicker a food spoils, the more nutritious it is. You should look to eat food in its natural state.

- If you look at the explosion of gastrointestinal and mental health problems that we face today, there is no doubt that gluten (wheat protein) has become a significant contributor to these health issues.

- For example, recognized world authorities on gluten sensitivity have reported that gluten sensitivity can be primarily and, at times, exclusively a neurological disease. That is, people can manifest gluten sensitivity by having issues with brain function without any gastrointestinal problems whatsoever. The antibodies that a person has when they are gluten sensitive can be directly and uniquely toxic to the brain.

- I believe that the reason for the problems many people face with gluten is not the gluten itself, it is simply that we are eating gluten on an enormous scale that we have not ever been exposed to during our evolution. Most people have not adapted to this. You will see throughout this book the problems that both gluten and casein have on human health.

- If you look at the typical breakfast in the UK, I would estimate that 95% would consist of both gluten and casein (milk protein). This simply would not have been the case even as little as 80 years ago. These 2 proteins can, no doubt, increase your likelihood of becoming overweight.

- An Italian study found that those with a significant allergy to gluten also developed a significant allergy to their own thyroids, which disappeared when the gluten was removed for three to six months.

- Gluten & Casein proteins are known to exert opioid-like effects on the brain. These proteins attach to receptors in the brain. They are nearly identical in structure to natural opioid-binding peptides. (Can have morphine-like effects)

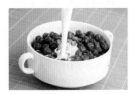

Feeding our children breakfast cereals everyday is a great way to fatten them up for the future

- You must remember that wheat and dairy are very new to the human diet and we are now eating it on a mass scale and it is undoubtedly causing us MULTIPLE HEALTH PROBLEMS both physical and mental.

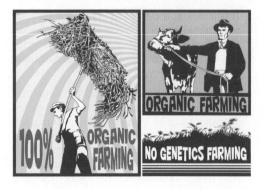

Toxins

- There are two things which can either make us fat, tired and depressed or lean, energised and happy?

- The answer is very simple: hormones (the body's chemical messengers) & mitochondria (cells energy burning furnaces)! When these are not working efficiently they can make us fat, tired and depressed. On the flip side, when they are functioning optimally you will be lean, energised and happy.

- Why is it that two people can eat the same amount of food and yet one gains weight while the other one does not?

- Its METABOLISM. What regulates metabolism? Your HORMONES & MITOCHONDRIA.

- The problem we have today is that the further we move away from nature the less efficient our hormones & mitochondria become and the fatter and more tired we become!

- This is why I can not stress enough, you must stick as close as you can to a natural diet and a natural lifestyle.

- For example, a person whose thyroid gland reduces the production of thyroxine (T4) will experience as much as a 40% drop in metabolism, or basal metabolic rate (the rate at which the body spends energy for maintenance activities). And it doesn't matter how much exercise you do, how much you live off lettuce leaves trying to reduce food intake, you will usually become fatter not to mention exhausted. The point that I am making here is that something as simple as an hormonal problem, like an under-active thyroid, can cause a severe weight gain. I cover hormones & mitochondria in great depth in this book so that you can get them working at full efficiency to enhance health and fat loss.

- Hormones tell your body whether to burn fat or to store fat. They also tell your body either to build muscle or cannibalise muscle. Understanding how to get hormones on your side, if losing fat and gaining lean muscle tissue is your goal, is essential in your ability to lose body fat safely, efficiently and for the long term.

- Most fat utilization occurs in the cell's mitochondria. The greater the number of mitochondria, the more efficient fat utilization will be. Because muscle is the largest mitochondria containing tissue, muscle composition directly effects fat utilization.

- This is why a well structured strength and conditioning program is incredibly important in your quest to be lean and healthy as they can have a positive impact on both of these, if planned correctly.

- Mitochondria are known as the powerhouses of the cell. They are organelles that act like a digestive system that takes in nutrients, breaks them down, and creates energy for the cell. The process of creating cell energy is known as cellular respiration. Most of the chemical reactions involved in cellular respiration happen in the mitochondria

- Endocrine (hormone) disruptors interfere with the way hormones communicate with cells

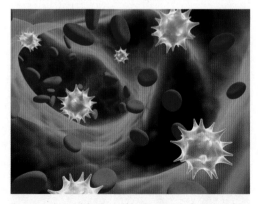

It is now understood that "toxic" blood triggers the formation of new fat cells. This is because the endothelial cells of your circulatory system directly communicates with your baby fat cells and can tell them what to do. Keeping your blood as clean as possible and supporting your liver are vital steps to ensure that this process goes smoothly.

and so can lead to many health disasters. This makes it difficult to lose weight, especially for the long term. Endocrine disruptors are found in many everyday products we use, including: some plastic bottles and containers, tinned foods, detergents, flame retardants, toys, cosmetics, pesticides and many more.

- I first became alerted to the effects that cosmetics can have on my athlete's body fat levels when I was consulting for a number of elite teams. I was researching this subject of endocrine disruptors whilst carrying out around 5000 body composition tests. I became suspicious that, due to the amount of training they were doing on a daily basis which saw them showering 8-12 times a week and using these products which, I found out could increase oestrogen levels. I could see the effect this was having on the players as some of their body fat percentage increased as the season progressed.

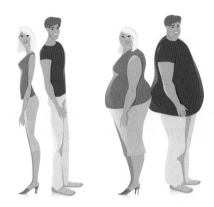

We are always being told that genes control us when, in reality, this is only partially true. Really, perception, nutrition, lifestyle and environment control our genes.

The following study magnifies the simplicity of this concept. Twenty pairs of identical twins who differed by more that 37lbs in weight were studied. The overweight twins had higher levels of stress hormones adrenaline and cortisol and poorer quality sleep, drank more alcohol and had higher levels of perceived stress. There was no difference in their genes only their lifestyles and stress levels.

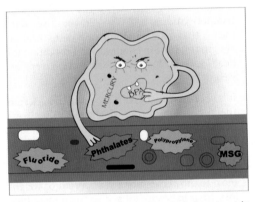

There are a variety of reasons toxins pose a major challenge to weight loss. A person who has too many toxins to process will make new fat cells and store those toxins along with fat in them. This is first a form of self-defense against being poisoned, and second, a strategy to get toxins out of the circulation and away from major organs. This means that some people will not be able to lose any weight at all, regardless of how little they eat, until the acute nature of their detoxification problems are addressed

- The cell-to-cell signalling system that is hormonal communication was firmly established long before plants and animals split off from each other on the evolutionary path millions of years ago and it has remained basically the same ever since.

- Because the obesity epidemic occurred relatively quickly, it has been suggested that environmental causes instead of genetic factors maybe largely responsible. What has, up to now, been overlooked is that the earth's environment has changed significantly during the last few decades because of the exponential production and usage of synthetic organic and inorganic chemicals.

- Your body's ability to process toxins is an essential factor in your ability to lose weight and reach a healthy goal weight. Struggling with this issue activates backup strategies for dealing with toxic overload, which include expanding the number of fat cells and stuffing them with toxins as well as fat. This is likely done to get the toxins out of your circulation and away from key organs. It causes easy weight gain and complicates weight loss because your body does not easily give up the toxic fat it has stored.

- So which organ is primarily responsible for dealing with all of these toxins? The liver. And, what happens when the liver's detoxification system is overloaded? The answer is simple: when the liver does not function properly, toxins that we are exposed to accumulate in the body.

- When the liver cannot process (detoxify) toxins fast enough, because of overload, the toxins have to be stored in the body to be dealt with later. Guess where it is stored?

IN OUR FAT!!!

- The more toxins in your body, the more fat you will lay down to absorb the toxins. It is almost impossible to be lean with a high content of toxins in the body.

Scientists estimate that everyone alive today carries within her or his body at least 700 contaminants, most of which have not been well studied. This is true whether we live in a rural or isolated area, in the middle of a large city, or near an industrialized area.

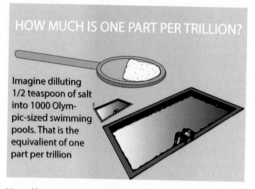

HOW MUCH IS ONE PART PER TRILLION?

Imagine dilluting 1/2 teaspoon of salt into 1000 Olympic-sized swimming pools. That is the equivalient of one part per trillion

Natural hormones are so potent that they can produce very dramatic changes in cell activity with very small amounts known as part-per-billion, or even parts-per-trillion, so minute that only extremely sensitive tests can measure them.

- In many ways, our polluted world is a true test of genetic survival of the fittest. The number of toxic chemicals now threatens the reproductive ability of the human race and is also a large part of the obesity epidemic. These chemicals contribute to weight gain in various ways, including disruption of the hormone signalling system that regulates your metabolism, damage to and accumulation in your adipose tissue (stored fat), and increased risk for poisoning during weight loss. It is absolutely vital that you understand this subject.

- The scientific theory of how these chemicals cause weight gain and difficulty losing weight has now been established. They bind to gene signalling within adipose tissue and induce new fat cells to form while simultaneously increasing inflammation. Often, the newly formed fat cells are themselves damaged by the toxins so that they cannot metabolically perform, which includes an inability to make leptin normally (an appetite regulating hormone that will be discussed more in Habit 6)

- These damaged fat cells can fill up with excess fat and toxins, but are not able to efficiently carry out normal functions of fat cells, leading

directly to increased risk for type 2 diabetes via the suppression of the important fat cell hormone known as adiponectin, a protein hormone that modulates metabolism including glucose and fatty acid catabolism. High levels are associated with low body fat.

- Several human studies confirm that polychlorinated biphenyls (PCBs) increase diabetes risk. These chemicals pose a serious problem to the thyroid gland and the efficient utilization of thyroid hormone throughout your body. Furthermore, they can cause either hypothyroidism (low thyroid function) or hyperthyroidism (over active thyroid). Trying to get the fat and toxins out of these damaged fat cells is no small challenge in terms of successful weight loss, yet it is vital to restore normal metabolism.

- Scientists have shown that such toxins can interfere with thyroid hormone function during weight loss. Human data shows that as the toxins go up in the blood during weight loss the levels of biologically active thyroid hormone triiodothyronine (T3) go down. This data means that your plumbing and detoxification systems must be in good working condition for healthy weight loss – or possibly even to engage weight loss.

- It is very clear that toxins are released back into the circulation during weight loss. This is especially the case during significant weight loss. In one study, during a weight loss of 12% of body weight, toxins in the blood increased 23-51%, with the heaviest individuals releasing the most toxins. Over a one year period of weight loss, toxic exposure ranged up to an incredible 388%.

- "Toxic" blood triggers the formation of new fat cells. This is because the endothelial cells of your circulatory system directly communicate to your baby fat cells and can tell them what to do. Keeping your blood as clean as possible and supporting your liver are vital steps to ensure that this process goes smoothly. I will cover how you can improve the health of your blood, in great detail, in Habit 8, "Nutritional Cardiology"

- Dr. Paula Baillie-Hamilton, an expert on metabolism and environmental toxins, was one of the first to make a link between the obesity epidemic and the increase in environmental chemicals. Baillie-Hamilton argued that exposure to chemicals can damage your body's natural weight-control mechanisms. She calls toxic chemicals that act as endocrine disruptors "chemical calories." Environmental researchers now call these chemical calories "obesogens."

- It is very important to understand how the organisations that produces the masses of man-made toxins found in our food, water, air & homes will stamp their feet and say very convincingly, usually whilst wearing a white coat to give them more credibility, that the amounts found in our food, water, air & homes is so small it would have very little or no effect at all. Well when you understand the concentrations that hormones work within the body then you realise that this simply isn't true.

- A review of 450 studies found that exposure to certain endocrine-disrupting chemicals is associated with an increase in body size in humans. Of particular concern was the chemical dichlorodiphenyldichloroethylene (DDE), which is a metabolite of DDT, and the form of DDT most often detected in foods and people. As the study's abstract noted: "Nearly all the studies investigating dichlorodiphenyldichloroethylene (DDE) found that exposure was associated with an increase in body size …"

- In the past 60 years around 87,000 man-made chemicals have been introduced into our food and water supply. Can you imagine the combined effect they may have on our body? What about prescription medications and their toxic effect on our liver and our body?

- It has been postulated by a number of studies that less than 5% of all cancers are genetically driven, whilst 95% or more are nutrition, lifestyle and toxicity driven.

- Toxins stockpile in your body! Studies reveal that 100% of those studied for toxins showed dioxins, PCB's, dichlorobenzene, and xylene. These toxins cause problems with our hormones and inhibit mitochondria and can contribute to obesity.

- The world wildlife foundation environmental group conducted a series of blood tests on people from all walks of life in the UK. In 2003, they tested the blood of individuals across the UK and found an average of 27 chemicals in every one of them. These compounds included long banned DDT and PCB's, from old electrical equipment and building materials, as well as more common chemicals found in every day materials such as paints, glues, toys, electrical goods, furniture, carpets and clothing.

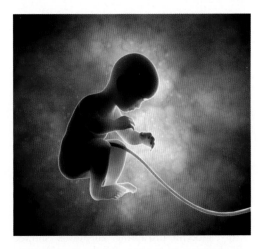

- As these chemicals build up, they can alter our metabolism, cause enzyme dysfunction and nutritional deficiencies, create hormonal imbalances, damage brain chemistry, and cause cancer. Because the chemicals accumulate in different parts of the body, at different rates and in different combinations, this can result in a disturbingly large variety of different chronic illnesses.

There is now very strong evidence that our bodies mistake certain man-made chemicals used in plastics, food, wrappers, and fragrances, and many more items, for naturally occurring hormones that regulate the production and storage of fat cells.

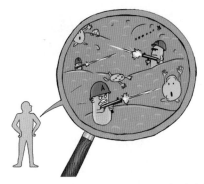

Expanding waistlines may be caused by more than bad diets and sedentary habits. Antibiotics could be disrupting our gut bacteria, helping people pack on fat like farm animals.

Are we programmed to be fat from the early life?

- *"Evidence has been steadily accumulating that certain hormone-mimicking pollutants, ubiquitous in the food chain, have two previously unsuspected effects. They act on genes in the developing foetus and newborn to turn more precursor cells into fat cells, which stay with you for life. And they may alter metabolic rate, so that the body hoards calories rather than burning them..."* —Retha Newbold of the National Institute of Environmental Health Sciences.

- Disconcertingly, studies on prenatal exposure to endocrine-disrupting chemicals showed that exposure in-utero (in the womb) could cause permanent changes that could predispose you to weight gain later in life.

- Infants are exposed to include pesticides, phthalates, bisphenol-A, flame retardants, and heavy metals such mercury, lead, and arsenic. These compounds have a broad range of negative effects on human biology. They damage the nervous system, increase your risk of cancer, and now it has been shown they contribute to obesity.

- This is not a fringe idea of radical environmentalists. The National Institutes of Health, the Food and Drug Administration, the Environmental Protection Agency and the National Academy of Sciences recently convened to examine this new phenomenon of "obesogens" - the toxins that cause obesity.

- A review in Current Diabetes Reviews (Nov 1;8(6):413-8) by a scientist at Classen Immunotherapies provides evidence that the epidemics of type 1 diabetes, obesity, metabolic syndrome, and type 2 diabetes may be caused by vaccines.

- The paper provides a review of evidence that the vaccines are causing the epidemics of insulin dependent diabetes (type 1 diabetes), obesity and non insulin dependent diabetes (type 2 diabetes). Upon receiving a vaccine some individuals' immune system becomes hyper active leading to autoimmune destruction of insulin secreting cells.

- Other individuals produce increased cortisol and other immune suppressing molecules, to suppress the vaccine-induced inflammation. The increased production of cortisol and other molecules leads to type 2 diabetes, obesity and metabolic syndrome.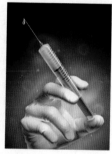

- I am not advocating that you do not vaccinate! I am simply showing you the evidence of the multiple causes of today's obesity epidemic. Vaccines should always be an individual choice. I would always suggest that each person does their own research and look at both sides of the fence.

- Expanding waistlines may be caused by more than bad diets and sedentary habits. Antibiotics could be disrupting our gut bacteria, helping people pack on fat like farm animals. This scenario is, for now, a hypothesis, but one that's fleshed out in two new studies. In the first, mice given antibiotics experienced profound changes to internal microbe communities that process food and regulate metabolism. In the other study, body weight in children rose with antibiotic exposures as infants.

- "Early life antibiotics are changing the microbiome (the totality of microbes, their genetic elements and environmental interactions in a particular environment), and its metabolic capabilities, at a critical time in development," said microbiologist Martin Blaser of New York University. "These changes have downstream effects on metabolism, including genes related to energy storage." For some reason, animals given steady low doses of antibiotics grow larger and faster than usual. Blaser wondered why this was, whether it was related to the animals' microbiomes, and whether something similar could happen in humans.

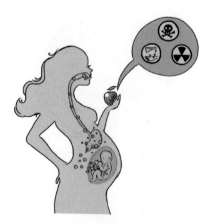

- In the Nature journal, researchers led by Blaser and fellow microbiologist Ilseung Cho, stated that steady, low doses of antibiotics to the diets of lab mice, mimicking the exposures received by farm animals.

- Their mice didn't gain weight, but their body fat swelled by 15 percent, an effect that held for different types of antibiotics. When the researchers looked at their microbiomes, they found markedly different types of bacteria. Changes were also found in the genetic profiles of their mice, with unusual activity in genes linked to breaking down carbohydrates and regulating cholesterol levels.

- According to Blaser, this could be a version of what happens inside people. That's difficult to study in gut-level detail, but an Aug. 21 International Journal of Obesity paper by Blaser and NYU paediatrician Leonard Trasande looked for population-level trends in 11,000 British children.

- Among children exposed to antibiotics before they were six months old, the researchers found small but consistent average increases in body mass years later. Antibiotics appeared to have altered their metabolic trajectories. Blaser called the data preliminary, but said it fits the patterns seen in both farm animals and his mice.

- It is estimated that the amount of antibiotics used in animal farming has sky-rocketed in the last few years. In just over a decade it is estimated that their use has increased eight-fold in the UK.

Could cow's milk be making you fat?

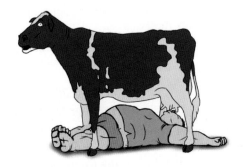

- *"In lieu of the recent evidence that cow's milk protein may be implicated in the pathogenesis of diabetes mellitus, we believe that the Committee on Nutrition should clarify whether cow's milk is ever appropriate for children and whether or not infant formulas that are based on cow's milk protein are appropriate alternatives to breast milk."*

  Paediatrics, July, 1992: 89

- *"Introduction of dairy products and high milk consumption during childhood may increase the child's risk of developing juvenile diabetes."*

  Diabetologia 1994;37(4):381-387

- Researchers in Maine report a new explanation for the mysterious link between consumption of cows' milk protein in infant formula early in life and an increased risk of later developing Type-1 diabetes. A protein in cow's milk that triggers an unusual immune response appears to be the main culprit, they say.

- In the study, Marcia F. Goldfarb points out that several studies have reported a possible link between the early introduction of cow's milk protein into an infant's diet and subsequent development of the disease. In Type-1 diabetes, the immune system erroneously appears to attack and destroy insulin-producing cells in the pancreas. It usually begins in childhood.

- A meta-analysis of case-control studies by Professor Gerstein of the University of McMaster implied that early exposure to cow milk proteins (<4 month old) was a risk predictor of type 1 diabetes. Early exposure to cow milk is related to shorter duration of breastfeeding. In a Finnish national case-control study, when both the duration of breastfeeding and the age at introduction of cow milk were studied, ear-

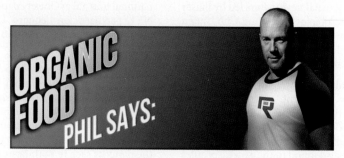

ORGANIC
FOOD
PHIL SAYS:

I always strive to buy organic fruits, vegetables, meats and fish wherever possible and advise my athletes to do the same and have done so for the last 20 years. With meat I also always look to buy grass-fed and always wild, not farmed, fish.

ly exposure to cow milk turned out to be the dominant risk determinant of type 1 diabetes

- A new intriguing hypothesis was proposed by the Finnish group, arguing that an early exposure to cow's milk formula results in an immune response to bovine insulin present in minute amounts in such formulas and that this could trigger an immune response to insulin, a key beta-cell antigen. The cow's milk theory is also compatible with the high diabetes incidence in milk-consuming countries such as Finland, Sweden, and Norway. The UK is now the 5th leading country in the World for type 1 diabetes.

- Remember, cow's milk is best kept for baby cows. However, I do believe that raw milk from a cow could be a nutritious food source for humans, due to its high enzyme content which have not been destroyed by pasteurisation and homogenisation.

- DDT, PCBs, trichloroethylene, perchlorate, dibenzofurans, mercury, lead, benzene, arsenic...all found in breast milk. Because breasts store fat, they store toxic, fat-loving chemicals. When we nurse our babies, we feed them, in albeit minuscule amounts, paint thinners, dry-cleaning fluids, wood preservatives, toilet deodorisers, cosmetic additives, gasoline by-products, rocket fuel, termite poisons and flame-retardants.

- The amount of chemicals that infants suckle through milk is not insignificant. Recent studies show that lactating mothers offload about 14% per month for dioxins, and up to 8% per month for PCBs, of their total body burden per month to their offspring, or about 30% if they nurse for a year. Bottle-feeding small babies

can set them up for a life of heart disease and obesity, according to a new study.

- While breastfed babies limit their own intake of milk because they have to work hard to get it, bottle-fed babies lie back and swallow what they are given. The danger, according to Singhal, is that they will be offered more than they need, building up an appetite for the future.

- "When they are exposed to high-protein, high-fat foods, they are more likely to become obese," he said

At least 20% of adult obesity is caused by over-feeding in infancy, according to Professor Atul Singhal from the MRC Childhood Nutrition Research Centre at the Institute of Child Health in London.

- Singhal and colleagues followed up children who were involved in two studies from the 1990s when they were new born babies. Some were given nutritionally enriched baby milk – now only ever given to weak, premature babies – and others were given standard formula.

- Those who were given the extra nutrition had a fat mass by the age of five to eight that was 22%-38% greater than those who were fed standard formula. Increased fat in childhood is a known risk for being overweight in adulthood.

- "This study robustly demonstrates a link between early nutrition and having more fat in later life in humans – a finding suggested by previous studies and confirmed in many other animals. Our findings are strong, consistent, show a dose-response effect, and are biologically plausible," said Singhal.

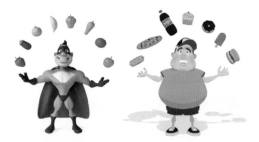

A picture tells 1000 words! Always eat fresh foods where ever possible.

- But the implications of the study go beyond the use of enriched formula milk, to the over-feeding of any baby. "In public-health terms, it supports the case in the general population for breastfeeding – as it is harder to overfeed a breastfed baby," Singhal said.

- He pointed out that formula milk is based on cow's milk – and that cows gain weight much faster than humans.

- Protein is a prime example of how human milk is unique nutrition for human babies. Human milk is low in protein, at least when

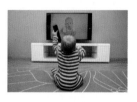

compared with the milk of other species, especially cow's milk. This isn't a nutritional deficiency; there are good reasons for this. Human infants are designed to grow slowly. While it's important for humans to develop strong bodies, even more important is brain development and the learning of social skills. The experiences that shape the brain come from close contact between mother and baby, when baby is held and carried. If human infants doubled their birth-weight in less than 50 days the way baby calves do, and then continued growing, how could their mothers carry them and talk to them and keep them close? Baby cows need to learn where to find the best grass in the meadow; baby humans need to learn how to turn the T.V. to the cartoon channel.

- The most recent example of how toxins make us fat can be seen in the dramatic increase in obesity in babies. In 2006, Harvard scientists from the School of Public Health found that the rate of obesity in infants less than 6 months old has risen 73% since 1980!

- It appears it may be the load of environmental toxins they are exposed to in the womb which contributes to their obesity.

Pesticides

- Studies suggest that every single one of us in the Western world may consume around 4.5 litres of pesticides a year.

- According to researchers at Purdue University in Indiana, apples now top the list as the most contaminated by pesticides (see the table below), even after they are peeled and washed.

- Strawberries are the third most contaminated fruit and veg, and other popular fruits such as grapes, blueberries are not that far behind. According to the group, eating five servings a day of the most contaminated fruits and vegetables is akin to ingesting 14 different pesticides per day. This is why consuming organic foods is so important in our quest for long term health and fat loss.

The 12 best and worst foods in regards to pesticide levels. (2012 results)	
Worst Offenders (Buy Organic)	Cleanest of the Bunch
1) Apples	1) Onions
2) Celery	2) Sweetcorn
3) Sweet Bell Peppers	3) Pineapples
4) Peaches	4) Avocado
5)Strawberries	5) Cabbage
6) Nectarines	6) Sweet Peas
7) Grapes	7) Asparagus
8) Spinach	8) Mangoes
9) Lettuce	9) Eggplant
10) Cucumber	10) Kiwi
11) Blueberries	11) Cantaloupe
12) Potatoes	12) Sweet Potatoes

- Not only have we introduced an estimated 87000 man-made chemicals to the environment, we have also decreased the nutrient content of our soil leaving us with foods that are deficient in vital detoxification nutrients which organs such as the liver require. The nutrient content of UK soil, between1939-1991, fell, in some cases dramatically.

- Vegetables: Sodium 49%, Potassium 16%, Magnesium 24%, Calcium 46%, Iron 27%, Copper 76%, Zinc 59%

- Fruit: Sodium 29%, Potassium 19%, Magnesium 16%, Calcium 16%, Iron 24%, Copper 20%, Zinc 27%. The only mineral to rise was phosphorous, by 2%

- Organophosphates are synthetically manufactured chemicals developed as a nerve gas and used in WW2. Since then, they have been used extensively in many different areas of manufacturing, food production and even medicine. At low doses, they have also been used to fatten up animals by severely reducing their ability to use up existing fat stores. As the animal's fat burning abilities slow down, they gain weight. Though the use of organophosphates as growth promoters has now been banned, they are still one of the most common pesticides and therefore continue to be found as residues in many of our foods.

- Another group of chemicals with very powerful weight gaining effects are the organochlorines. Studies show that the higher the level of these chemicals in the body, the greater the body weight will be. One animal study, found that one type of organochlorine, the pesticide and widespread pollutant, hexachlorobenzene (HCB), to possess such extreme fattening effects that when they're food intake was cut by 50%, animals treated with HCB still managed to gain more weight than did untreated animals on full rations!!!

- Organochlorine pesticides are insecticides composed primarily of carbon, hydrogen, and chlorine. They break down slowly and can remain in the environment long after application and in organisms long after exposure. Organochlorine pesticides are mostly used as insecticides. Specific uses take a wide range of forms, from pellet application in field crops, to sprays for seed coating and grain storage. Some organochlorines are applied to surfaces to kill insects that land there.

- Many organochlorines are known or suspected hormone disruptors, and recent studies show that extremely low levels of exposure in the womb can cause irreversible damage to the reproductive and immune systems of the developing foetus.

- Dr Annette Pernille Hoyer, who has worked on many studies looking at pesticide use, said: "I fear that the link is significant. The use of pesticides should be reduced as much as possible in general. Human beings are naive when they do not believe that a poison designed to kill living organisms does not harm them".

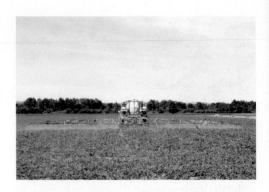

- Approximately 95% of the pesticide residue we are exposed to in our food comes not from fruits or vegetables, but from the meat we eat.

- Many pesticides are deliberately designed to target mitochondria as the stronger the ability of a chemical to poison the mitochondria, the more effective it is in killing. Organochlorines are also big players in the energy lowering chemical league. They actually reduce tissues ability to convert food into readily usable energy in the form of ATP. Not only does this effect energy production in our mitochondria, but it effects all of the mechanisms used by our body's to produce energy.

- One endocrine-disrupting chemical that may be linked to obesity include Bisphenol A (BPA). It is used to make polycarbonate plastic water bottles, baby bottles, the linings of metal food and soft-drink cans, thermal receipt paper, and dental sealants. Studies show that mice and rats fed low doses of BPA during early development became more obese as adults than those that weren't fed the chemical. BPA leaches from food and beverage containers into what we eat and drink.

- BPA first caught researchers' attention after normal mice began to display uncommon genetic abnormalities. The defects were linked to plastic cages and water bottles that had been cleaned with a harsh detergent, causing BPA to leach out of the plastic. After determining how much BPA the mice had been exposed to, the researchers realized even an extremely small dose of 20 parts per billion daily, for just

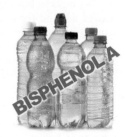

Bottled water can absorb the BPAs from the plastic

five to seven days, was enough to produce effects.

- Phthalates are also endocrine disrupting chemicals and are commonly found in personal care products such as moisturisers, nail polishes, soaps, hair sprays and perfumes. They are also used in adhesives, electronics, toys and a variety of other products.

- Researchers, lead by Tamarra James-Todd, Ph.D., a researcher in the Division of Women's Health at BWH, analysed urinary concentrations of phthalates in 2,350 women who participated in the National Health and Nutrition Examination Survey. They found that women with higher levels of phthalates in their urine were more likely to have diabetes.

- Another study linked a type of phthalate that leaches into processed food with abdominal obesity and insulin resistance in men.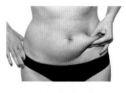

- Phthalates or plasticizers have an affinity for the testicles, which accounts for the ever worsening levels of testosterone in males. It is no surprise that the average male is producing less testosterone than 20 years, and it is getting worse. Phthalates are also known to block the receptor sites for thyroid.

- One type of phthalate, called DEHP, blocks estradiol production in the ovaries. This causes an ovulation, or lack of egg production in the ovaries, which in turn leads to oestrogen dominance. This can also lead to other problems, such as build up of the uterine lining, with subsequent excessive bleeding and infertility.

- Unfortunately the chemistry of phthalates resemble that of many hormones. As hormone mimickers, they are potent environmental endocrine disruptors. They can for example damage hormone receptors the place on the cell membrane where our endogenous (produced within the body) hormones get transported into the cell to do it's work. By blocking the action of our natural hormones this often makes hormone replacement ineffective, that's why a lot of people for example on thyroid medication feel no difference when they are on the medication.

- One study of more than two thousand adults found at least 80% had detectable levels of six persistent organic pollutants that can remain in our tissues for up to ten years. Those people whose bodies had high levels of persistent organic pollutants such as dioxin, PCB's, and chloradane were thirty eight times more likely to be insulin resistant than people with low levels - this is a recipe for obesity.

Cooking and Digestion

- Perfluorooctanoic acid (PFOA) is used to make non-stick cookware, found in grease-proof food packaging, and stain-proof coating on clothing and carpeting. Several studies show that PFOA exposure results in reduced birth weight followed by weight gain after puberty.

- Toxic (cookware) gases can also threaten hormonal balance. A recent study has shown a link between thyroid disease, cancer and non-stick cookware. The study was published in the journal Environmental, which is affiliated with the National Institutes of Health, and reported that people with high levels of PFOA, were more likely to develop thyroid problems, as well as various types of cancers.

- Professor Bernard Blanc of the University of Lausanne, and an independent researcher, Dr. Hans U. Hertel concludes "Food, heated by microwaves, causes pathogenic changes in the blood of individuals who consume such food, similar to what is seen in the initial stages of cancer."

- Microwaving food leads to unhealthy clumping, or agglutination, in the blood. Each time, the effect can last up to two hours or longer.

TOXIC COOKWARE

Perfluorooctanoic acid

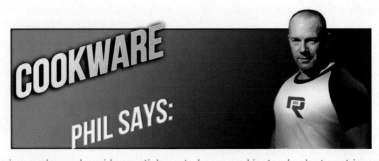

COOKWARE
PHIL SAYS:

When I'm buying cookware I avoid non-stick coated pans and instead select cast-iron or ceramic pans. I also always advise all of my athletes to do the same.

- Another problem with microwave ovens is that carcinogenic toxins can leach out of your plastic and paper containers/covers, and into your food.

- The January/February 1990 issue of Nutrition Action Newsletter reported the leakage of numerous toxic chemicals from the packaging of common microwavable foods, including pizzas, chips and popcorn. Chemicals included polyethylene terpthalate (PET), benzene, toluene, and xylene. Microwaving fatty foods in plastic containers leads to the release of dioxins (known carcinogens) and other toxins into your food.

- One of the worst contaminants is BPA, or bisphenol A, an oestrogen-like compound used widely in plastic products. In fact, dishes made specifically for the microwave often contain BPA, but many other plastic products contain it as well.

- A study published in the November 2003 issue of The Journal of the Science of Food and Agriculture5 found that broccoli "zapped" in the microwave with a little water lost up to 97% of its beneficial antioxidants. By comparison, steamed broccoli lost 11% or fewer of its antioxidants.

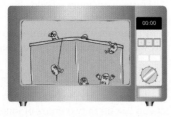

Microwaving your food can reduce the nutrient density of your food. It can also cause chemicals to leach out of plastic containers

Chemicals in Everyday Products

- Petrochemical compounds are found in general consumer products such as creams, lotions, soaps, shampoos, perfumes, hair sprays and room deodorizers. Such compounds often have chemical structures similar to oestrogen and indeed act like oestrogen in the body.

- Parabens are chemical preservatives that have been identified as oestrogenic and disruptive of normal hormone function and can be found in multiple beauty products.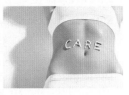

- As much as 60% of any substance applied to the skin or scalp is absorbed into the body. This is facilitated further as there are detergents present in many products which improve skin absorption. These toxins go straight into the bloodstream and put tremendous strain on the kidneys and liver as they work to rid our bodies of these harmful chemicals. The use of these harsh chemicals would not be such a problem if the skin did not readily absorb them. Some chemicals can penetrate the skin in significant amounts, especially when left on the skin. A recent case that made headline news found traces of 350 man-made chemicals, including residues from personal care products, in human breast milk.

- Even in most commercial tampons there are some other ingredients including;

- Dioxin and disinfection-by-products (DBPs) such as trihalomethane. These chemicals are present when the tampon is bleached, and are very toxic. Dioxin is also a hormone disruptor and a known carcinogen.
- Oestrogen. This encourages heavier flow.
- Pesticides, herbicides and synthetic fertilizers that are used in non-organic cotton.
- Phthalates. These are chemical plasticisers that are used in plastic tampon applicators and cardboard applicators.
- Polypropylene. This is a type of plastic which can withstand very high temperatures.
- Rayon. Made from wood or cotton pulp, rayon is an artificial fibre that is highly chemically processed and highly absorbent, making it particularly dangerous when used in a tampon as it can lead to Toxic Shock Syndrome.
- Viscose. Another type of wood pulp that is treated with toxic chemicals such as caustic soda and sulphuric acid.

The average woman absorbs 4lb 6oz of chemicals from toiletries and make-up every year, the industry magazine In-Cosmetics recently reported.

The Dangers of Sunscreen and the Benefits of Sunlight

- Many common sunscreen chemicals are strong. Margaret Schlumpf and her colleagues (Institute of Pharmacology and Toxicology, University of Zurich, Switzerland) have found that many widely-used sunscreen chemicals mimic the effects of oestrogen and trigger developmental abnormalities in rats. Her group tested six common chemicals that are used in sunscreens, as well as lipsticks and facial cosmetics. Five of the six tested chemicals (benzophenone-3, homosalate, 4-methyl-benzylidene camphor (4-MBC), octyl-methoxycinnamate and octyl-dimethyl-PABA) behaved like strong oestrogen in lab tests and caused cancer cells to grow more rapidly.
- A recent study has shown that a potent sunscreen ingredient, oxybenzone, may be a cause of endometriosis. This condition occurs when uterine tissue grows in abnormal sites in the abdomen and causes severe pain. Women are usually diagnosed because of severe cramping

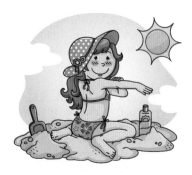

during their periods. In this study of 600 women, those with the highest levels of a form of oxybenzone in their urine had a 65% increased risk of endometriosis. Oxybenzone, like bisphenol-A (BPA), is a chemical that mimics oestrogen. And, endometriosis growth is fed by oestrogen.

- This study should be another warning sign that oxybenzone should not be put on the skin. The highest levels of oxybenzone in the urine of women in this study occurred in the months of July and August, proof that the sunscreen ingredient is readily absorbed into the bloodstream.
- Exposure to sunlight promotes good health. The more sun exposure we get, the better our bodies function. Preventing sunburn during the hottest part of the day is a good idea. Sun-

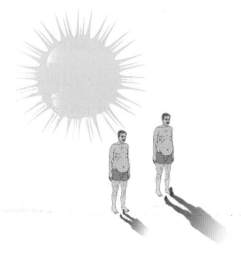

If your shadow is longer than you are tall (an indicator of the oblique angle of the sun), you are not making much vitamin D. Factors that affect vitamin D production from the sun including angle of the sun, time of day, season and latitude where you live, skin type, and others.

Other than those regions situated close to the equator, there are only between 4-8 months during the year when vitamin D synthesis is impossible.

burn damages the skin. But with all of the evidence that sunlight is beneficial in the prevention of cancer and heart disease, maintaining a strong immune system, and building bones, no one should be using sunscreens on a routine or daily basis.

- This doesn't mean you should never wear a sunscreen product, of course. If your skin is really pale and you're planning a day on the beach in Spain, you will obviously benefit from some level of sun protection using a truly natural sunscreen product. But an informed health-conscious person would try to allow their skin to achieve a natural, healthy tan (yes, a tan truly is healthy if it's combined with good nutrition,) through sensible exposure levels that activate vitamin D production in the skin.

- It has also been shown in many studies that as body fat increases, active levels of vitamin D decrease. This leaves many people feeling weak, tired and with sore muscles. A US study in 2000 found that as body fat increases, more vitamin D is stored in fat tissue making less available to the body compared to non obese individuals.

- Our skin was designed to produce vitamin D through UVB exposure from the sun, as there are few natural food sources of vitamin D. Most fortified dairy products usually contribute only around 100 IU per serving. If we rely on food alone, most of us are going to fall short of the daily goal and potentially end up with suboptimal or deficient levels. When you read the literature from experts on vitamin D, they usually advise that you consume between 2000-4000IU a day. We will cover this in more detail in habit 7.

- In one study, 32% of healthy physicians, students, and residents at a hospital in Boston who reported drinking a glass of milk daily, eating salmon once a week, and taking a supplement daily still had deficient vitamin D levels.

- Until a few generations ago, most humans walked and slept in direct contact with the surface of the earth. Our modern life style involves wearing insulating shoes and sleeping in buildings that electrically isolate the body from the ground plane.

- Our planet is a sextillion metric ton battery that is continually being replenished by solar radiation, lightening, and heat from its deep molten core. Exposure to the ground provides electrical nutrients in the form of electrons,

which recharge our batteries and keeps us connected with mother earth.

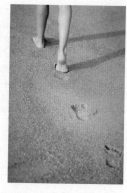

- I regularly use grounding with myself and my athletes on a regular basis as the scientific literature has also shown that it is a great anti-inflammatory. What do I mean by grounding? Grounding is simple walking barefoot on grass or sand and absorbing the energy from the earth.

Xenoestrogens and Their Effects on Oestrogen Levels

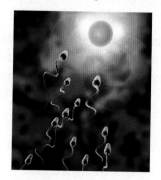

- According to the British Association of Aesthetic Plastic Surgeons, there has been an abrupt rise in the number of men popping in for a breast reduction procedures in recent years. It is now the second most common cosmetic procedure for UK men. Again, the offender seems to be alterations in hormone levels, notably an increase in .

- Xenoestrogens have shown the ability to induce aromatase activity. Aromatase is the enzyme responsible for synthesis of oestrogen from the androgens (male hormones).

- What exactly are xenoestrogens? Xenoestrogens are man-made chemicals that can enter the body and mimic the effects of the female hormone oestrogen.

- We have to consider the population-wide drop in sperm concentration which has plummeted, according to the British Fertility Society, by about 30%, as well as the fact that Britain seems to be gripped by a fertility crisis.

Is What You're Drinking Making You Fat?

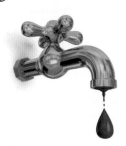

- Robert Carton, former president of the Union of Government Scientists at the US Environmental Protection Agency – the body that oversees drinking water quality in the US – has described fluoridation as "the greatest case of scientific fraud of this century, if not of all time."

- It is now known - thanks to the meticulous research of Dr. Jennifer Luke from the University of Surrey in England - that the pineal gland is the primary target of fluoride accumulation within the body.

- Britain's tap water should be monitored for powerful medicines after traces of cancer and psychiatric drugs were detected in samples, a report has warned. The 100-page statement, commissioned by the drinking water watchdog, the Drinking Water Inspectorate (DWI), reveals that pharmaceuticals are finding their way into the water supply despite extensive purification treatments used by water companies.

- Our water and food supply is loaded with halogens, which are elements that can replace iodine in the thyroid gland. They mainly include

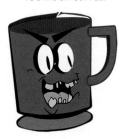

TOO MUCH COFFEE?

Too much coffee can definitley be a bad thing. The caffeine and CGA's can have detrimental effects in you quest for fat loss

fluorides, chlorides, and bromides. These elements compete with iodine for absorption and utilization in our bodies. When they replace iodine, the thyroid gland simply stops working properly. Tap water contains always chloride and in many places fluoride which decrease thyroid function.

- Fluoride, a common additive to your water supply, and ingredient in the toothpaste you and your children use may be contributing to the increased rates of hypothyroidism -- and other health concerns -- in the UK without improving dental health. Fluoride is an element from the halogen group, as are iodide and chloride. It is commonly added to the water supply as hydrofluosilicic acid, silicofluoride or sodium fluoride. Fluoride is also found as an additive in toothpastes and some mouthwashes.

- Dr. John Yiamouyiannis examined the raw data from a large study that was conducted by the National Institute for Dental Research (NIDR). He concluded that fluoride did not appear to have any decay preventing success, as there was little difference in the DMFT values (the mean number of decayed, missing or filled teeth) for approximately 40,000 children. It did not matter whether they grew up in fluoridated, non-fluoridated or partially fluoridated communities. (Yiamouyiannis, J.A. "Water Fluoridation and Tooth Decay: Results from

Fizzy drinks in Britain have been found to contain pesticides at up to 300 times the level allowed in tap or bottled water.

A worldwide study found pesticide levels in popular fizzy orange and lemon drinks sold, which are popular with children, were at their highest in the UK.

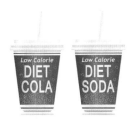

the 1986-87 National Survey of U.S. School-children", Fluoride, 23, 55-67, 1990).

- A larger study has been conducted in New Zealand. There, the New Zealand National Health Service plan examines the teeth of every child in key age groups, and have found that the teeth of children in non-fluoridated cities were slightly better than those in the fluoridated cities. (Colquhoun, J. "Child Dental Health Differences in New Zealand", Community Healthy Services, XI 85-90, 1987).

- If you are not familiar with the controversy surrounding the use of fluoride in water, toothpaste and numerous other products and industries, your mouth will drop as you read the book "The Fluoride Deception" by Christopher Bryson. You'll read how a leading Harvard toxicologist who found that fluoride in water produced nervous system changes in rats that resemble attention deficit hyperactivity disorder (ADHD) was fired just days before his research was accepted for publication.

- Bryson cites numerous, and specific, scientific studies linking fluoride, which he describes as "so potent a chemical that it's also a grave environmental hazard and a potential workplace poison," to numerous health ills including arthritis, bone cancer, emphysema and nervous system disorders like Alzheimer's disease and attention deficit disorder (ADD). In fact, the evidence is so compelling that you will likely find yourself reading and rereading in disbelief.

- Research carried in the American Journal of Clinical Nutrition. Eight men were given two drinks of vodka and sugar-free lemonade separated by 30 minutes. Each drink contained just under 90 calories. Fat metabolism was measured before and after consumption of the drink. For several hours after drinking the vodka, whole body lipid oxidation (a measure of how much fat your bod by a massive 73%.

- A 2008 report by PAN Europe found that 100% of conventionally produced wines that they analysed, including wines made in France, Germany, Austria, Italy, Portugal, South Africa, Chile and Australia, were shown to contain

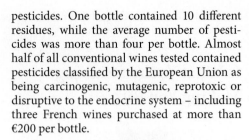

pesticides. One bottle contained 10 different residues, while the average number of pesticides was more than four per bottle. Almost half of all conventional wines tested contained pesticides classified by the European Union as being carcinogenic, mutagenic, reprotoxic or disruptive to the endocrine system – including three French wines purchased at more than €200 per bottle.

- The European Commission published a 10 year overview of the use of pesticides in European agriculture. The EU study shows that grapes receive 4.7kg of synthetic pesticides per hectare – a higher dose than any other crop except potatoes. In fact despite accounting for 3.5% of the total EU agricultural area, grapes receive 15% by weight of the synthetic pesticides applied to all major crops.

- Australian researchers found that over consumption of certain polyphenols found in coffee called chlorogenic acid (CGA) could prevent fat loss and lead to insulin resistance.

- The study, which was published in the Journal of Agricultural and Food Chemistry, tested CGA's effects on obese mice, which were given different doses of the compound.

- The mice that were given doses equivalent to five or six cups of coffee per day showed retention of fat within cells.

- The obese mice also showed more glucose intolerance, a pre-diabetic condition, and increased resistance to insulin regulation.

- Caffeine intake from all sources is linked with higher oestrogen. Studies have shown that women who consumed at least 500 milligrams of caffeine daily, the equivalent of four or five cups of coffee, had nearly 70% more oestrogen than women who consume no more than 100 mg of caffeine daily, or less than one cup of coffee.

GM Foods

- A new study by the EU's official food watchdog, the European Food Safety Authority (EFSA), has revealed that the international approval

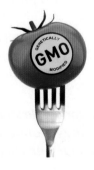

process for GM crops failed to identify a viral gene.

- As a result, watchdogs have not investigated its impact on human health and the plants themselves when assessing whether they were safe.

- The findings are particularly powerful because the work was carried out by independent experts, rather than GM critics.

- It was led by Nancy Podevin, who was employed by EFSA, and Patrick du Jardin, of the Plant Biology Unit at the University of Liege in Belgium.

- They discovered that 54 of the 86 GM plants approved for commercial growing and food in the US, including corn and soya, contain the viral gene, which is known as 'Gene VI'.

- Significantly, the EFSA researchers concluded that the presence of segments of Gene VI 'might result in unintended phenotypic changes'.

- Such changes include the creation of proteins that are toxic to humans. They could also trigger changes in the plants themselves, making them more vulnerable to pests.

- Director of the campaigning group, GM Freeze, Pete Riley, said the discovery of the gene, 'totally undermines claims that GM technology is safe, precise and predictable'.

- He said: 'This is a clear warning the GM is not sufficiently understood to be considered safe. 'Authorisation for these crops must be suspended immediately, and they should be withdrawn from sale, until a full and extended review of their safety has been carried out.'

- In global terms the use of GM crops has increased steadily since the first commercial plantings in North America in the late 1990s. By 2012 over 17 million farmers in 28 countries were growing GM crops on 170 million hectares, which is more than 12% of the world's arable land, an area of land more than 5 times the size of the UK.

- As this goes to print, no GM crops are currently being grown commercially in the UK, but imported GM commodities, especially soya, are being used mainly for animal feed, and to a lesser extent in some food products.

- As part of a long-term project studying the health effects of GM foods, researchers from Norway fed food containing GM corn to one group of rats and food containing non-GM corn to another group. Over the course of 90 days, the rats on the GM-corn diet grew fatter and consumed more food than the rats on the non-GM diet. The researchers also noticed that rats got fatter when they ate fish that had been raised on GM corn.

- They also tried the experiment on salmon and saw similar results: Fish eating GM corn grew faster, and they ate more, than fish eating non-GM corn. The salmon on GM corn were also less able to digest proteins, and experienced immune-system changes that didn't occur in non-GM-fed fish.

- I personally, from my research on GM foods, would never consume these products or give them to anyone in my family. However, I would like to see studies done on with politicians who push these Frankenstein foods on their citizens. I would like to see them eat these foods every day for a minimum of 3 years and see the effects that this would have. If they are proven to be in a fit and healthy state, then I might consider GM foods occasionally, so long as there was nothing left to eat on this earth.

Monosodium Glutamate (MSG) and Artificial Sweeteners

- MSG is found in almost all convenience foods, fast foods and processed foods. It is used as a flavour enhancer in cheap, processed foods to make their taste more appealing. While making bland foods taste more appealing, this chemically structured ingredient is shown to cause neurotransmitter damage and is also linked to the sky-rocketing cases of obesity we see today.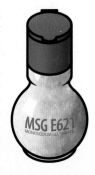

- A team of scientists in the Faculty of Medicine at the Complutense University of Madrid has discovered that when given to rats, E-621 (AKA MONOSODIUM GLUTAMATE) produces a massive 40% increase in appetite. The scientists think the additive affects the arcuate nucleus area of the brain and so prevents proper functioning of the body's appetite control mechanisms. According to this hypothesis, people (and children) who consume foods with large quantities of MSG just feel more and more hungry, the more they eat.

- By directly stimulating the pancreas to release insulin, which drops the blood sugar, MSG can be considered an "anti-appetite suppressant". In other words, eating MSG makes you hungrier than you would have been, sooner than you would have been. Over-release of insulin can lead to obesity and insulin resistance - the start of Type II Diabetes.

- Obesity, and Type II diabetes are now epidemic in children. Before the introduction of MSG into the Western diet, these diseases were rare in children. Based on these simple facts, doctors are now questioning if the rising use of MSG had a hand in creating these two new "epidemics".

- People who use MSG as a flavour enhancer in their food are more likely than people who don't use it to be overweight or obese even though they have the same amount of physical activity and total calorie intake, according to a University of North Carolina at Chapel Hill School of Public Health study published in the journal Obesity.

If fried snack crisps had a warning printed right on the bag that said, "Warning: these chips will make you obese," would you still buy them? Would you still eat them?

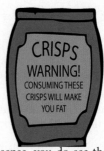

- Well, in a sense, you do see that warning on chips; just read the ingredient list. Research suggests that MSG causes obesity, making unhealthy snacks even unhealthier than you may have suspected.

- Rats are not normally fat. When scientists inject the rodents at birth with MSG, like magic, they produce obese test subjects. Because MSG triples the amount of insulin the rat's pancreas creates, the results are perfect....MSG Treated Rats = Fat Rats. These findings are substantiated in over 100 studies and can be found at the National Library of Medicine, at www.pubmed.com. All you have to do is search under "MSG Obese."

- Researchers at UNC and in China studied more than 750 Chinese men and women, aged between 40 and 59, in three rural villages in north and south China. The majority of study participants prepared their meals at home without commercially processed foods. About 82 percent of the participants used MSG in their food. Those users were divided into three groups, based on the amount of MSG they used. The third who used the most MSG were

MSG masquerades on food ingredient labels under many names including of the following;	
• glutamic acid	• sodium caseinate
• glutamate	• calcium caseinate
• autolyzed yeast	• natrium glutamate
• autolyzed yeast protein	• flavours
• yeast extract	• so-called `natural` flavours
• textured protein	• hydrolyzed corn
• monopotassium glutamate	• yeast food
• ultra-pasteurized and any enzyme-modified ingredients.	
• Many manufacturers of medications use MSG as a filler ingredient in tablets and other medications.	

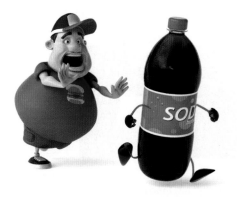

Aspartame is found in many drinks, foods and even childrens' multi vitamins. You, and your children, should be very cautious of this ingredient and avoid it at all costs.

nearly three times more likely to be overweight than non-users.

- "Animal studies have indicated for years that MSG might be associated with weight gain," said Ka He, M.D., assistant professor of nutrition and epidemiology at the UNC School of Public Health. "Ours is the first study to show a link between MSG use and weight in humans."

- Because MSG is used as a flavour enhancer in many processed foods, studying its potential effect on humans has been difficult. He and his colleagues chose study participants living in rural Chinese villages because they used very little commercially processed food, but many regularly used MSG in food preparation. "We found that prevalence of overweight was significantly higher in MSG users than in non-users," He said. "We saw this risk even when we controlled for physical activity, total calorie intake and other possible explanations for the difference in body mass. The positive associations between MSG intake and overweight were consistent with data from animal studies."

Contrary to popular belief, studies have found that artificial sweeteners such as aspartame can:

- *Stimulate your appetite*

- *Increase carbohydrate cravings*

- *Stimulate fat storage and weight gain*

- Now, yet another study has been published showing that saccharin and aspartame cause greater weight gain than sugar and increases insulin resistance.

- The featured study, published in the January 2013 issue of the journal Appetite, was done by a Brazilian research team with the Faculty of Medicine of the Federal University do Rio Grande do Sul. Rats were fed plain yogurt sweetened with either aspartame, saccharin, or sugar, plus their regular rat chow, for 12 weeks.

- "Results showed that addition of either saccharin or aspartame to yogurt resulted in increased weight gain compared to addition of sucrose, however total caloric intake was similar among groups," the researchers write.

- The reason for the similar calorie consumption between the groups was due to increased chow consumption by the rats given artificially sweetened yoghurt. This type of compensation has been found in previous studies as well, indicating that when your body gets a hit of sweet taste without the calories to go with it, it adversely affects your appetite control mechanisms, causing increased food cravings. The authors concluded that: "Greater weight gain

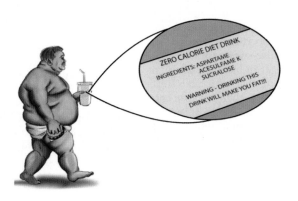

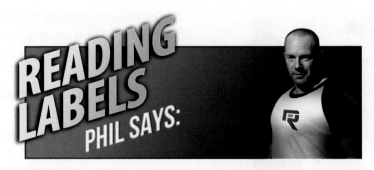

READING LABELS
PHIL SAYS:

If you are buying packaged food/drink products, I strongly suggest that you become vigilant in reading labels. This is why I am a strong advocate of only buying foods in their natural state as most processed foods are loaded with an array of flavourings, artificial sweeteners, trans fats and a host of other nasties.

was promoted by the use of saccharin or aspartame, compared with sucrose, and this weight gain was unrelated to caloric intake. We speculate that a decrease in energy expenditure or increase in fluid retention might be involved."

- Diet fizzy drinks can raise the risk of diabetes by 60%, startling research has revealed.

- A study of more than 66,000 women found those who drank artificially sweetened drinks were more likely to develop the disease than those who indulged in regular, 'full fat' versions.

- The findings, published in the American Journal of Clinical Nutrition, fly in the face of conventional thinking that regular versions of fizzy drinks are always worse for our health.

- Studies have began to show that drinking these low calorie, sugar free drinks are linked to increases in weight.

- The San Antonio Heart Study looked at over 5000 men and found that those who drank these drinks had BMI's over 40% higher than those who didn't even when other factors were taken into account.

- Food additives and sweeteners are able to augment the addictive properties of food. As an example, on the relative sweetness scale, glucose the primary sugar in blood weighs in at a measly 0.8. Compare that with table sugar (sucrose) that is rated 1.0. High fructose corn syrup is 1.2 and fructose is 1.4 almost twice as sweet as glucose. Food manufacturers understand this addiction all too well and that's why thousands of foods are loaded with artificial sweeteners to get us addicted to this junk food which makes the junk food industry billion's of

pounds whilst we also gain pounds unfortunately around our waistlines.

- Where do artificial sweeteners fall on this same scale? Aspartame is listed 180, acesulame K at 200, and saccharin at 300, while sucralose weighs in at 600. This means Splenda is 750 times as sweet as glucose. No wonder so many of us are addicted to foods containing these super sweet additives, many of which are already loaded with sugar and high-fructose corn syrup (HFCS). The sweet taste products deliver can change the way we perceive food, think about food, crave food and they can increase appetite and the secretion of the hormone insulin.

- A 2010 scientific review published in the Yale Journal of Biology and Medicine (YJBM) discussed the neurobiology of sweet cravings and the unexpected effect of artificial sweeteners on appetite control. It cites several large scale prospective cohort studies that found positive correlations between artificial sweetener use and weight gain, which flies in the face of "conventional wisdom" to cut calories in order to lose weight.

- For example: The American Cancer Society study conducted in early 1980s included 78,694 women who were highly homogeneous with regard to age, ethnicity, socioeconomic status, and lack of pre-existing conditions. At one-year follow-up, 2.7-7.1% more regular artificial sweetener users gained weight compared to non-users matched by initial weight... Saccharin use was also associated with eight-year weight gain in 31,940 women from the Nurses' Health Study conducted in the 1970s."

- Research published in the Journal of Toxicology and Environmental Health in 2008 found that Splenda can also reduce the amount of good bacteria in your intestines by 50%.

- Fructose is a cheap form of sugar used in thousands of food products and soft drinks, which can damage your, or your child's, metabolism. More than any other form of sugar, heavy fructose consumption can cause dangerous growths of fat cells around vital organs and can trigger the early stages of diabetes, heart and liver disease.

- Fructose, usually derived from corn, is fuelling the obesity crisis in a big way due to its heavy use by the food and beverage industry in the form of high-fructose corn syrup (HFCS) and crystalline fructose. If you or your child are consuming excess fructose daily, it can result in damage to your liver.

- Dr. Richard Johnson's book, The Fat Switch, dispels many of the most pervasive myths relating to diet and obesity. He discovered the method that animals use to gain fat prior to times of food scarcity, which turned out to be a powerful adaptive benefit. His research showed that fructose activates a key enzyme, fructokinase, which in turn activates another enzyme that causes cells to accumulate fat.

- Since all fructose gets shuttled to your liver, and, if you eat a typical Western-style diet, you consume high amounts of it, fructose ends up taxing and damaging your liver in the same way alcohol and other toxins do. And just like alcohol, excess fructose is metabolised directly into fat – not cellular energy, like glucose. While in times of complete glycogen depletion (i.e. post work-out or true hunger), fructose can be used to replenish these stores, any excess will mostly be converted to fat. So, eating fructose in excess of the very small amount our body can handle is really like eating fat – it just gets stored in your fat cells, which leads to mitochondrial malfunction, obesity and obesity-related diseases.

- Two new studies have added more reason for concern that high-fructose corn syrup causes significantly more harm to the body than its mere sugar content would suggest.

- High-fructose corn syrup contains 55% fructose and 45% glucose. In contrast, table sugar (also known as sucrose) contains a 50-50 split.

- In the first study, published in the journal Pharmacology, Biochemistry and Behaviour, researchers from Princeton University found that rats consuming high fructose corn syrup gained more weight and developed more cardiovascular risk factors than rats consuming equivalent amounts of sucrose.

"Some people have claimed that high-fructose corn syrup is no different than other sweeteners when it comes to weight gain and obesity, but our results make it clear that this just isn't true," researcher Bart Hoebel said.

- Hoebel and colleagues fed two groups of rats an identical diet, supplemented with one of two sweetened beverages. One beverage consisted of a sucrose solution in concentrations similar to those found in many sweetened beverages. The other consisted of a high-fructose corn syrup 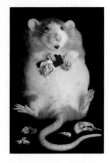 solution at roughly half the concentration of a typical soda. The researchers found that the rats consuming the corn syrup solution gained significantly more weight than the rats consuming the sucrose solution.

- After six months, the rats in the corn syrup group had gained 48% more weight. They also underwent an increase in fat deposition (especially in the abdomen). Every rat consuming high-fructose corn syrup became obese. In

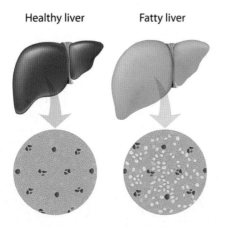

Healthy liver   Fatty liver

contrast, rats fed a high-fat diet did not become obese in all cases.

- After eating fructose, 100% of the metabolic burden rests on your liver - ONLY your liver can break it down. This is much different than consuming glucose, in which your liver has to break down only 20%, and the remaining 80% is immediately metabolised and used by the rest of the cells in your body.

- Fructose is converted into fat that gets stored in your liver and other tissues as body fat. Part of what makes excess fructose so bad for your health is that it is metabolised to fat in your body far more rapidly than any other sugar. For example, if you eat 120 calories of fructose, around 40 calories are stored as fat. But if you eat the same amount of glucose, less than one calorie may get stored as fat. Consuming fructose is essentially consuming fat!

Plastic Fats

- Trans fats (artificial fats) make you fatter than other foods with the same number of calories - but that's not all. Researchers at Wake Forest University find that trans fats increase the amount of fat around the abdomen. They do this not just by adding new fat, but also by moving fat from other areas to the abdomen.

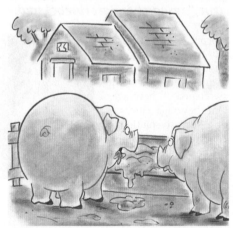

"Do you think this has any trans fat?"

- "Trans fat is worse than anticipated," Wake Forest researcher Lawrence L. Rudel, Ph.D. says. "Diets rich in trans fat cause a redistribution of fat tissue into the abdomen and lead to a higher body weight even when the total dietary calories are controlled."

- The Nurse's Health Study of 80,000 women found that a 2% increase in trans fat consumption increased a woman's risk of heart disease by 93%.

- Just a 2% increase in trans fats calories has been found to boost your risk of diabetes by 39%.

- In the UK hydrogenated vegetable oil, otherwise known as trans fat, doesn't even have to appear clearly on ingredients labels (at the time of printing). Have a look, and you might find it called 'shortening', or 'hydrogenated fats', maybe 'hydrogenated vegetable oils' (HVOs), perhaps 'partially hydrogenated vegetable oils' (PHVOs), or not mentioned at all.

EMFs

- EMFs are electrical magnetic frequencies and come from things such as wi-fi and mobile phones.

- Perhaps, one of the most serious consequences of EMFs exposure is its effects on our hormonal systems. Artificially created EMFs are estimated to be 100-200 million times greater than what existed just two generations ago. Every minute of every day, whether we are awake or asleep, we are exposed to a constant barrage of man-made EMFs

- Rajkovic et al. (2003) showed that after three months exposure to power line frequencies, the thyroid glands of rats showed visible signs of deterioration. They also lost their ability to produce the thyroid hormones, which they did not recover even after the fields were switched off. Esmekaya et al. (2010) found a similar visible deterioration of the thyroid gland in rats exposed to simulated 2G cell phone radiation for 20 minutes a day for three weeks. Eskander et al. (2012) found that people living for six years

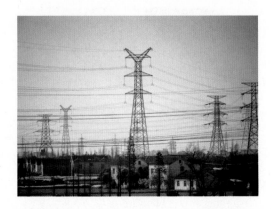

within 100 metres of a cell phone base station showed a significant reduction in the release into the blood of a number of hormones, including ACTH from the pituitary gland, cortisol from the adrenal glands, and prolactin and testosterone from organs elsewhere. However, the most highly significant loss was in their ability to produce the thyroid hormones. The expected consequence of this is hypothyroidism, the most frequent symptoms of which are fatigue and obesity.

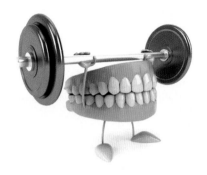

Dental Health

- Your dental health can make you fat, sick and tired. Amalgam fillings should be called DEATH by slow poison fillings. 50% of these are made from mercury, the 2nd most toxic poison known to man after plutonium. This is a tragedy and the dental profession should hold their head in shame in allowing this health tragedy to take place. Approximately 8 million amalgam fillings are placed in our mouths every year in the UK.

- Scientific research has demonstrated that mercury, even in small amounts, can damage the brain, heart, lungs, liver, kidneys, thyroid gland, pituitary gland, adrenal gland, cells, enzymes and hormones and suppress the body's immune system.

The height of irony is that dental amalgam is shipped as a hazardous material to the dental office, and any amalgam leftover is also treated as hazardous and requires special precautions to dispose of. Yet most dentists will readily implant this hazardous material directly into your mouth, with assurances that it's perfectly safe and harmless!!!

- Mercury is continually released from mercury dental fillings in the form of mercury vapour and abraded particles. These mercury vapours can increase as much as 15-fold by chewing, brushing, drinking hot liquids, etc.. The World Health Organization recently concluded that the daily intake of mercury from amalgam dental fillings exceeded the combined daily intake of mercury derived from air, water and food (including fish).

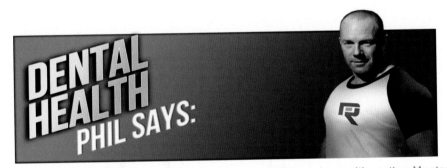

"If you have mercury fillings and want to remove them as I did then do so with caution. My story was a mercury disaster as the dentist removed 7 fillings, one root canal and a decayed back molar all in one sitting which took approximately 6 hours. What happened over a 5 year period after this was a health disaster. Everyday I genuinely thought I was going to die and that is no exaggeration. So learn from my lesson; DO NOT remove more than 1 – 2 fillings per month. I've also put a detoxification nutrition and supplement plan together from my extensive research in this area which thankfully has allowed me to regain my health. Do not remove amalgam fillings without a proper detoifification before, during and after. You will find these plans in habit 9 on detoxification."

- Mercury is a potent neurotoxin that can damage your brain, central nervous system and kidneys, and mixing it with other alloys and placing it in your mouth does NOT all of a sudden render it harmless. Children and foetuses whose brains

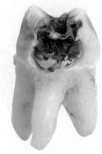

Posion in your mouth

are still developing are at greatest risk, but anyone can be affected. Naturally, the more amalgams you have, the greater your risk of experiencing health problems as a result of this mercury toxicity.

- For many years the dental community maintained that mercury was tightly bound with other metal components and did not escape from amalgam fillings. This is a lie research has proven that mercury vapours do escape during chewing, brushing and when contacted with hot or acidic foods.

- One study reported on levels of mercury vapour measured in the mouth after chewing. The mercury level was 54 times higher in the mouth of an individual with amalgams than in the mouth of an individual without amalgams. It is physically impossible for mercury to be "locked in" the amalgam fillings once they are placed in the teeth.

- Mercury can inhibit the action binding of happy hormones like serotonin at the synapse (nerve to nerve connection) leading to depression & carbohydrate cravings.

- Methyl mercury has been shown to accumulate in the testosterone-producing Leydig cells of the testes decreasing production of testosterone. Several studies have shown workers occupationally exposed to mercury have lower testosterone levels.

- The enzyme thyroid peroxidase, converts T4 (inactive form of thyroid hormone) to T3 (active form of thyroid hormone) and this can be blocked by mercury in the body.

- Today as well as being described the second most toxic chemical in the world, mercury has been categorised by Dr. Lars Friberg, M.D., Ph.D., a former head of toxicology of the World Health Organization (WHO), in this way: "There is no safe level of mercury and no one has actually shown there is a safe level and I would say mercury is a very toxic substance."

- Researchers at New England Research Institutes and the Harvard School of Public Health studied more than 500 children with different types of dental fillings to investigate the health impacts of mercury amalgam fillings. What they discovered was surprising…at the five-year follow-up, children with white composite fillings displayed more behavioural problems than the children with silver fillings containing mercury.

- Many white fillings contain bisGMA, a synthetic material that is created using bisphenol-A, or BPA, a hormone-disrupting chemical linked to many health problems, including autism and temper tantrums in kids. The new

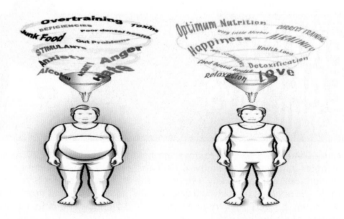

When we fill our body & mind with hate, anger, jealousy, poor foods, alcohol, caffeine & toxins, losing body fat becomes an impossibility. Why? You have to be healthy before you can lose weight. The body can't and won't release fat until it is at a certain level of health. And this is why so many diets fail.

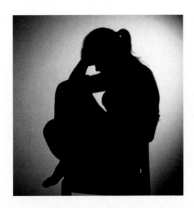

study published in Paediatrics suggests that as the composite fillings on chewing surfaces degrade, more BPA is released. Kids with BPA-containing composite fillings were more likely to suffer from social stress, anxiety, depression, and difficulty forming relationships. These are similar problems previous researchers have associated with BPA exposure early in life.

Mental Health

- With all this toxicity going on today within our body it's enough to make you depressed and, unfortunately, our society as an epidemic of mental illnesses including depression on a huge scale. You must ask the question, why? Did our ancestors have this problem on the scale we do today? I very much doubt it you only got to look at the remaining few indigenous tribal people today depression would simply not be on the percentage it is in modern society. Mental illness is, in my opinion, worse than physical illness as it is invisible and unless you are suffering with it or have suffered with it you will usually have very little time for someone with a mental illness.

- I have suffered from depression and a personality disorder for over 25 years. Thankfully though, I have now resolved many of the problems I faced, through applying a lot of the information that I have gained over the years, in researching for this book, which I would now like to share with you.

5 Biggest Regrets of People on their Death Beds

When one is faced with imminent death, there are always the expected regrets as to how one has lived life. A nurse by the name of Bronnie Ware, who worked for many years in palliative care, composed a list of the five largest regrets that people have on their death beds. "Some incredibly special times were shared," Ware said. "I was with them for the last three to twelve weeks of their lives."

1. I wish I'd had the courage to live a life true to myself, not the life others expected of me.

- "When people realize that their life is almost over and look back clearly on it, it is easy to see how many dreams have gone unfulfilled. Most people had not honored even a half of their dreams and had to die knowing that it was due to choices they had made, or not made," Ware says.

2. I wish I didn't work so hard.

- "This came from every male patient that I nursed. They missed their children's youth and their partner's companionship . All of the men I nursed deeply regretted spending so much of their lives on the treadmill of a work existence."

3. I wish I'd had the courage to express my feelings.

- "Many people suppressed their feelings in order to keep peace with others. As a result, they settled for a mediocre existence and never became who they were truly capable of becoming. Many developed illnesses relating to the bitterness and resentment they carried as a result," Ware warns.

4. I wish I had stayed in touch with my friends.

- "Often they would not truly realize the full benefits of old friends until their dying weeks and it was not always possible to track them down. Many had become so caught up in their own lives that they had let golden friendships slip by over the years. There were many deep regrets about not giving friendships the time and effort that they deserved. Everyone misses their friends when they are dying."

5. I wish that I had let myself be happier.

- "This is a surprisingly common one. Many did not realize until the end that happiness is a choice. They had stayed stuck in old patterns and habits. The so-called 'comfort' of familiarity overflowed into their emotions, as well as their physical lives. Fear of change had them pretending to others, and to their selves, that they were content. When deep within, they longed to laugh properly and have silliness in their life again."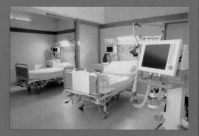

Conclusion

- Now you can see that there is no single cause of obesity. There are unfortunately multiple causes, from constant stress, drinking water, EMFs, dental products, medications, pesticides, herbicides, fungicides, MSG, aspartame, trans fats, high fructose corn syrup, vaccinations, antibiotics, processed foods, phthalates, xenoestrogens, beauty care products, cookware and a host of other hormone disrupting products. Now you can see, when you move away from nature, the fatter you become!

- So what is important from our first habit is to stay as close to mother nature as we possibly can as our ancestors have done for over 100,000 generations. Habit 2 will concentrate on detoxification which will help us rid the body of the multiple factors that are making it 100% impossible to have vibrant health and to maintain a healthy body fat %.

- Some authors that I recommend are Robb Wolf, Loren Cordain, Lindsey Berkson, Nora Gedgaudas and Dr Walter Crinnion

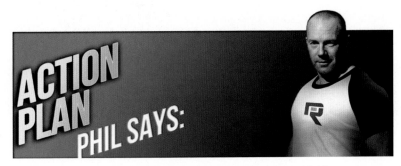

Eat organic foods, get a reverse osmosis water filter fitted for clean drinking water, use chemical-free washware produts, use safe cookware, throw your microwave away, minimise mobile phone use (if at all), reduce stress as much as possible.

Make sure that you surround yourself with very positive, loving and caring people. This will have an incredible effect on your health and well-being.

These simplistic measures alone will have a monumental effect on your health and your ability to lose body fat safely, efficiently and for the long term.

Please enjoy the rest of the habits as all of the information you need are contained within these.

HABIT 2

DETOXIFICATION IS ESSENTIAL FOR OPTIMUM FAT LOSS

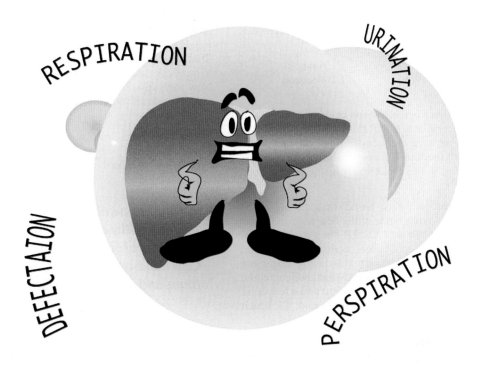

Since I first met Phil I have changed so much as an athlete. Not only am I getting stronger, but I'm also now much more aware of the food I use to fuel my workouts and training.

Due to a knee injury, there was a stage where I had to limit my training. However, with Phil's guidance and nutritional approach, I still managed to race at the European age group championships and win a silver! I was the top British finisher! My nutritional plan is now very different compared to before and I feel so much better. As I write this I am eating a chickpea salad – so much more nutritionally beneficial than my old breakfast of muesli and weetabix!

Nick Dunn (World Triathlete Champion)

- Before we start looking at the pathways of detoxification, I want you to understand that one of the biggest toxins we face everyday are our thoughts. You must ensure that you do not fall into the trap of negative thinking. At every opportunity you get, think good thoughts. This will be one of the most powerful detox tools that you can have and one of the most important factors in your quest to lose fat. Do not under-estimate the power of your thoughts.

Detoxification Pathways

- Physically, we get rid of toxins through four pathways:

  1. Perspiration   3. Urination
  2. Respiration   4. Defecation

- The liver is the nucleus of detoxification and must make sure that this is working efficiently. As we have just seen from habit 1, we are hit with thousands of chemicals that our liver has never, in our evolutionary history, had to cope with.

- Researchers have found that dieting without detoxing is one of the best ways to poison yourself and get FATTER. In a study at Laval University, in Quebec, scientists showed that the rise in circulating toxins during weight loss led to a drop in the resting metabolic rate (the energy we expend during rest) and a reduction in the most active form of thyroid, T3, which drives metabolism!

- Another study from Lavel University, Quebec, found that those who released the most pesticides (organochlorines) from their fat stores during weight loss had the slowest metabolism after weight loss.

- A study published in Obesity review 2003 concluded that pesticides (organochlorines) and PCBs (from industrial pollution) are released from the fat tissue, where they are stored, and poison our metabolism preventing us from losing weight.

- A study that was published in the American Journal of Physical Endocrinology Metabase, 2002, said that the increase in toxins during weight loss in men inhibited normal mitochondrial function and reduced the subjects ability to burn calories, retarding further weight loss. Now you can see why detoxification needs to run in parallel if you want long term successful weight loss.

- Toxins block nutrients from adequately nourishing the cells of your body. This can have a devastating effect on the energy & health of the cells.

You must remember that you are only as healthy as your cells. You are a mass of 60 trillion plus cells. Cells make tissues, tissues make organs and organs make humans.

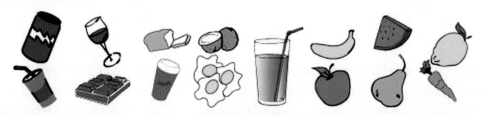

The following table will give you an idea of which foods are acidic and which are alkaline. A more comprehensive list can be found at the end of the chapter.							
fizzy drinks carbonated water energy drinks	cheese pork chocolate beer pasta wine vinegar roasted nuts	coffee beef white bread	fruit juice eggs cocoa liver salmon coconut	water	apple pineapple apricot cherries banana quinoa	pear grape melon green beans green tea	carrot lemons cucumber onions spinach cabbage raw broccoli cauliflower
3	4	5	6	7	8	9	10
Acidic pH				Neutral pH		Alkaline pH	

0   7   14

NEUTRAL

ACID   ALKALINE

pH: What does it mean? pH is the abbreviation for potential hydrogen. The pH of any solution is the measure of its hydrogen-ion concentration. The higher the pH reading, the more alkaline and oxygen rich the fluid is. The lower the pH reading, the more acidic and oxygen deprived the fluid is. The pH range is from 0 to 14, with 7.0 being neutral. Anything above 7.0 is alkaline, anything below 7.0 is considered acidic.

- There are two sides of detoxifying: the first is to reduce the toxins your body is exposed to, and the second is to improve your body's ability to detoxify.

- Detoxification supports a healthy metabolism. By removing toxicity, you allow the cells to process nutrients in a more efficient way. This will significantly boost the rate at which you metabolize the foods you eat. When you clean up your diet at the same time as you detoxify, metabolism is further enhanced.

The importance of pH in our detoxification

- First, let's look at the importance of pH levels whilst detoxifying as this should never be overlooked.

The majority of the foods and drinks we consume are acidic, such as meat, grains and sugar, with colas, alcohol, coffee and other soft drinks being highly acidic. So unless you have been eating a very healthy diet, full of fresh fruit and vegetables, your body is more likely to be acidic, which creates an environment where disease can manifest.

- Detoxing in our incredibly polluted environment is not an occasional endeavour. In order to maintain a healthy immune system with a slightly alkaline pH, we need to consider detoxification to counter the "slow kill" from the myriad of toxins pervading every element of our environment which we saw from habit 1.

- Arthur C. Guyton, M.D., who is considered one of the world's most recognized author on human physiology, has spent the better part of his life studying the pH or, acid/alkaline balance, of the body. In his "Textbook of Medical Physiology", which is used to train medical students, he states that the first step in maintaining health is to alkalise the body.

- Rudolph Virchow (Father of Pathology), said: "If I could live my life over again, I would devote it to proving 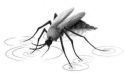 that germs seek their natural habitat, diseased tissue, rather than being the cause of the diseased tissue; e.g., mosquitoes seek the stagnant water, but do not cause the pool to become stagnant."

- In the 1860's Louie Pasteur's theory became cemented in our minds, that germs cause disease. Hailed as one of the most important discoveries of modern science, we supposedly had found the real cause of disease. Disease arises from micro-organisms outside the body. These

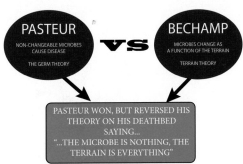

PASTEUR — NON-CHANGEABLE MICROBES CAUSE DISEASE — THE GERM THEORY

VS

BECHAMP — MICROBES CHANGE AS A FUNCTION OF THE TERRAIN — TERRAIN THEORY

PASTEUR WON, BUT REVERSED HIS THEORY ON HIS DEATHBED SAYING... "...THE MICROBE IS NOTHING, THE TERRAIN IS EVERYTHING"

HOWEVER, THE ROAD WAS SET FOR THE GERM THEORY AND AS A RESULT, MEDICINE TODAY ALLEVIATES THE SYMPTOMS OF DISEASE BUT RARELY THE CAUSE

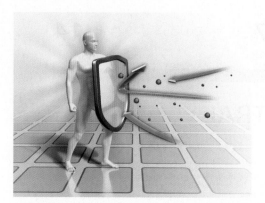

Raising pH increases the immune system's ability to kill bacteria, concludes a study conducted at The Royal Free Hospital and School of Medicine in London. Viruses and bacteria that cause bronchitis and colds thrive in an acidic environment.

micro-organisms do not change, and anybody can be a victim of disease.

- Antoine Bechamp was a French Physician and Biologist Professor of Medical Chemistry and Pharmacy at the Montpellier University and University of Lille.

- From examinations of an amputated arm and many examinations of frozen plants during a cold winter, these convinced him that, upon injury, bacteria developed internally without any outside influence due to terrain changes.

- Bechamp believed that germs where pleo-morphic, that they changed depending on the terrain. This means that disease usually arises from within the body, that healthy micro-organisms exist within the body, and micro-organisms change and transform based on their environment.

- When you think logically about the biggest killers in the western world, e.g. heart disease and cancer, you realise that you do not catch

these diseases. These diseases are built from within.

- What determines the state of micro-organisms in the body is a very simple matter. If you are continually acidifying your system, and if you have habits whereby you are acidifying your systems constantly, (heavy metals, toxins, downing coffee, tea, coke, acid thoughts, meat, dairy, pharmaceuticals, alcohol, pollution, pastries, relationship stress etc..) then you are creating an environment where disease can thrive.

- As our bodies become acidic, their oxygen level begins to drop, leaving us tired and fatigued and this is what allows fungus, mould, parasites, bad bacteria, and viral infections to flourish and gain a hold throughout the body which can then cause disease.

- The health of the cell depends on the quality of the nutrients that it takes in, how well the nutrients are assimilated, the effectiveness of the cells detoxification and the fluids that which the cell is bathed in. The following example by Nobel Prize winner Dr. Alexis Carrol is a perfect example of cell health & environment.

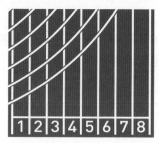

If I threw a grass seed onto a running track, it is 100% impossible for the grass seed to take root. Why? Because the environment is not conductive for growth. However, if i threw that grass seed onto a lush patch of grass, it will inevitably take root. The environment allows this to happen. It is the same with us - we can only catch disease from outside sources if our internal environment is right for disease/germs to get a foot hold due to an acidic terrain.

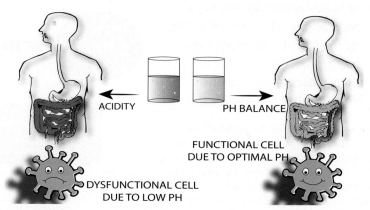

ACIDITY   PH BALANCE

FUNCTIONAL CELL
DUE TO OPTIMAL PH

DYSFUNCTIONAL CELL
DUE TO LOW PH

Creating the optimum pH levels within the body creates the right environment for cells to thrive

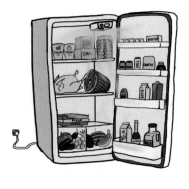
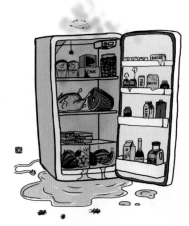

It has been demonstrated that an acidic, anaerobic (lacking oxygen) body environment encourages the breeding of fungus, mold, bacteria, and viruses.

Let's look at an example.

If we were to seal the door to our freezer which is full of frozen food and then unplug it, come back and open the door in four weeks, what would we find? Mold, bacteria, microscopic bugs. Things will be growing and multiplying. Where did they all come from? They did not sneak in - remember the door was sealed. The answer is . . . "they were always there". It is simply that the environment changed to a more inviting and healthy one for the "critters" to live in.

- Nobel Prize winner Dr. Alexis Carrel did an experiment [1912-1940] to keep cells from a chicken's heart alive and reproducing new cells for 28 years! A chicken's lifespan is far less than this. So why did these chicken cells live so well and so long?

- Dr Carrel did this by placing the cells in a saline solution that was the perfect temperature, pH, and nutrient/mineral balance.

- He and his co-workers replaced this solution daily (cleaning away the toxic [acidic] wastes). Eventually, after 28 years the purpose of the experiment was achieved.

- The cells did not die of aging they simply stopped the experiment and Dr. Carrel concluded the following;

"The cell is immortal. It is merely the fluid in which it floats which degenerates. Renew this fluid at intervals, give the cells what they require for nutrition and, as far as we know, the pulsation of life may go on forever."

- Bruce Lipton cell biologist & author; "I will never forget a piece of wisdom I received in 1967, on the first day I learned to clone stem cells in graduate school. It took me decades

to realize how profound this seemingly simple piece of wisdom was for my work and my life. My professor, mentor, and consummate scientist Irv Konisberg was one of the first cell biologists to master the art of cloning stem cells. He told me that when the cultured cells you are studying start ailing, you look first to the cell's environment, not to the cell itself, for the cause."

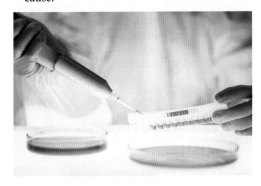

- Dr. Otto Warburg, winner of the 1931 Nobel Prize for his studies in cell respiration, believed that a person's level of health and vitality has a direct correlation to the levels of oxygen in his or her blood stream. Proving that: viruses, bacteria and cancer cells can not survive in an oxygenated environment. Dr Otto Warburg noted that alkaline bodies absorb up to 20 times more oxygen than acidic bodies.

Detoxification Through Respiration

- The lungs are the organ responsible for bringing oxygen to the blood. It plays the crucial role of the first detox organ to get in contact with airborne toxins, chemicals, viruses, bacteria, and allergens. The lungs oxygenate the veins to bring new oxygen to the heart for distribution while removing toxic waste like carbon dioxide from the arteries to be expelled from the body.

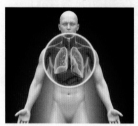

The lungs play a role in eliminating toxins from the body

- A poor diet, air pollution, shallow breathing and habits like smoking all contribute to make our lungs less efficient and decrease its natural detoxification ability. Supporting our lungs with proper breathing techniques increases its effectiveness. A more efficient lung provides more oxygen for our bodies resulting in increased energy levels and a clear state of mind.

- Breathing Exercise for lung detox: Learning deep breathing is an important aspect of lung detoxification. Proper breathing techniques allow more air into the lungs and improves its efficiency. This is another reason why exercise is so important during detoxification.

Detoxification Through Perspiration

- Sweating is one of the most effective methods for getting the most damaging toxins out of the body. There are no drugs, no surgery, no chelation, nor other detoxification methods with before and after measurements that compare to sweat. The skin is the largest organ of the human body. Usually nobody thinks of skin being an organ. Skin is very thin and it takes only a few moments, for some kind of liquid substance to be absorbed. Make a little experiment with garlic. You can rub it into your foot and wait. Very soon you can taste the garlic in

your mouth. Here is the proof that skin easily absorbs most things.

- So, our skin not only absorbs well, it excretes toxins as well. The human body has an important ability to sweat, which is a natural body reaction to expel various sorts of toxins, including heavy metals.

- There are between 10-100 times more toxins in your fat than in your blood, so one of the best ways to remove toxins is to decrease your body fat. That really is your first defence. Choosing the right foods and exercise are key here. After that, one of the most effective detoxification strategies I know of is the use of an infrared sauna.

- This can be done for about 30 minutes to one hour daily. Remember, it's important to hydrate well before and during the sauna treatment to avoid dehydration. Also, check with your health care provider you are fit enough to use the sauna.

- Additionally, you can exercise for 30-60 minutes immediately prior to help liberate some of the toxins from your fat. I suggest that you do aerobic exercise to increase blood flow and perspiration.

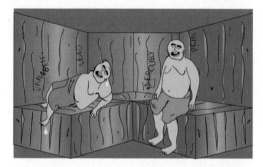

Infrared saunas are an amazing way to help detoxify through perspiration and because of the softer heat, they are more tolerable than regular saunas

- Far infrared rays are part of the sun's natural spectrum. The radiant energy produced by an infrared sauna is the same as heat from the sun, with the exclusion of the ultraviolet rays. A heat source, (usually ceramic heating elements), emits infrared waves that penetrate and relax the body as increased blood circulation warms the skin.

- Sweat and toxins are released through the skin's open pores as the warm blood circulates deeper throughout the body. The infrared sau-

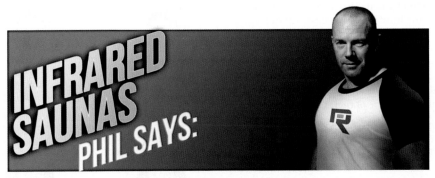

INFRARED SAUNAS
PHIL SAYS:

I use the infrared sauna 4 – 5 times per week and have personally had outstanding results. I usually do 30 minutes after I've done an hours training in the morning. Before I begin, I take 1 teaspoon of alkalising salts in 1 pint of water - this is loaded with electrolytes. When my sauna is finished, within ten minutes I then drink 1 pint of water with a tablespoon of heavy metal chelator to ensure that I pull as many toxins out of my system as possible. Since I've done this my body fat as reduced significantly. Remember before trying any supplements, exercise plan or use of modalities like sauna consult with a qualified medical practitioner. I am simply sharing with you what works for me.

na is a powerful means of cellular cleansing as it increases metabolism and blood circulation. In addition to its use for detoxification it also relaxes muscles and rejuvenates the body.

Far-Infrared Versus Steam Saunas

- The far infrared sauna is far safer and infinitely more tolerable, because it uses a heat energy that penetrates tissues, triggering mobilization of chemicals from subcutaneous fat storage, directly into the sweat. This activating penetration allows for a much lower overall temperature to be used.

- Infrared saunas warm the body instead of heating the surrounding air. Traditional steam saunas heat the air and require temperatures ranging from 150 – 200 degrees Fahrenheit to promote perspiration, whereas a heat range of 110 – 140 degrees in an infrared sauna produces the same results. The cooler air temperature is more tolerable to heat-sensitive individuals and allows for sessions of up to 45 minutes, nearly twice as long as in a typical steam sauna session.

- The softer heat of an infrared sauna also penetrates deeper into the skin - as much as 1 ½ inches - and draws out more toxins than a steam sauna, according to Dr. Aundrea Adams of the International Institute of Holistic Healing, who compared the detoxification findings of the two sauna types.

- Dr. Adams summarizes a report which concludes that sweat from a traditional sauna was up to 97% water, while the sweat released in an infrared sauna was only 80 – 85% water. The remaining 15–20% was comprised of heavy metals, sulphuric acid, sodium, ammonia, uric acid and fat-soluble toxins .

- The deep penetration of infrared heat activates and releases debris from the subcutaneous fat just beneath the skin. It also allows the body to gradually free stored toxins from organs and tissues, which eventually make their way to the fat tissue under the skin, finally to be purged through perspiration.

- In a two week study of twenty five obese adults, body weight and body fat were reduced after sauna therapy for fifteen minutes at 60 degrees Celsius daily in a far-infrared sauna. Researchers reported on another obese patient who couldn't exercise because of knee arthritis and lost 17.5 kilograms, decreasing body fat from 46 to 35 % after ten weeks of sauna therapy. Saunas and steam rooms help rid the body of toxins which could be choking your ability to lose weight.

- Clearly the therapeutic advantages of the infrared sauna are considerable. In her book Detoxify Or Die, Sherry Rogers, M.D. extols the benefits of the far-infrared sauna. She cites a study done by specialists at the Mayo Clinic which proves the effectiveness of therapeutic infrared sauna use for patients of end-stage congestive heart failure.

- The individuals in this three-week study tolerated the infrared sauna heat without side effects, and experienced significant chemical detoxification. The toxic load was the underlying cause of their condition and the heart function of each of these patients improved as a result of the therapeutic cleansing. They were also able to eliminate some of their medications.

- Of course there are many other ways to sweat other than sitting in an infrared sauna. I regularly run most days, not only for fitness but especially for sweating it's a great way for detoxing both chemically and emotionally. Try to run as close to nature as you can this gives you a good karma and clears your head, I often get my best ideas whilst running.

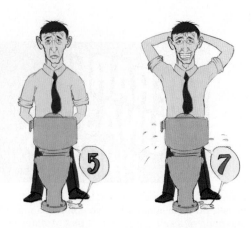

One of the best ways to assess whether your body has healthy pH levels is to check your 2nd urine of the day. A good reading would be between 6.8-7.2. Remember, the urine pH indicates the acidity of your tissues, nots your blood.

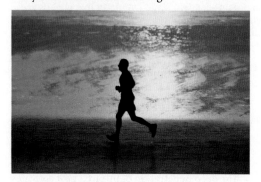

Detoxification Through Urination

- The kidneys play an important role as a detoxification organ. One way to ensure that the kidneys are functioning to their maximum level is to drink around 8-10 glasses of clean, filtered water daily and to pass out urine when the bladder is full, without holding or controlling the need to pass urine.

- Nothing supports the body's cleansing and elimination like clean drinking water. Water is the ultimate detoxification tool because releasing toxins without being able to flush them from the body accomplishes little. These toxins will be deposited in other areas. During detoxification, wastes that have been stored in fatty tissue are dumped into the bloodstream and lymph and many are then sent to the liver and kidneys to neutralize and break down these toxic compounds.

- Water is also very important during the final stage of elimination, lubricating the intestines and providing the basis for urine. Drinking more clean water during detoxification therefore is an obvious must. I strongly recommend reverse osmosis as the cornerstone of your drinking water, you can get RO water machines which also re-mineralises the water.

Detoxification Through The Liver

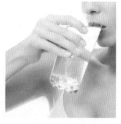

- The liver is the largest glandular organ of the body. It weighs about 3 lb (1.36 kg). The liver lies on the right side of the abdominal cavity beneath the diaphragm.

- The liver's ability to function and to rebuild and repair itself is absolutely dependent on the quality of nutrients

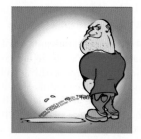

Once toxins have been removed from fat cells, they need to be eliminated from the body. Chelating agents can help remove these toxins to be excreted from the body via the urine.

that you consume and the less toxins consumed the quicker the liver can detoxify YOU!

- The liver can become congested from chemicals, alcohol, toxins, drugs and heavy metals. Evidence of a "fatty liver" is often shown by a roll of fat at the waistline, which happens because the liver has stopped breaking down fat and started storing it.

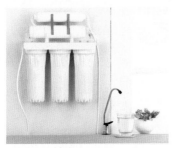

- So, can you remember from habit 1 what happens when the liver's detoxification system is overloaded?

When the liver does not function properly, toxins that we are exposed to accumulate in the body.

- The hands down fastest and most effective way to lose excess weight is to cleanse your liver. Why? Your liver is your prime fat burning organ and it's also your prime detoxification organ. So, when your liver is overwhelmed with toxins - which is incredibly common these days - it makes it challenging for your liver to get around to burning fat. And when this is the case, weight loss is very difficult - no matter what you do. This is exactly why most people struggle when trying to lose weight, and this is the reason it so often seems like an uphill battle.

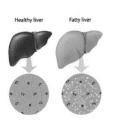
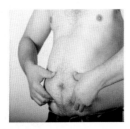

Healthy liver   Fatty liver

- It is the external environment that contributes most to the load of toxins that the liver has to detoxify. Today, the burden on the liver is heavier than ever before in history. Additionally,

nutritional deficiencies and imbalances from unhealthy eating habits add to the production of toxins, as do alcohol and many prescription drugs, further increasing stress on the liver and requiring a strong detoxification capacity.

- Many of the toxic chemicals that enter the body are fat-soluble, which means they dissolve only in fatty or oily solutions and not in water. This makes them difficult for the body to excrete. Fat soluble chemicals have a high affinity for fat tissues and cell membranes, which are composed of fatty acids and proteins. In these fatty tissues of the body, toxins may be stored for years, being released during times of exercise, stress or fasting. During the release of these toxins, several symptoms such as headaches, poor memory, stomach pain, nausea, fatigue, dizziness and palpitations can occur.

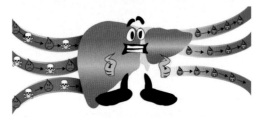

The liver is responsible for removing toxins from the blood. Without a clean, efficient liver and healthy kidneys, blood is not filtered clean. "Dirty" blood, loaded with toxins or waste products, is heavier and more sluggish. This causes poor circulation and reduced capacity to carry oxygen and nutrients. A clean and efficient liver which produces cleaner blood would help energy production because clean blood can carry more oxygen and nutrients. Clean blood is also lighter; it flows better and results in better blood circulation.

- The following are the most common symptoms of a toxic liver; being edgy, easily stressed, elevated cholesterol, skin irritation, depression, sleep difficulties, indigestion, kidney damage, heart damage, brain fog, hypothyroidism, chronic fatigue, weight gain, poor memory, PMS, blood sugar imbalances, allergies, or obesity.

- Nutrition is the most critical factor where detoxification is concerned. Like any of the body's functions, detoxification requires nutrients. If these nutrients are not present in sufficient quantity, detoxification is hindered or stalled completely. One reason many toxins are stored is because the nutrients are not available to complete the process of detoxification. The other difficulty is that the number and amount of toxins are greater today than at any other time in human history.

- When the liver gets damaged over the years, toxins that are normally filtered out can recir-

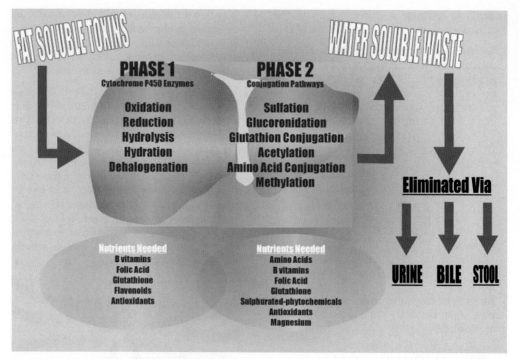

FAT SOLUBLE TOXINS   WATER SOLUBLE WASTE

PHASE 1
Cytochrome P450 Enzymes

Oxidation
Reduction
Hydrolysis
Hydration
Dehalogenation

PHASE 2
Conjugation Pathways

Sulfation
Glucoronidation
Glutathion Conjugation
Acetylation
Amino Acid Conjugation
Methylation

Eliminated Via

URINE   BILE   STOOL

Nutrients Needed
B vitamins
Folic Acid
Glutathione
Flavonoids
Antioxidants

Nutrients Needed
Amino Acids
B vitamins
Folic Acid
Glutathione
Sulphurated-phytochemicals
Antioxidants
Magnesium

Here's how the two phase process works in the liver:

Phase 1: Toxins such as environmental chemicals, drugs, and metabolic end products enter the body and activate a group of enzymes called cytochrome P450 mixed function oxidases. In this phase, the toxins are transformed into an intermediate state that can be broken down in phase 2.

Phase 2: in this step, the body adds specific nutrients to transform the toxin into a water soluble compound for a safe exit via urination or bowel movements.

culate through the body, re – exposing glands to harmful compounds, triggering a toxic overload. Every fat burning hormone works through the liver providing it is clean.

• The liver plays a key role in breaking down hormones, such as oestrogen. When the liver is overloaded, oestrogen dominant conditions can occur: PMS, hot flushes, fibrocystic breast disease, difficult periods, breast and other gynaecological cancers. And, remember oestrogen in excess can cause weight gain.

Alcohol and the Liver

• Alcohol is detrimental to the health of your liver and is also a notorious oestrogen increaser. It does this by affecting the liver's P450 enzyme subsystem in a negative way. Basically, it slows down your body's ability to process oestrogen, allowing it to build up in your blood stream. That means that testosterone will be reduced because oestrogen is a testosterone reducer.

• The strain that alcohol also puts on the liver is well known. The liver detoxifies alcohol by a few enzymes to break it down into harmless chemicals that can be excreted from the body. However, stores of these enzymes are not unlimited and the liver can become overburdened quickly. If too much alcohol is consumed then it cannot be broken down properly and acidic metabolites are formed.

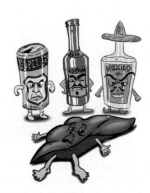

Alcohol is terrible for our liver. Overwhelming evidence has proven that alcohol itself is toxic to the liver, even when nutrition is adequate. Alcohol interferes with the liver's ability to metabolize hormones.

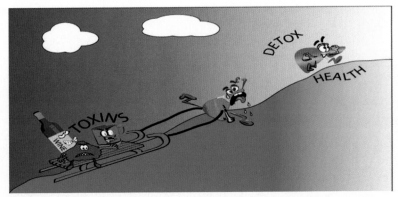

There are many things today that accumulate and eventually over-burden the liver. Once this happens more fat cells are laid down in order to store excess toxins

- In one study volunteers consumed the equivalent of at least a six-pack of beer a day, along with high protein diets enriched in minerals and vitamins. After one "weekend" of drinking, fat accumulation in the liver was already detectable by chemical analysis. In another study, baboons were given an adequate diet, but had alcohol as 50% of their total calories. All developed fatty liver.

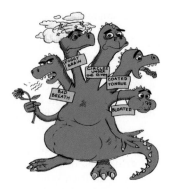

Five signs of a toxic or dysfunctional liver.

Caffeine and the Liver

- Caffeine reaches its peak concentration thirty to sixty minutes after consumption, after which it is inactivated by the liver, with only half its peak level left four to six hours. However, during this time, the liver has to work very hard to detoxify the caffeine and is consequently less efficient at detoxifying other toxins. If you are lean and healthy having a cup of organic coffee with your breakfast every day is like throwing a marble at an elephant's ass trying to get it's attention, in other words it isn't going to have any effect on your already super efficient liver. However if you are obese and tired constantly give coffee a miss until you can see your toes again whilst standing!

Thyroid Hormones and Liver

- Your thyroid gland produces two main hormones: T4 (also called thyroxine) and T3 (also called triiodothyronine). These hormones help to control your metabolic rate, that is the rate at which your body burns calories. They also have a huge bearing on your energy levels and maintenance of normal body temperature.

- T4 is not the active thyroid hormone; it must be converted into T3 in your body in order to exert its effects. The majority of this conversion does not occur in your thyroid gland. Most T4 to T3 conversion happens in your liver, kidneys and muscles. In fact, 60% of T4 is converted into T3 in the liver providing it is functioning at full effectiveness. Now you can see why a dysfunctional liver can lead to a cascade of hormonal problems.

- If you are taking thyroid hormone medication in the form of thyroxine, it too must be converted into the active form in your body. Therefore if you are taking thyroid medication but still not feeling much better, your liver could be to blame! It is vital that you work on improving the health of your liver if you want healthy thyroid hormone levels.

- Thyroid hormones affect the liver cells responsible for detoxification. When thyroid function is low due to hypothyroidism the enzymes that carry out detoxifying tasks simply can't do their job efficiently. We will cover thyroid function more in habit 5.

- If you have a fatty liver or a sluggish liver, this conversion will not be effective. This can leave you feeling tired, depressed, puffy, overweight and with dry skin and thinning scalp hair. Indeed you would have a thyroid problem caused by a faulty liver.

Sugars, Insulin and the Liver

- Insulin is also a fat storing hormone. So high levels of insulin can promote the storage of fat, especially in the abdominal area. The high levels of insulin also send a message to the liver to store more fat, so many people with a high insulin level develop a fatty liver.

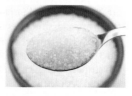

- Avoid eating large amounts of sugar, especially refined sugars, as the liver will convert sugar into the unhealthy type of fat called triglycerides. These fats can build up inside our cells causing fatty degeneration of organs or will be transported to areas for storage, such as the hips, thighs and stomach. This is why many people become fat on a high carbohydrate/low fat diet.

- "Avoid the artificial sweetener aspartame found in diet drinks and diet foods as aspartame is also toxic to the liver. When you ingest the toxic chemical aspartame it is absorbed from the intestines and passes immediately to the LIVER where it is taken inside the liver via the liver filter. The liver then breaks down or metabolises aspartame to its toxic components – phenylalanine, aspartic acid and methanol. This process requires a lot of energy from the liver which means there will be less energy remaining in the liver cells. This means the liver cells will have less energy for fat burning and metabolism, which will result in fat storing. Excess fat may build up inside the liver cells causing "fatty liver" and when this starts to occur it is extremely difficult to lose weight. In my vast experience any time that you overload the liver you will increase the tendency to gain weight easily". Sandra Cabot, M.D.

Human Liver Anatomy

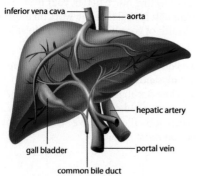

inferior vena cava
aorta
hepatic artery
gall bladder
portal vein
common bile duct

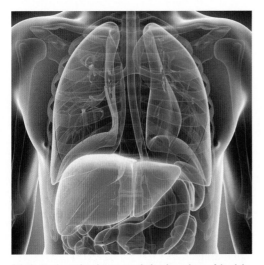

"The liver is located in the upper right-hand quadrant of the abdomen (in the front part of the body), up under the rib cage."

- Many substances inhibit cytochrome P450 (part of the first phase of liver detoxification). This situation can cause substantial problems as it makes toxins potentially more damaging because they remain in the body longer before detoxification. For example, grapefruit juice decreases the rate of elimination of drugs from the blood and has been found to substantially alter their clinical activity and toxicity. Eight ounces of grapefruit juice contains enough of the flavonoid naringenin to decrease cytochrome P450 activity by a remarkable 30%.

- The liver's second detoxification process involves the synthesis and secretion of bile. Each day the liver manufactures approximately 1 litre of bile, which serves as 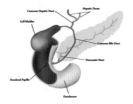 a carrier in which many toxic substances are dumped into the intestines.

- In the intestines, the bile and its toxic load are absorbed by fibre and excreted. However, a diet low in fibre results in inadequate binding and re-absorption of the toxins.

Things the Liver Loves

- There are certain foods that help to protect and detoxify the liver itself so that it can perform better to detoxify the entire body:

- Apples contain pectin which helps to bind and excrete heavy metals through the intestines. This directly helps to reduce the load of filtration on the liver.

- Beets, carrots, red onions and aubergine (eggplant) contain flavonoids and beta-carotene which are potent antioxidants.

- Garlic contains allicin and the mineral selenium, both antioxidants. It assists the removal of heavy metals from the liver.

- Eggs, brown rice and whole grains, broccoli and spinach contain B-complex vitamins which improve liver function and promote liver de-congestion.

- Vitamin B12 helps to metabolize fats and improves liver health.

- Cruciferous vegetables such as cauliflower, broccoli, cabbage, brussel sprouts, Bok Choy, kale, radishes, and turnips contain glucosinolates which help the liver produce enzymes for detoxification.

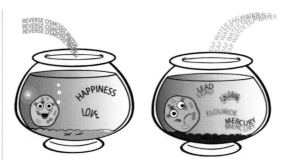

The health of the cell is determined by it environment. When the cell is sick, change the enviroment it is in to a healthier one. Everything from the type of water you drink, the pesticides in the food you eat, the toxins in your cosmetic products and your emtions can all impact the health of the environment.

45

Liver herbs to aid detoxification (traditionally known as 'blood cleansing' herbs):

- Dandelion root, beet leaf & Yellow Dock: (stimulates liver secretions and bile flow)

- Artichoke leaf: promotes regeneration of the liver and promotes blood flow in that organ, stimulates bile flow

- Silymarin (bioflavonoid found in Milk Thistle): according to research, this herbal extract stabilizes the membranes of liver cells, preventing the entry of virus toxins and other toxic compounds including drugs. Supports the protection of the liver and promotes it's regeneration.

- Turmeric, one of the most powerful foods for maintaining a healthy liver, has been shown to actively protect the liver against toxic damage, and even regenerate damaged liver cells. Turmeric also boosts the natural production of bile, shrinks engorged hepatic ducts, and improves overall function of the gallbladder, another body-purifying organ.

- Taurine plays a major role in good liver function via detoxification and the formation of bile. Taurine is the major amino acid required by the liver for the removal of toxic chemicals and metabolites from the body.

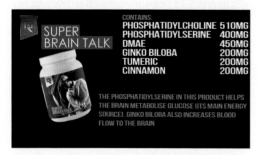

- Recent findings are demonstrating that taurine is one of the major nutrients involved in the body's detoxification of harmful substances and should be a part of any liver detox plan. Taurine is found in high amounts in animal protein, organ meats and invertebrate seafood and is often deficient in vegetarians. When glutathione encounters toxic compounds in the liver, it attaches onto them in a process called S-conjugation which makes the toxin more water soluble. That allows the toxins to be flushed out through the kidneys. Alpha Lipoic Acid (ALA) promotes the synthesis of glutathione in the body and can increase glutathione levels by as much as 30%.

- Mercury interferes with sulphur bearing compounds throughout the body, and can block the ability of the body to synthesize glutathione. Selenium is not only essential for activation of glutathione but it also helps rid the body of deadly mercury. Mercury can bind to selenium, making it useless for this protective purpose.

- For every molecule of chemical that is detoxified, we use up deplete, or lose forever a molecule of glutathione, plus a molecule of ATP. This is one reason why, today we have people who are constantly tired as they are using their valuable energy stores detoxing instead of rebuilding.

- Vitamin C is also a very powerful antioxidant for the liver and reduces toxic damage to the liver cells from chemical overload. It neutralises free radicals generated during the phase 1 detoxification pathway in the liver. Toxic chemicals are far less dangerous if there is plenty of vitamin C in the liver.

- In a study on guinea pigs short term vitamin C deficiency reduced the levels of vitamin C in the liver by 25% and led to a 50% reduction in both the amount produced and the effectiveness of the bile.

- Among foods, the brassica family, i.e. cabbage, broccoli, and Brussels sprouts, contains chemical constituents that stimulate both phase I and phase II detoxification enzymes. One such compound is indole-3-carbinol, which is also a powerful anti-cancer chemical. It is a very active stimulant of detoxifying enzymes in the gut as well as the liver.

Guinea pigs, like humans, can not produce any vitamin C.

- Oranges and tangerines contain limonene, a phytochemical, a strong inducer of both phase I and phase II detoxification enzymes that neutralize carcinogens.

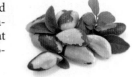

- Beetroot contains betaine which pro-

Brazil nuts are one of the richest sources of selinium

motes the flow of fat and bile from the liver. Betaine also protects the liver from the toxic effects of alcohol.

- Lecithin is one of the best supplements to thin the bile so that toxins and chemicals can flow out of the liver more readily.

- To date, findings from all of nine double-blind trials indicate phosphatidylcholine (PC) clinically supports liver recovery from toxic chemical attack or acute or chronic viral damage! The liver is the workhorse organ of the body, and its parenchymal cells depend heavily on the membrane phospholipids to optimally process newly absorbed nutrients, assemble circulating lipoproteins (LDL and HDL cholesterol, among others) and detoxify thousands of potentially toxic incoming chemicals.

- Other organs such as the lungs, skin and kidneys also have phase 1 and 2 enzymes. This is one of the reasons that deep breathing, sweating and drinking lots of water help the body detoxify.

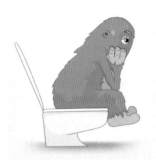

- The body depends on a clean bowel. Remember, the cleanliness of any tissue in the body depends upon the condition of the bowel. It is the source of most internal toxic material, which makes its way into the blood and the lymph through the bowel wall and is then carried to and deposited in the cells and tissues. A cleaner bowel leads to cleaner blood, which leads to cleaner cells and then onto cleaner tissues allowing metabolism to function optimally.

Detoxification Through Defecation

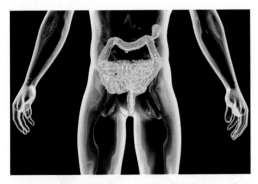

Your bowel health is critical for your fat loss goals. Ensure you have a good supply of pro- and prebiotics, keep hydrated and have a good supply of fibre in your diet

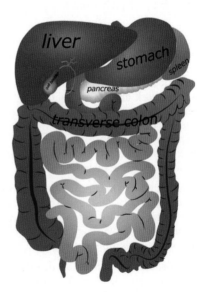

Our digestive system

- When the bowel becomes under-active, toxic wastes are more likely to be absorbed through the bowel wall and into the blood stream. The blood then circulates these toxins to every cell in the body potentially altering cellular function. As the body becomes increasingly toxic, proper oxygenation cannot take place in the tissues. Without oxygen, the body loses energy and this becomes a downward spiral of health. A tired body has reduced ability to throw off toxins, which is why toxic, sick people are always tired people.

- The bowel is considered to be a part of the digestive or gastrointestinal system. It is designed to help the body absorb nutrients and fluids from the foods we eat and drink. After taking out everything the body needs, the bowel then expels the leftover waste.

- The beginning of the bowel is the small intestine, sometimes referred to as the small bowel. This is where the useful nutrients are absorbed from what you eat. If the small intestine was to be laid out, it would be more than 20 feet long. The small intestine delivers the waste to the colon. The small intestine can deliver up to 1 litre of waste to the colon per day.

- The colon is a 5-6 foot long muscular tube that delivers stool to the rectum. As the stool moves through the colon, the fluids are removed and absorbed into the body. The consistency of the stool is dependent upon many things, including how long the stool sits in the colon, how much of the water has been absorbed from the waste, and the amount of fibre and fluids in your diet.

- Stool consistency can vary from hard lumps, mushy, very loose to watery stool. The best and easiest consistency of stool is mushy, like toothpaste; this consistency may be attained by adding fibre to your diet preferably from fruits and vegetables.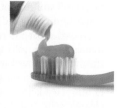

- Fibre helps move waste through the colon because it is indigestible by the human body. In other words, fibre adds 'bulk' to the stool. It is important to eat a diet high in fibre; however, most of us lack fibre in our diet. About 25-35 grams of fibre is required by the body to keep the bowels healthy and moving. If your bowel movements are too loose, fibre can make them firmer; on the other hand, if your stools are too hard, fibre can make them softer.

- Another factor that helps to control the consistency of your stool is fluid. If the colon does not have enough fluids to absorb from the waste, the stool will be dehydrated, resulting in hard, lumpy stool that is difficult to pass.

- In most adults without bowel disease, a diet high in fibre and drinking 1-2 litres of water a day will produce soft stools that are easy to pass. Fluid and fibre work together to encourage healthy bowel habits. You must eat a diet high in fibre and drink plenty of water. Remember, "healthy" stools should be the consistency of toothpaste being squeezed from the tube – soft and free flowing.

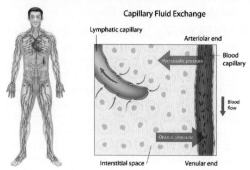

The body also eliminates waste via the lymphatic system which runs in parallel to your bllod stream. Waste is exchanged from capillaries into lymphatic capillaries

- One of the most frequent bowel problems that people experience today is constipation. A constipated system is one in which the transition time of toxic wastes is slow. The longer the "transit time," the longer the toxic waste matter sits in our bowel, which allows them to putrefy, ferment and possibly be reabsorbed. The longer your body is exposed to putrefying food in your intestines, the greater the risk of developing disease.

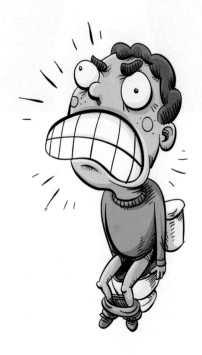

Examples of prebiotic foods include;	
• Oats	• Bananas
• Tomatoes	• Cottage cheese
• Onions	• Goats milk
• Almonds	

- A highly processed diet and an unhealthy lifestyle can cause a dysfunctional bowel leading to intestinal toxaemia. When the intestinal tract is the recipient of an improper diet or when the colon is not evacuated in a timely fashion, the normal intestinal flora are replaced by more harmful bacteria, and intestinal toxaemia is the inevitable consequence.

- In modern civilization, the greatest numbers of bowel disturbances are found in industrialized countries. Modern societies who still live as hunter/gatherers very rarely if ever encounter bowel problems, for example the research by British surgeon Denis P. Burkett M.D., has confirmed the lower incidence of several types of cancer amongst Eastern African natives eating a high fibre diet which reduces bowel transit time.

- One of the main differences between the African natives and the British, he also found, was the fact the British had much slower transit time through the colon compared to that of the African natives due to less fibre in the diet of the British.

- The average Western diet contains 11.0 grams of fibre, as compared to 24.8 grams of fibre in the diet of Bantu tribesman. In rural eastern Africa and other primitive societies there is virtually no incidence of diverticulitis or colon cancer, unless the natives adopt a modern "civilized" diet, as they do when they move to urban areas.

- ly and enjoy your food, chewing it thoroughly and focusing on the nutrients and energy your meal is providing you.

- I also suggest that whilst eating your food, you do not watch anything stressful on the TV(like the news) as this will increase your stress hormones. This will take blood from the gut and to the muscles as the body prepares for fight-or-flight. This will decrease you ability to digest foods.

- Our emotions (that is our feelings and mental state have a great effect on the bowel), so much so that the bowel in ancient times was called the seat of emotions. The colon is extremely sensitive and is influenced greatly by every emotion, both positive and negative. It has been proven that unpleasant emotions can interfere with peristalsis (Peristalsis is the process of wave-like muscle contractions of the alimentary tract that moves food along).

- Try not to let yourself dwell on stressful thoughts or situations during this time. Simply enjoy your mealtime and allow your body to utilize the nourishment it needs.

- Begin transitioning to a diet which also includes plenty of raw fruits & vegetables (steamed). This will keep your digestive system in a healthier state.

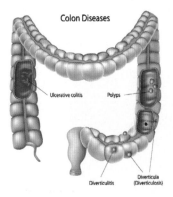

- I strongly suggest that you relax before you eat any meal. When you sit down for a meal, instead of digging right in, perform a little relaxation ritual to start your digestion off right and be very grateful. Before you even pick up your fork, take a slow, deep breath and try to release any tension in your muscles. Eat slow-

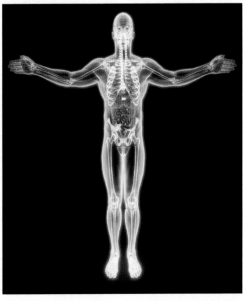

The brain comminicates with the gut and the gut comminicates with the brain. We will discuss this more in habit 3.

- Chew your food thoroughly this is very important for better absorption from foods and will allow regular and easy elimination.

- The human body consists of over 100 trillion micro-flora (bacteria), 80% of which live in our intestines and weighing between 1-2kg.

- The micro-flora in our gut can be good for the body (such as probiotics which can increase immune function) or potentially harmful to the body by causing illness and infections.

It is suggested that we should have between 50-85% "good" bacteria. Although, worryingly, those on a high meat diet have been found to have only 5%, meaning it is outnumbered by the "bad" bacteria 20 to 1.

- Your diet plays a large role in determining the ratio of good and bad bacteria. Sugary foods help many harmful bacteria to thrive. A diet high in fibre (and therefore prebiotic, which feed good bacteria) gives probiotics the edge as they can digest fibre whereas many harmful bacteria cannot.

- Microbes survive longer when they stick to cells of the intestine, and so escape being swept away by peristalsis (wave-like contraction of muscles which squeezes food through the digestive tract). Probiotics regulate peristalsis and compete with harmful microbes for access to these cells, which means more harmful microbes leave the body.

- A study published in Environmental Health in 2005 randomly gave workers either drinking straws with probiotics or a plain straw. Over the next 80 days those with the plain straws had around 80% more days off due to illness. This occurred even though all those who took part described themselves as "healthy".

- A double-blind study in Germany with around 500 people looked at the effect of supplementing with vitamins or vitamins plus probiotics in preventing colds over winter. Those who took the probiotics not only had fewer colds, their colds lasted for less time. And, when blood samples were analysed, it was found that their white blood cells numbers had increased from the start of the study. This is due to the fact that around 80% of the immune system is found in the digestive tract.

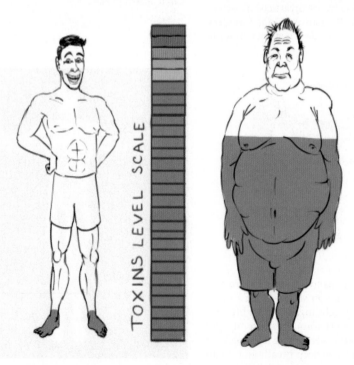

Remember, toxins are stored within our fat cells. If you exposed to high levels of toxins, then you will have to lay down fat cells for these to be stored in.

- Probiotics thrive when fibre is present. The reason for this is that many fibrous foods have prebiotic qualities and so can be digested by probiotics but not by many harmful bacteria. Therefore it is essential that we get enough prebiotic foods . The prebiotic part of foods avoids digestion in the small intestine and is passed on to the large intestine where it is fermented by the probiotic bacteria.

- Wheat fibre can cause bloating, hinder weight loss and is high in phytic acid, which has a negative effect on the absorption of vitaminB3 and certain minerals. This is why I have not advocated high fibre breakfast cereals to anyone in over 20 years!

- One of the reasons why it is difficult for an overweight person to lose body fat may be because of their gut bacteria. Analysis of the microbiota of obese mice and humans have been shown to increase the number of short-chain fatty acids, which increase the energy harvest from food and promote fat storage as adipose tissue.

- Put simply, the gut bacteria in obese people may make them absorb more energy from food and store more of this energy as fat.

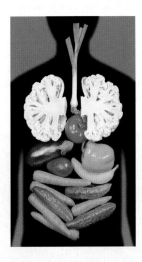

- From the research I've done for this book, I can't recommend colonics. I believe a more sensible way to live is to eat more raw foods, chew the food thoroughly, take digestive enzymes, take a good probiotic every day and stay well hydrated. This will regenerate a colon and beats having a tube shoved up your ass where there really hasn't been any scientific evidence to show any benefits of colonics.

Detoxification of heavy metals

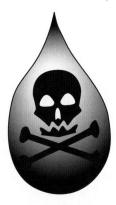

- I had many mercury fillings for 30+ years and then had them removed without any detoxification protocol in place; I was on my knees. This led me to develop my Heavy Metal Chelator, which contains cilantro, chlorella, spirulina and modified citrus pectin.

- Now let's look at these nutrients and why I included them in this product.

- Cilantro is capable of mobilizing mercury, cadmium, lead and aluminium in both bones and the central nervous system.

- It is probably the only effective agent in mobilizing mercury stored in the intracellular space (attached to mitochondria, tubulin, liposomes etc.) and in the nucleus of the cell (reversing DNA damage of mercury). It mobilizes mercury so well, it could overwhelm your liver if you don't use one to five grams of chlorella daily to help flush the mercury out.

- Chlorella is a "green food," a single-celled, micro-algae that is about two to ten microns in size. It's very small. It is this small size combined with its unique properties that make it such a useful detoxification tool. Its molecular structure, allows it to bond to metals, chemicals and some pesticides.

- When chlorella is taken into your body, its natural action will bind it to lingering heavy metals, chemicals and pesticides found in your digestive tract, which is your body's pathway to your bloodstream where these harmful toxins are delivered and deposited into your body's cells.

- So chlorella first and foremost will help your body eliminate unwanted metals and toxins.

- Studies in Japan have shown chlorella may help reduce body fat percentage and may be useful in fighting obesity and weight related diabetes. It may also help reduce both cholesterol and hypertension. Chlorella's cleansing action on your bowel and other elimination channels, as well as its protection of your liver, also helps promote clean blood. And clean blood helps assure metabolic waste get efficiently carried away from your tissues.

- A three year double blind metal detoxification study with over 350 people participating was undertaken at a Russian metal foundry, where more than 20 natural compounds were used in trials to remove heavy metals from people who had been exposed at very high levels to four main metals -- antimony, lead, cadmium and arsenic.

- What were the results of testing chlorella as a heavy metal detoxification agent?

- The Russian trial using chlorella combined with cilantro eliminated ALL heavy metals, including mercury! With no reported side-effects alone.

- Chlorella appears to bind to heavy metals as well as other toxic substances in the bowel and help with the detoxification process. Chlorella also increases serum albumin levels necessary for optimum health. Many reports have come from Japanese research studies that followed the nuclear catastrophe resulting from atomic bombs being dropped on Hiroshima and Nagasaki in 1945. In a report on animals, authors noted that chlorella (8 grams daily) increased elimination of cadmium: 3-fold in faeces and 7-fold in urine (Ichimura 1973). Other researchers from Japan showed that chlorella helped detoxify uranium and lead (Horikoshi 1979). Chlorella has detoxification potential for similar compounds, such as dioxin and poly-chlorinated biphenyls (PCBs) (i.e., chemical compounds used in plastics, insulation, and flame retardants, with potential to cause cancer and liver damage). Other research indicates that chlorella is useful in detoxification of high levels of mercury in the body caused by removal of mercury amalgam. Some dentists recommend chlorella to patients having mercury amalgams replaced (as well as to themselves

and staff who can incur accidental exposure from day-to-day exposure to amalgam filling procedures) (O'Brien 2001).

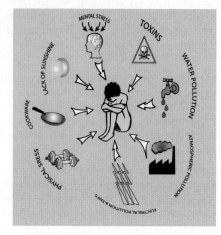

We face toxic stress from numerous places in our everyday lifes.

- In addition to its detox abilities, chlorella is one of nature's best super foods. It contains all the amino acids, providing easy-to-digest protein. It also contains vital minerals such as magnesium and iron. The high level of chlorophyll in chlorella helps optimize oxygen into blood intake.

- Spirulina has been shown as an effective chelating agent for removing toxins such as mercury, and radioactive substances from the body. It has also been used to remove cadmium and lead from waste water.

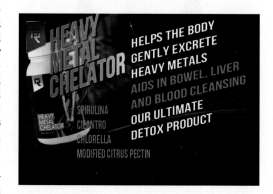

Conclusion

- Detoxification is simply about keeping the elimination channels operating efficiently. Eating nutrient dense foods and drinking plenty of clean reverse osmosis water. Taking sensible exercise in the fresh air with sunshine and getting a good sweat on whilst opening the lungs. Use infrared saunas to enhance the detoxification and eliminate as much as you can all man made toxins from multiple sources which we looked at in habit 1.

- Some of the books that I have read in learning about detoxification, and which you may find helpful are;

  - "The 7 Principles of Fat Burning" by Eric Berg
  - "The Pure Cure" by Sharyn Wynters & Burton Goldberg
  - "The pH Miracle for Weight Loss" by Robert Young & Shelly Young
  - "The Detox Solution" by Dr Patricia Fitzgerald
  - "Toxic Dentistry Exposed" by Drs Graeme & Lilian Munro-Hill
  - "Detoxify or Die" by Shelly Rodgers

HABIT 3

CHANGE YOUR BRAIN
CHANGE YOUR THOUGHTS
CHANGE YOUR WEIGHT

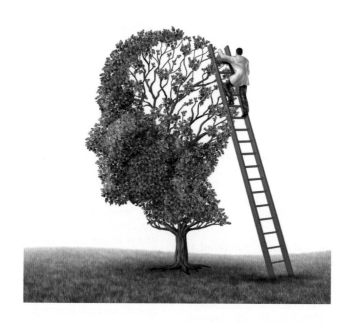

"I have come across a great many people who say that they are an expert in nutrition, yet often they disappoint. Phil Richards however, has spent an enormous amount of time researching and developing his knowledge. I can say without hesitation that you will hear from him absolute cutting edge information. In fact, if you want to become the person that you dream about, you'll be seriously missing an opportunity if you do not look at what Phil delivers."

Dr Karl Morris
World Leading Golf Psychologist

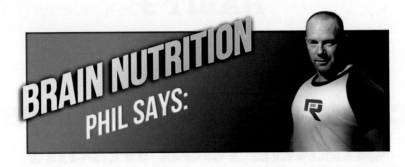

BRAIN NUTRITION
PHIL SAYS:

I have personally been fascinated with brain nutrition for many years and have developed a number of nutritional products to enhance my own brain function. When your brain is working at optimum efficiency, life is 100% more enjoyable.

When your brain is broken you will struggle with emotion, addictions, relationships and life in general. This is why you need to know what's breaking your brain and how to rebuild it. I personally suffered over for 30 years with depression, suicidal thoughts, self sabotage and a host of other mental health problems.

My life changed almost over night at the age of 45 when I realised I had become a prisoner of my own thoughts and had caused every bit of chaos in my life up until that point. Realising that if I can control my thoughts, instead of my thoughts controlling me, has meant that I can have the life I want. Now, I never allow any negative thinking to enter my head, I have massive gratitude for life and I nourish my brain every day. I can now honestly say hand on heart I now love my life.

- In this habit, we are going to discuss how you can develop a high-functioning brain. Remember, it is the brain that makes the choices in your life and can help you achieve not only a better quality of life, but also help make the correct food choices, which will allow you to build a lean, healthy body.

- Your brain is flesh and blood. The mind is simply a function of the brain. For you to understand this point with more clarity, think of someone with Alzheimer's. This terrible disease will cause this person to lose their mind. Why? Because their brain has become diseased and, therefore, dysfunctional

- Paul MacLean, the former director of the Laboratory of the Brain and Behaviour at the United States National Institute of Mental Health, developed a model of the brain based on its evolutionary development. It is referred to as the "triune brain theory" because MacLean suggests that the human brain is actually three brains in one. Each of the layers, or "brains", were established successively in response to evolutionary need. The three layers are; the reptilian system (or R-complex), the limbic system, and the neocortex. Each layer is geared toward separate functions of the brain, but all three layers interact substantially.

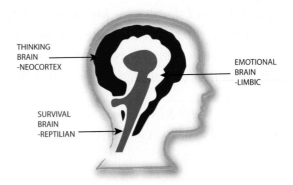

THINKING BRAIN -NEOCORTEX

EMOTIONAL BRAIN -LIMBIC

SURVIVAL BRAIN -REPTILIAN

The brain has 3 major components; the neocortex, the limbic complex and the reptilian complex

The Reptilian Complex

- The Reptilian complex consists of the brain stem and the cerebellum. Its purpose is closely related to actual physical survival and maintenance of the body. The cerebellum orchestrates movement. Digestion, reproduction, circulation, breathing, and the execution of the "fight or flight" response in stress are all housed in the brain stem. Because the reptilian brain is primarily concerned with physical survival, the behaviours it governs have much in common with the survival behaviours of animals. It plays a crucial role in establishing home territory, reproduction and social dominance. The overriding characteristics of R-complex behaviours are that they are automatic, have a ritualistic quality, and are highly resistant to change.

The Limbic System

- The limbic system, the second brain to evolve, houses the primary centers of emotion. It includes the amygdala, which is important in the association of events with emotion, and the hippocampus, which is active in converting information into long term memory and in memory recall. Repeated use of specialized nerve networks in the hippocampus enhances memory storage, so this structure is involved in learning from both commonplace experiences and deliberate study.

- However, it is not necessary to retain every bit of information one learns. Some neuroscientists believe that the hippocampus helps select which memories are stored, perhaps by attaching an "emotion marker" to some events

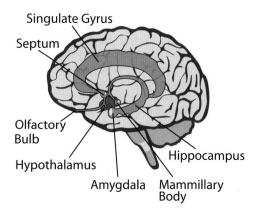

so that they are likely to be recalled. The amygdala comes into play in situations that arouse feelings such as fear, pity, anger, or outrage. Damage to the amygdala can abolish an emotion-charged memory. Because the limbic system links emotions with behaviour, it serves to inhibit the R-complex and its preference for ritualistic, habitual ways of responding.

- The limbic system is also involved in primal activities related to food and sex, particularly having to do with our sense of smell and bonding needs, and activities related to expression and mediation of emotions and feelings, including emotions linked to attachment. These protective, loving feelings become increasingly complex as the limbic system and the neocortex link up.

The Neocortex

- Also called the cerebral cortex, the neocortex constitutes five-sixths of the human brain. It is the outer portion of our brain, and is approximately the size of a newspaper page crumpled together. The neocortex makes language, including speech and writing possible. It renders logical and formal operational thinking possible and allows us to see ahead and plan for the future. The neocortex also contains two specialized regions, one dedicated to voluntary movement and one to processing sensory information.

- All three layers of the brain interact. The layers are connected by an extensive two-way network of nerves. On-going communication between the neocortex and the limbic system

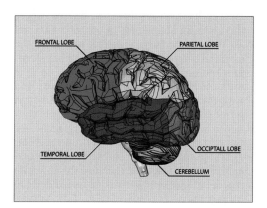

The cerebral cortex of the brain. This is the part which seperates us from other species

57

links thinking and emotions; each influences the other and both direct all voluntary action. This interplay of memory and emotion, thought and action is the foundation of a person's individuality. The full extent of this interconnectedness is unclear. However, it is entirely incorrect to assume that in any situation one of our three "brains" is working and the others are not. What we can do, tentatively, is assume that at times one particular focus may be dominant while the rest of the brain acts in support and that education can influence which focus dominates.

- When you look to the fact that our brain is what will tell us what to eat and drink or how we feel, then doesn't it make sense to look first at brain health if we want to maintain a healthy weight? For it will be the brain that will decide if you have a piece of chocolate cake over an apple or whether you dwell on past hurts or move on with hope. It will be your brain that decides whether you stick to your exercise regime or watch TV while munching on junk food.

Your brain is the most complex, mind blowing organ in the universe. It weighs only about three pounds, usually around 2 percent of the body's weight. Unbelievably it is 80% water. The brain uses 25 percent of the oxygen we breathe and up to 70 % of the glucose we consume when at rest.

- The brain is connected to every cell in the body through the nervous system. The signals and messages of the nervous system consist of chemical "runners" who deliver messages to and from the brain. These chemical runners are known as neurotransmitters.

- Our thoughts are transmitted by neurons. They gather information by transmitting electrical impulses along their elongated bodies. These impulses can cause chemical reactions. If you have lots of depressing thoughts you will experience depression. Similarly, lots of happy thoughts will help you experience happiness.

Why we went from dumb arse to smart arse

- Your brain is a maze of trillions of connections capable of performing 20 million – billion calculations per second. It has 3 major components.

  - Neurons: brain cells that power the communication message. Neurons need an abundance of essential fatty acids and phospholipids.
  - Neurotransmitters: chemicals that create the message, e.g. serotonin. Neurotransmitter are primarily amino acids therefore quality protein is required.
  - Receptors: proteins that receive the message.

- So it is clear what you eat determines who you are!

- Somewhere in the evolutionary backwoods of the brain, something unprecedented happened in the story of life on Earth. The human brain changed and was suddenly able to compute, manage and store information like never before. Why did this happen? Scientists think they have found the answer:-

- Human life first originated in the sea, where there was an abundance of omega-3 fatty acids – the same fatty acids that now form the essential components of our eyes' photo receptors and our brain's cell membranes. As time went on, flowering seed plants appeared and with them a brand new fatty acid family was introduced. The seed oils of these plants contained what we call omega-6 fatty acids. For the first time, the omega-3 and omega-6 fatty acid families existed on earth together and apparently this opened the door for an entire new set of species to arrive that would develop bigger brains.

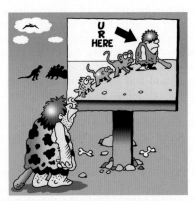

A lot of the knowledge that I have gained on brain fats has been from Michael Schmidt and Dr Barry Sears and their excellent books.

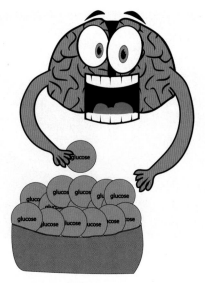

The brain is a glucose hog requiring around 120g of glucose per day

- How did the new species develop bigger brains? Human beings are thought to have lived on earth for millions of years, however the big brain change happened only in the last 200,000 years or so. What could have caused the change in human brains? And why did some human brains change and others stay the same? Could it have been what they ate?

- The puzzle of the big brain change involved scientists putting together pieces that, at first look, had no relation. The first piece of the puzzle involved discovering early human populations that demonstrated greater intelligence. They found evidence in the East African Rift Valley and on the southern Cape of South Africa.

- The second piece of the puzzle was the discovery that docosahexaenoic acid (DHA) was a large contributor to brain growth. The third piece was the discovery that DHA was found in seafood.

- When scientists put all the pieces together they found that the early humans who lived near water sources and ate seafood experienced the big brain change!

- People collecting shellfish could have easily provided themselves with a plentiful source of brain-specific nutrition, and their children would have naturally participated in the exploitation of this extremely rich resource.

- There must have been enough omega-3 and omega-6 fatty acids available in their diet to provide many generations with fuel for fetal/infant development as well as childhood and

adult needs for the cardiovascular system and the brain.

- This increase in the consumption of algae derived fats, coupled with a consistent supply of blood glucose for a constantly glucose – hungry brain, laid the foundation for the emergence of a new species: modern humans.

- Dr Donald Rudin, author of "The omega 3 phenomenon", has estimated that, over the past seventy five years, we have reduced our omega 3 fatty acid consumption by 80%. This explains why we are getting dumber, fatter and sicker. You must fully understand that without EPA & DHA primarily derived from fatty fish (salmon, mackerel, sardines, anchovies & tuna) or pharmaceutical grade fish oil your brain cannot function at full efficiency it is 100% IMPOSSIBLE.

- Remember from Habit 1, the diet that made us human is the one that will keep us human. That diet was one rich in fruits, vegetables, nuts, seeds and high quality animal protein, especially offal & fish.

- Your brain orchestrates the symphony of consciousness that gives you purpose and passion, motion and emotion.

- The brain is critically dependent upon abundant blood flow, because it requires about 25% of all blood pumped by the heart. Therefore, any disruption of cerebral circulation has a profoundly negative effect upon the brain. Vascular plaque, caused by excessive inflammation, contributes to decreased blood flow to brain cells

- Both the heart and lungs must be healthy for optimal brain function. If the function of either organ is inadequate, then brain dysfunc-

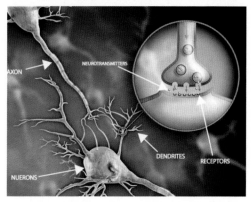

What our neurons look like. This is one way the brain communicates.

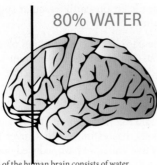

80% WATER

About 80% of the human brain consists of water

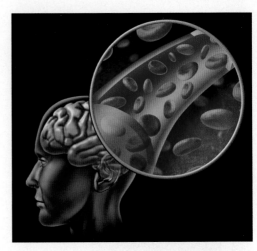

The brain needs a huge supply of blood. Around 25% of blood flow is directed to the brain

tion will be the consequence. With roughly 400 miles of blood vessels, the human brain also needs healthy blood vessels if it is to function efficiently.

Your brain runs almost EXCLUSIVELY on glucose and uses more than 20% of your body's total energy even though it only weighs a few pounds, yet your brain has no place where it can actually STORE glucose. We use approximately 120 grams of glucose per day for just brain function alone.

- When insulin levels are high, glucose the main fuel for the brain, is directed away from the brain and into other tissues, such as muscle. This elevation of insulin not only starves the brain of glucose but it keeps the fat switch well and truly on. So it is imperative for optimum functioning of the brain, and to keep lean, to maintain a steady blood glucose supply.

- Phosphatidylserine is a phospholipid which enables your brain cells to metabolize glucose and to release and bind with neurotransmitters, all of which is important to learning, memory and other cognitive functions.

- Ginko biloba is a herb that has been shown to increase blood flow to the brain. This was one of the reasons why I added this herb to super brain talk.

- Over the past ten years, neuroscientists have identified an inability of the brain in Alzheimer's patients to properly use glucose. This has been documented by sensitive brain scans called positron emission tomography, or PET, scans. In certain instances, these changes can be seen decades before a diagnosis of Alzheimer's disease is made, which suggests to experts in this field that the inability of the brain to

properly use glucose might be a key factor in the development of the disease.

- There is actually another fuel that the brain can readily use and stop your food cravings almost instantly. Any absence of fuel for your brain's function is perceived correctly by your body as a code red emergency. Powerful biochemical messages then order you immediately to eat refined carbohydrates to fuel your brain quickly. The amino acid L- glutamine reaches the starving brain within minutes and can often immediately put a stop to even the most powerful sweet and starch cravings. The brain feeds on L-glutamine instead of glucose and is satisfied and prevents you hopefully from destroying the chocolate cake in the fridge.

- When you have extreme carb cravings, which usually happen late in the evening, towards bed time, you will find that glutamine will help curb these cravings. Glutamine has also been shown to increase growth hormone release. This is one of the reasons why I included it in my Nitric Oxide Generator

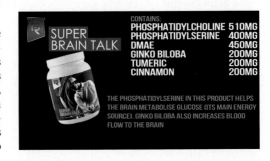

SUPER BRAIN TALK

CONTAINS:
PHOSPHATIDYLCHOLINE 510MG
PHOSPHATIDYLSERINE 400MG
DMAE 450MG
GINKO BILOBA 200MG
TUMERIC 200MG
CINNAMON 200MG

THE PHOSPHATIDYLSERINE IN THIS PRODUCT HELPS THE BRAIN METABOLISE GLUCOSE (ITS MAIN ENERGY SOURCE). GINKO BILOBA ALSO INCREASES BLOOD FLOW TO THE BRAIN

Dehydration & Brain Function

- About 80% of the human brain consists of water.

- Water intake is very individualised. I am not going to tell you how much is optimum for you but, I have found that if I consume at least 1 litre of alkalised, filtered water for each 25kg of my body weight, then this is optimum for me. When I exercise, I will obviously then take on extra fluids, which I will go into further in Habit 9.

- At 4–5 % below optimal fluid intake, you could experience a 20–30% decline in cognitive function.

- The decline in blood volume that occurs with even slight dehydration impedes the transport of oxygen and nutrients to the brain.

- A study in which men were subjected, on separate occasions, to each of three test conditions:

1. 40 minutes of walking on a treadmill with quite a steep incline (5%) at a speed of 5-6 km/hr in a temperature of about 28 degrees centigrade. The men were also treated with the drug frusemide – a diuretic that speeds dehydration.
2. Same conditions as above, but instead of being given frusemide, the men were treated with a placebo.
3. Same conditions as above, while the hydration status of the men was maintained (in other words, they were not allowed to become dehydrated).

- Basically, conditions 1 and 2 were designed to induce dehydration of two severities (the one with frusemide being more severe), and condition 3 was designed to act as a control (where individuals expended about the same amount of energy in the same heat but did not suffer dehydration). The participants were then subjected to tests of mental function, fatigue and mood.

Dehydration was found to reduce vigilance and working memory (the ability to actively hold information in the mind needed to do complex tasks such as reasoning, comprehension and learning). Fatigue during exercise was worse during dehydration. Measures of tension and anxiety were greater too.

- What this study shows is that dehydration does indeed have the capacity to affect brain function and mood, and therefore it pays to stay topped up with water. Our requirements for water vary according to a variety of factors including weather, temperature, how active we are, how much we sweat and how much water we get via what we eat. A good guide, in terms of water intake, is to drink enough to keep urine pale yellow in colour throughout the course of the day.   Ganio MS, et al. Mild dehydration impairs cognitive performance and mood of men. British Journal of Nutrition. 7 June 2011

Brain Destroyers

- Britain has one of the highest suicide rates in Europe. Around the world, around one million people commit suicide each year, including more than 6,000 in the UK and Ireland, of whom around 1,500 are women and 4,500 men.. The Samaritans estimate that in the UK there is a suicide every 82 minutes. At least 140,000 people in England and Wales attempt suicide every year, and this number is rising dramatically, particularly among the young. There are many factors that will cause someone to suffer with mental illnesses and suicidal thoughts or suicide itself. Let's look at 5 brain destroyers which can effect brain function.

Mobile Phones

- A Swedish study indicates that mobile phone use can raise the risk of brain tumours. In the study, 2,200 cancer patients, and an equal number of healthy control cases, were examined for mobile phone use. Among the cancer patients, about a tenth of the nearly 1,000 with malignant brain tumours were also heavy mobile phone users. Heavy use was defined as 2,000 or more hours, or about 10 years' use at an hour per day. Brain cancer patients also showed a significant increase in risk of tumour for the side of the head where they generally used the mobile phone. The researchers who conducted the study said that the figures demonstrate a 240% increased risk of a malignant tumour on that side of the head.

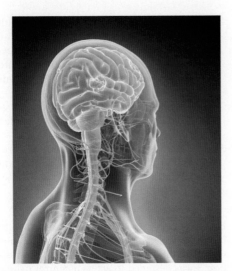

Use of mobile phones, (especially from a young age) has been linked to an increase risk in brain tumors

"people who started mobile phone use before the age of 20" had more than five-fold increase in glioma, a cancer of the glial cells that support the central nervous system.

- The risk to young people from household cordless phones was almost as great. Cordless phones caused a fourfold increase in risk. Young mobile phone users were also five times more likely to get acoustic neuromas, disabling tumours of the auditory nerve that often cause deafness.

- On June 1st, 2011 Scientists at WHO (World Health Organisation) classified mobile phones as carcinogenic: In a debate that has been ongoing with divisive opinions and inconclusive evidence, the WHO has come out and stated that the radiation emitted from mobile phones can "possibly" boost the risk of brain cancer.

- Research has also indicated that children and teenagers are five times more likely to get brain cancer if they use mobile phones. Such studies are raising fears that today's young people may suffer an epidemic of the disease in later life. Swedish research has also reported more worrying news on mobile phone use and brain health at the first international conference on mobile phones and health. It came from a further analysis of data from one of the biggest studies carried out on the mobile phone/cancer link, headed by Professor Lennart Hardell. Professor Hardell told the conference that

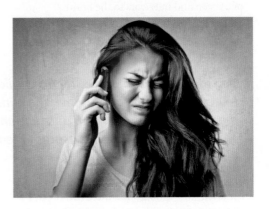

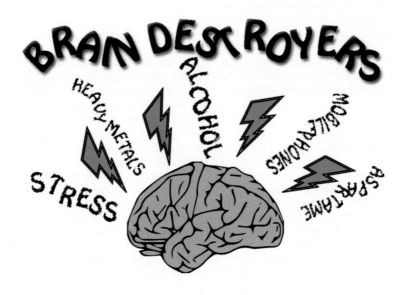

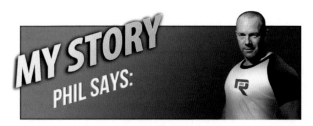

MY STORY
PHIL SAYS:

From my life's experience, I feel as if I have a phd in emotional management. For me, it started from a very young age where I was raised in family where the word "love" was never mentioned. I cannot ever recall having fun times as a child. However, I must say that my mother worked very hard to raise me and my brother.

My parents got divorced when I was very young. This is where I feel that my instability began. I could not decide which parent to live with. I probably moved house around 20 times from the ages 6-16. Living with my father at about 9 years old, I was beaten up by my father as I walked through the living room on my way to the toilet and, as I walked through the living room, he was having sex, which obivously, as a 9 year old, I did not realise. Looking back, I have realised that that must have been trigger as why he decided to beat me up. To this day I look back with total disbelief at how someone could do that to thier son. I kept going back from pillar-to-post, mother-to-father until eventually I joined the Army, at 16, to get away!

My grandfather then became like a father figure to me. He played a huge role in my life. I was seeing pyschaitrists at the age of 14 and many things were just put down to teenage blues. I then joined the army at the age of 16, which I thrived upon. I loved the discipline, freindship and having 3 square meals a day. I was the model solider, the fittest in my regiment. In fact, I was put forward for special forces selection at the age of 19, but my behaviour was always unpredictable as I became bored very quickly. This often got me onto trouble with the military.

In 1986, at the age of 19, my regiment was called upon to do a tour of duty, the preperation for which was incredible. I thrived on this, the more pressure and stress there was, the more I shone. We did an intense period of training before departing for active service. Before we left we were given 3 days leave. As I was based in Germany I decided to come home and see my family. On ariving home, I had a bottle of whiskey for my grandfather as this was his favourite drink. When my mother opened the door to me, she informed me that my grandfather was dead. I was devastated. She had informed my regiment that he had died, but they hadn't informed me. I was angry. Then, I was deployed into active service, holding onto this anger.

After 4 months of active service, I was sent back to Germany as I was, in the eyes of the military, "too mentally unstable" to hold a weapon. Shortly after this, I was diagnosed with a personality disorder. Thankfully, I have now managed to get this under control after many years of self-destruction.

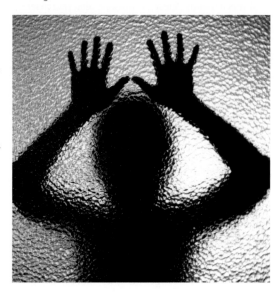

Many years ago, when I was married, I found out that my wife at the time was having an affair with someone who I considered to be a good friend and somebody that I had trained in professional sport for many years. What made things even more unbearable was that this person, who I considered a friend, had a wife who, at the time, was heavily pregnant, and my eldest son had just turned 2.

My exercise tolerance, like myself, was on its knees. During this difficut period, spanning around 18 months, I put on around 40lbs in weight, even though I continued doing the same amount of exercise as I had previously.

From this experience, I seriously considered taking my own life multiple times. Thankfully I didn't (obviously). What this unpleasant situation taught me was that; dishonesty is ugly and that you must learn to forgive, otherwise anger will kill you.

I can honestly say that it took me over 10 years to get over this. I did it after a lot of self-help, but the most important thing was realising that I deserve to be happy.

"The purpose of our lifes is to be happy."
Dalai Lama

When my youngest daughter was born, I was told she had Down's Syndrome. There was no warning that this would be the case. I was 45 years old at the time and, while being told this news, felt that someone had just ripped my heart out. I remember walking around the hospital feeling sorry for myself and then, thankfully, the reality of the situation hit me; I believed that with my expertise on health and nutrition, I could research this condition and no doubt find many new exciting discoveries that could not only help my daughter, but also many others with Down's Syndrome, over the years to come.

So, if you are in a dark place, trust me, there is hope. You must never give up. You must realise that you deserve to be happy and healthy. Never give up on your dreams.

Stress

- Nothing kills brain cells (especially those in the hippocampus where memories are stored) faster than excess cortisol. Look after your stress levels if you want to look after your brain. Enduring a high stressor for over 30-60 minutes at a time has been shown to negatively impact the hippocampus in various ways. Sustained exposure to higher than normal levels of cortisol results in the pruning back of the number of branches and synaptic connections of hippocampal neurons. By a variety of mechanisms, these conditions also increase the rate of cell death in this region of the brain. As if this wasn't bad enough, research is also demonstrating that sustained increases in glucocorticoid levels also has negative effects, impairing the hippocampus' ability to create new neurons. All of this could result in the shrinking in size of the hippocampus, with associated declines in cognitive function, including the ability to retain new information and adapt to novel situations.

- Even for healthy people, stressful moments can take a toll on the brain, a study from Yale University suggests. Researchers reported in the journal Biological Psychiatry that stressful occasions (like going through a divorce or being sacked) can actually shrink the brain by reducing gray matter in regions tied to emotion and physiological functions. This is important because these changes in gray matter could signal future psychiatric problems, researchers warned.

Aspartame

- The phenylalanine in the artificial sweetener aspartame depletes serotonin, leading to panic attacks, manic depression, rage and violence. There are over 92 different symptoms associated with aspartame consumption which is found in most diet products. Small amounts of aspartame can lead to the build up of formaldehyde (bound to protein) in the liver, kidneys, brain and soft tissues. Tests on rats show that they developed unusually high numbers of brain tumours when exposed to aspartame.

- One study concluded that "Compared to other environmental factors putatively linked to brain tumours, the artificial sweetener aspartame is a promising candidate to explain the recent increase in incidence and degree of malignancy of brain tumours. Evidence potentially implicating aspartame includes an early animal study revealing an exceedingly high incidence of brain tumours in aspartame-fed rats compared to no brain tumours in concurrent controls" J Neuropathol Exp Neurol. 1996 Nov;55(11):1115-23.

- It is interesting to note that the first experiments performed to test the safety of aspartame before its final approval in 1981 disclosed a high incidence of brain tumours in the animals fed the sweetener. This study was carried out by the manufacturer of nutrasweet®, G.D. Searle. In this study 320 rats were fed aspartame and 120 rats were fed a normal diet and used as controls. The study lasted two years. At the end of the study twelve of the aspartame fed rats had developed brain tumours, while none of the control rats had. This represented a 3.75% incidence of brain tumours in the rats fed aspartame, which was twenty-five times higher than the incidence of spontaneous brain tumours developing in rats (0.15%).

Heavy Metals

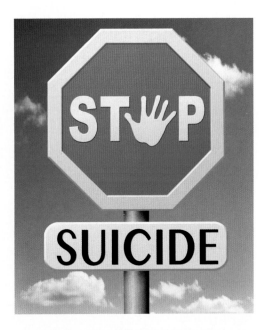

- Mercury causes damages to the brain and the central nervous system,causes psychological changes and can cause development changes in young children. Mercury is a toxic substance which has no known function in human biochemistry. It targets and kills neurons in specific areas of the nervous system.

- Several mechanisms have been proposed to explain how mercury kills neurons:

  - Protein inhibition
  - Disruption of mitochondria function
  - Direct affect on ion exchange in a neuron
  - Disruption of neurotransmitters
  - Destruction of the structural framework of neurons

- Methylmercury is especially dangerous to developing babies. This form of mercury is highly toxic and can cross the placenta and the blood-brain barrier. Mercury is concentrated in the brain of the developing foetus because the metal is absorbed quickly and is not excreted efficiently. Children exposed to mercury may be born with symptoms resembling cerebral palsy and other movement abnormalities, convulsions, visual problems and abnormal reflexes. The brains of children who have died as a result of mercury poisoning show neuron loss in the cerebellum and throughout the cerebral cortex. Mercury also appears to affect brain development by preventing neurons from finding their appropriate place in the brain. You have to question pregnant mothers being offered the flu jab which can contain thiomersal (mercury). In 2001, the European Agency for the Evaluation of Medicinal Products advised doctors to use only vaccines without thiomersal for toddlers and infants, who are thought to be more likely to suffer harm from exposure

to mercury. This followed a 1999 announcement by the U.S. Public Health Service and the American Academy of Paediatrics (AAP) that thiomersal should be reduced or eliminated in vaccines as a precaution.

- A study by the American Institute of Medicine concluded that a link between thiomersal in vaccines and neuro- developmental disorders was 'biologically plausible'. In a related U.S. study, researchers found a statistically significant association between thiomersal in vaccines and children with problems such as attention deficit disorder (ADD) and speech and language learning delays.

Alcohol

- Research from the University College of London has estimated that the average Briton consumes 20 units of alcohol every single week.

- Autopsy studies have shown that patients with a history of chronic alcohol consumption have smaller, lighter, more shrunken brains than non-alcoholic adults of the same age and gender. This finding has been repeatedly confirmed in living alcoholics using a variety of imaging techniques. Structural imaging reveals a consistent association between heavy drinking and physical brain damage, even in the absence of medical conditions previously considered to be clinical indicators of severe

Anthony's Story

Anthony (21 years of age) had several classic symptoms of depression. His sleep patterns were disrupted, he might go to sleep but then wake very early in the morning and not be able to get to sleep again.

He had lost his appetite and as a result, had lost weight. He found it difficult to concentrate on his work and as a result, was in danger of dropping out of college and most crucially, he frequently felt suicidal.

Anthony had visited many GP's and then on to a number of specialists who had prescribed several different types of anti-depressants, none of which had really helped.

It was clear that Anthony had what is known as resistant depression, the severest form of the illness and one that does not respond to treatment. Anthony was in imminent danger of killing himself and this is where Dr Basant K Puri comes into the picture.

The treatment that Dr Puri described was eicosapentaenoic acid or EPA, which is a derivative of a naturally occurring essential fatty acid found in fish/fish oil.

On this basis, Anthony was prescribed a highly purified form of EPA. Anthony also agreed to allow him to run several highly specialist tests, including brain scans, in order to observe the effects of the EPA.

9 months later, Anthony was transformed. He appeared a confident, self assured young man, who shook Dr Puri's hand warmly and who had no problem looking him in the eye. All the signs of depression had gone.

After analysing Anthony's brain scans, Dr Puri compared the brain scan he had taken after the course of EPA with the one taken 9 months earlier, before treatment began. The results were astonishing.

Because Anthony was already an adult, Dr Puri would not expect to see any change in the brain structure over a 9 month period. If he had started to develop a brain disease, such as dementia, in which he was losing nerve cells and cerebral tissue, then he would expect to see that the two largest brain ventricles had become larger as the brain deteriorated.

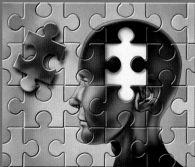

Anthony's brain ventricles had become smaller and parts of his cerebral cortex had become thicker. Both changes that pointed to the possibility that re-growth had taken place in parts of his brain.

The result of Anthony's brain scans led Dr Puri to believe in the possibility that EPA can in some way stimulate stem cells in our brains to produce new nerve cells, offering hope for a variety of conditions that adversely affect the brain.

alcoholism (e.g., chronic liver disease or alcohol-induced dementia).

- Imaging reveals shrinkage to be more extensive in the folded outer layer (i.e., cortex) of the frontal lobe, which is believed to be the seat of higher intellectual functions. Repeated imaging of a group of alcoholics who continued drinking over a 5-year period showed progressive brain shrinkage that significantly exceeded normal age-related shrinkage. The rate of frontal cortex shrinkage in this study correlated approximately with the amount of alcohol consumed.

- There are many alcohol-related brain disorders, some of which include:

  - Cerebellar atrophy – the cerebellum is the part of the brain responsible for muscle coordination. Damage results in difficulties with balance and walking, which is called 'ataxia'.

- Frontal lobe dysfunction – the brain's frontal lobes are involved in abstract thinking, planning, problem solving and emotion. Damage results in cognitive difficulties.

- Korsakoff's amnesic syndrome – this includes a loss of short-term memory, an inability to acquire new information and 'confabulation' (the person fills in gaps in their memory with fabrications that they believe to be true).

Your Brain Needs Nourishing to Function Optimally

- You must fully understand that when the brain is well nourished, well oxygenated, well hydrated and has a steady blood sugar supply, it is difficult to make the wrong food choices. We only choose the wrong foods when we have the wrong brain chemistry.

- Remember the brain has 3 major components which are totally dependent on what you eat and drink; neurons, neurotransmitters and receptors.

  - Neurons need an abundance of essential fatty acids and phospholipids.
  - Neurotransmitter are primarily amino acids therefore quality protein is required.
  - Receptors are proteins that receive the message.

- Nothing you put in your mouth is as agreeable or disagreeable to the intricate structures of your brain cells as fat. Your brain is the body's fattiest organ – 60% is made up of various fat like substances. This also makes the brain extremely vulnerable to toxins, as toxins have an ability for fat.

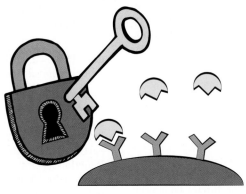

Each nuerotransmitter has to fit perfectly into the receptort of the nueron (much like a lock and key). If it does not fit exaclty will not activate a clear transmission

- A lack of omega 3, particularly DHA and EPA, combined with high levels of omega 6 is linked with deterioration of brain and visual function.

- Denied the right fats, and flooded with the bad fats, your cerebral tissue may become partly starved - not a good picture.

- The outer membranes of your brain cells may stiffen and shrivel the dendrite tentacles that reach out to form patterns of communication with other cells may become stunted, the rich chemical flood of neurotransmitters may dry up or become short circuited, unable to gain entry to neurons and carry messages from neuron to neuron. It is a mess that nature never intended yet that is the state of many people's brains today.

- We know that neurons can continue to grow and expand at all ages, even into old age. Such growth though requires rich supplies of essential fatty acids. Thus, the fat you eat throughout life is constantly moulding your brain. It's an exciting but sobering thought, considering that most brains are fed garbage fats throughout life. This usually results in garbage brains.

- The membranes of neurons – the specialized brain cells that communicate with each other – are composed of a thin double-layer of fatty acid molecules.

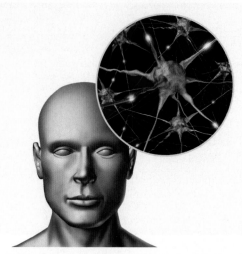

The neurons in our brain act like telephone lines, connecting to each other and sending messages all throughout the brain and the body.

Compelling research, in small laboratory animals, shows that excess saturated fat in the diet can actually change not just the function of brain cells, but also their very shape.

- Researchers have known for more than a decade that saturated fat does something awful to mammalian brains. Laboratory animals fed lots of saturated lard don't learn as quickly or perform as well on a wide spectrum of memory tests, including finding their way out of mazes, as do animals that are fed polyunsaturated fats.

- Indeed, lard-fed animals consistently display short and long term memory resulting in learning and memory dysfunction on a wide range of tasks and functions this indicates that dietary fat has sweeping effects on brain function.

- So the major villain is saturated fat. It predictably causes major detrimental effects on memory and learning. Mono-unsaturated fat may be beneficial to memory and polyunsaturated can both be beneficial or detrimental depending on the type and ratio of omega 3 to omega 6.

- Dr. Carol Greenwood from University of Toronto says, "the more saturated fats animals eat, the more severe their brain and memory malfunction." Dr Greenwood demonstrated that rats learning curves dropped in direct proportion to the amount of saturated fat they ate. On a diet of 10% saturated fat, the animals learned virtually nothing.

- Further, the harmful effects of saturated fat on the brain seem to be cumulative. The more years you eat a high animal fat diet, the more severe risk of dumbing down. In fact, it appears the brain over time begins to adapt to a high animal fat diet, resulting in impaired learning.

- Dr. Greenwood says animal studies suggest that a consistent high saturated fat diet seems to somehow exert a direct toxic anti-learning effect on the brain cells, regardless of the other types of fat you eat.

- In other words the danger comes from the saturated fat itself, not just an imbalance or lack of other beneficial fats.

- But now comes another astonishing discovery, showing that saturated fat may literally strangle brain cells. Ground breaking research by Patricia Wainwright and colleagues in the Department of Health Studies at the University of Waterloo in Ontario Canada, finds that saturated fat does more that influence the morphology, or shape of the brain cells themselves!

DENDRITES BRING INFORMATION TO THE CELL BODY

CELL BODY

AXONS TAKE INFORMATION AWAY FROM THE CELL BODY

An illustration of a nueron. There are over 100 billion of these in your brain alone.

- Analyses of the gray matter of the fat fed animals showed fewer and shorter dendrites with fewer branches needed to reach out to send and receive messages.

- Dr. Greenwood explains that stunted dendrites can cripple memory, because physical changes actually take place in brain cells during memory and learning.

- Many scientists have rallied around a theory, proposing saturated fat degrades memory and learning by affecting the hormone insulin. Both animals and humans who eat a lot of saturated fat tend to develop insulin resistance.

- Insulin is an important chemical that helps the body metabolize glucose in the body. However, it also helps the body metabolize fats as they travel throughout the body, including the brain.

- When a person's brain develops insulin resistance, it becomes unable to metabolize fats or lipids. The result is these fats build up, resulting in nerve stress and inflammation. These are common factors associated with the development of diabetes. They are also associated with developing dementia, a characteristic of Alzheimer's disease.

- There is another alarming way fat can harm your brain; overeating Omega 6 and under eating Omega 3. Most of us are filling our brain cells with the wrong kind of fat and ignoring the right type of fat - another reason why we are becoming dumbed down today!

- During prehistoric days when our brains evolved, our ancestors ate equal amounts of Omega 3 and Omega 6. Omega 3 is found in seafood and our Omega 6 at that time came mostly from meat, fruits, vegetables, eggs & nuts. Today, unfortunately, a high percentage of our Omega 6's come primarily from processed vegetable oils.

- One of the most fearful potential consequences of omega 6 dominance in brain cells is persistent inflammation of brain tissue. Such inflammation can injure cerebral blood vessels, set up processes that kill brain cells, warp nerve cell membranes disrupting normal functioning, interfere with neuronal message transmission, and promote strokes, Alzheimer's disease, and probably all degenerative brain diseases.

- In 1999 evidence of chronic inflammation increased the odds of stroke by nearly 500% in a large group of men observed for twenty years as part of the Honolulu Heart Study.

- What's critical to the brain is not just the total amounts of omega 3 & 6 you eat but the relative amounts of each or the ratio. In fact the ratio is the critical factor that determines how well information is transmitted from neuron to neuron.

What is a neuron?

- A neuron is a nerve cell. The brain is made up of approximately 100 billion neurons.

- Neurons are similar to other cells in the body in some ways such as:

- Neurons are surrounded by a membrane.

- Neurons have a nucleus that contains genes.

- Neurons contain cytoplasm, mitochondria and other "organelles".

In a perfect world you would eat no more than one molecule of omega 6 fatty acid for every one molecule of omega 3 fatty acid for optimum brain function. But in reality that isn't going to happen research is showing that you can maintain excellent brain function with a ratio of 4–1 omega 6 & 3.

- Your brain is the body's fattiest organ – 60% of the dry weight is made up of lipids (fat like substances). Making it very vulnerable to oxidative damage! It is because of this that I encourage you to eat a diet that is rich in anti-oxidants (e.g. berries, broccoli, peppers, beetroot).

- We can now see that the chemistry of the fat we eat can profoundly influence the very architecture of our brain cells; the profusion or scarcity of all-important dendrites and synapses the linchpins of intelligence, learning, memory, attention, concentration and mood.

- Essentially, the membrane consists of two layers of fatty molecules (phospholipids), and the membranes flexibility depends on the consistency of its fat. If the fat is hardened like lard, the membrane is stiff & rigid or if the fat is more fluid like fish oil, the membranes is soft and pliable.

- Cell membranes must be pliable and in constant flux to perform the communication miracles of the brain, says Dr. Joseph Hibben, a research psychiatrist at the National Institute Of Health in Bethesda, Maryland. That is especially true, he says, in the synapses of brain cells the junctions where nerve cells converge to pass their messages

- A single nerve cell may make up to 20,000 connections with other cells. The place where these cells connect is the synapse. The portion of the nerve making the connections is called the synaptic membrane. This part of the nerve has the highest concentration of DHA than almost any other tissue in the body..

- These synaptic gaps, where signals jump from one cell to another, are the source of the brain's awesome powers. The more of these transmission centres or synapses on brain cells and the smoother the communication between them, the better the brain functions and the better sense of well-being that you will feel.

How Much Omega-3 is in the Typical UK diet ?		
	Men	Women
Total omega-3	2.3g	1.7g
	(Henderson et al 2003)	
EPA + DHA (Estimate)		
Oily fish eaters (27%)		244mg
White fish eaters	113mg	
Non-fish eaters	46mg	
	(Givens & Gibbs 2006)	

- Moreover, the number and quality of synaptic connections determine intelligence and optimal brain function even more than the total number of brain cells.

Omega 3 fish oil, more precisely the part called DHA (docosahexaenoic acid) is the building material for synaptic communication centres. You can't create more synapses, dendrites, or receptors that increase your brain's potential without a robust supply of DHA.

- Before you start drinking fish oils by the litre, to jump start your deficient brain, let me first educate you on the fact that taking fish oils without any anti-oxidant protection added to them, during processing, will have less benefit than those that are protected. Those without anti-oxidant protection are very susceptible to going rancid and so may cause more problems than benefits. This is why I developed my Ultimate Fish Oils (liquid and capsules). They both have great levels of this anti-oxidant protection in the form of fat-soluble vitamins (A, D, E, K2) which are added during the processing method.

- Like a growing tree, any time a nerve cell makes a new branch it requires new raw materials. Without adequate DHA available, branching out cannot happen. If brain fats are not available in needed amounts you will not grow new dendrites & axons and have a very hard time learning new material.

- Millions of messages pass through the synapses of a cell hourly. To accomplish that, a chemical messenger a neurotransmitter is cast adrift into a watery void by one nerve cell to find its way into the receptors of a nearby nerve cell.

- If the neurotransmitter does not fit perfectly into the receptor of the waiting neuron, the attempted communication fails.

- When a neurotransmitter does lock in, it activates the cell to fire and release more neurotransmitters to traverse thousands of synapses in a perpetual chain reaction of tiny sparks amongst billions of brain cells that ultimately form our universe, our thoughts, actions and mood.

- Each neurotransmitter, such as serotonin or dopamine, has a unique shape that must fit into the receptor embedded in the cellular surface of the membrane. For the perfect fit needed to activate clear transmission, the receptor alters its shape slightly.

- If the membrane is made of fluid fat, such as fish oil, the receptor can easily change configuration. But if the membrane is made of rigid, hard fat, the receptor is immobilized, unable to wiggle or expand to let the neurotransmitter lock in. Then the communication between cells is not activated, in fact is short circuited, garbled, muted, or instantly terminated.

- Thus, how efficiently neurotransmitters pass from one neuron to another depends on the fluidity of the synapses. You can amplify message transmission across synapses a thousand fold by altering fat membrane consistency.

- Even if you have an ample supply of chemical neurotransmitters, the message can't get through if the receptors don't function properly. You can send out all the neurotransmitters you want but, if only 50% of the normally functioning receptors are in a state to activate the messengers, only 50% of the message gets through.

- In short, a receptor sitting in a cell membrane filled with rigid fat is a dead or mute receptor. It can't sense or transmit much of anything. That is something to remember the next time you set out to solidify your cell membranes with too much animal fat, omega 6 fats & trans fats.

- An intriguing way fish oil seems to influence mood and behaviour is by boosting brain levels of the feel good neurotransmitter serotonin.

- It's well documented that many people with abnormally low brain and blood levels of serotonin are depressed, at high risk of suicide, and criminally impulsive.

- However, if you have high levels of DHA fish oil in your blood, you're apt to have high amounts of serotonin in your brain. Precisely how fish oil manages to boost serotonin is not well understood currently, but scientists speculate it may happen in several ways:

- Changing the fat composition of membranes which alters the actions of critical enzymes that, for example, convert tryptophan (an amino acid) to serotonin and control its breakdown and reuse or re-uptake.

- There's also recent evidence that eating fish creates more serotonin simply because the body uses DHA to manufacture more synapses, with more nerve endings, that in turn produce more serotonin. It's like building more serotonin factories, instead of just increasing the efficiency of the serotonin.

- UCLA neuroscientists have shown that a diet high in the omega-3 fatty acid DHA helps protect the brain against the memory loss and cell damage caused by Alzheimer's disease. The new research suggests that a DHA-rich diet may lower one's risk of Alzheimer's disease. The journal Neuron reported the findings on Sept. 2004.

- "This is proof that our diets affect how our brain cells communicate with each other under the duress of Alzheimer's disease," said Greg Cole, senior author and a professor of neurology at the David Geffen School of Medicine at UCLA. "We saw that a diet rich in DHA, or docosahexaenoic acid, dramatically reduces the impact of the Alzheimer's gene."

- It used to be taught as fact, in medical schools, that the human brain in an adult is not capable of further growth. Since then, it has been proven that the adult mammalian brain does have

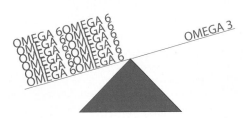

Our intake of omega-6 can often outweigh our intake of omega 3 which can have implications on our brain function

> **Gluten is a protein component of grains. The following grains contain gluten:**
>
> - Wheat (durum, semolina)
> - Rye
> - Barley
> - Spelt
> - Triticale
> - Kamut
> - Farina
> - Oats
>
> - Casein is a protein derived from dairy products: Includes milk, butter, cheese, yogurt, ice cream, etc.
> - Goat's milk has casein, but it may or may not be reactive (controversial).
> - *Elliott RB, Harris DP, Hill JP, Bibby NJ, Wasmuth HE. Type I (insulin-dependent) diabetes mellitus and cow milk: casein variant consumption. Diabetologia 1999 Mar;42(3):292-6*

the capacity to regenerate its cells though we still know little about this process.

- Neurogenesis is the term used to describe the recently discovered capacity of the human brain to grow new neurons.

- That's right, our brain is not physically fixed, it is constantly changing, losing some neurons, growing some neurons, making or deleting connections, and we all have the potential to achieve outstanding things in our lives, simply by nourishing and challenging our brains. This will force our brains to become smarter

- Cell Membranes are made of the following:
  - Fatty Acids from wild fish and fish oil, the omega 3 fats DHA and EPA.
  - Phospholipids from foods like egg yolk, liver, soya beans, sardines, lentils, sesame seeds, flaxseed.
  - Cholesterol from eggs, liver, poultry. This is the glue between molecules.
  - Protein from high quality meat sources etc.

> ### Gluten-Free Grains
>
> - Being gluten intolerant doesn't mean you have to eat a totally grain-free diet. Here are a few options you can still enjoy (in moderation) when grain-cravings strike:
>
>   - Rice
>   - Corn
>   - Quinoa
>   - Buckwheat
>   - Millet
>   - Amaranth
>   - Teff
>   - Sorghum
>   - Wild rice

- Receptors, transporters, gates, signal transducers etc. The most abundant fats in your cell membranes are the phospholipids. There are three main kinds of phospholipids - phosphatidylcholine, phosphotydylserine and dimethylaminolamine, abbreviated DMAE.

Super Brain Builder – Phosphatidylcholine

- Phosphatidylcholine is a substance which can be derived from the nutrient compound lecithin that consists of; phosphate, fatty acids and choline. The components of phosphatidylcholine, particularly the fatty acids and choline, make it valuable as a brain-promoting agent.

- Supplementing phosphatidylcholine has some very positive benefits for your brain. Research on rats at Duke University Medical Centre in the USA, demonstrated that giving choline during pregnancy creates the equivalent of super brains in the offspring.

- The researchers fed pregnant rats choline halfway through their pregnancy. The infant rats whose mothers were given choline had vastly superior brains with more neuronal connections and, consequently, improved learning ability and better memory recall.

- All of which persisted into old age. This research showed that giving choline during pregnancy helps restructure the brain for improved performance in the long term.

- "Choline does dramatically change the very structure of memory centres in the hippocampus of the developing foetal brain," declares Dr

Stephen Zeisel, a world expert on choline. Dr Zeisel and colleagues found that when choline is lacking, cell division in the foetal brain is reduced. Cells migrate abnormally. An increasing number of brain cells die prematurely.

- If your brain does not get enough phosphatidylcholine, nutritionally, it will literally cannibalise brain cells to obtain this nutrient according to Dharma Singh Khalsa, M.D., Brain Longevity: The Breakthrough Medical Program that Improves Your Mind and Memory.

Don't forget Phosphatidylserine

- Over 3,000 published research papers and more than 60 clinical trials have established that phosphatidylserine (PS) can help to rejuvenate your brain cell membranes.

- Phosphatidylserine increases communication between cells in your brain by increasing the number of membrane receptor sites for receiving messages.

- Phosphatidylserine modulates the fluidity of cell membranes - essential to your brain cells' ability to send and receive chemical communication.

- Phosphatidylserine also stimulates your brain to produce dopamine and this is likely why patients diagnosed with clinical depression have shown marked improvement in their symptoms as a result of taking phosphatidylserine daily.

- One of the best known and most effective ways to lower excess cortisol levels is with the nutrient phosphatidylserine. Phosphatidylserine is believed to facilitate the repair of the cortisol receptors in the hypothalamus.

- It is believed that the cortisol receptors get damaged by high cortisol levels reducing the ability of the hypothalamus to sense and correct high cortisone levels.

- Because phosphatidylserine helps repair the feedback control apparatus, it is useful in correcting both high and low cortisol levels.

- Phosphatidylserine can also help reduce increases in exercise-induced cortisol levels. In a double-blind, crossover study conducted at California State University, 10 men were given 800 mg of phosphatidylserine a day and then put through a vigorous whole-body workout (designed to elicit a cortisol response) four times a week.

- Each participant received phosphatidylserine for two weeks and then repeated the workout program for another two weeks with a placebo, after a washout period of 3 1/2 weeks. Blood samples were taken 15 minutes after each workout. This study found that phosphatidylserine reduced cortisol levels after exercise by 20%.

- The researchers also found that testosterone levels, which normally decline after intensive exercise, were not reduced.

- Phosphatidylserine also boosts acetylcholine levels and contributes to healthy brain cell membranes, with benefits for cognition and mood.

- Phosphatidylserine may be even more effective when combined with the omega-3 fatty acid DHA.

- Substantial laboratory research suggests that phosphatidylserine ability to improve cognitive skills is greatly increased in the presence of DHA.

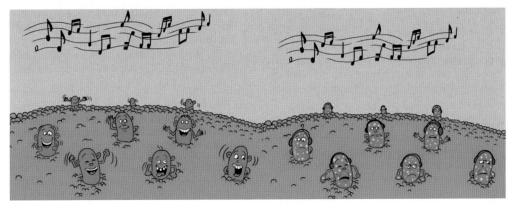

Phosphatidylserine helps to increase communication between cells. This is required by all cells, especially brain cells.

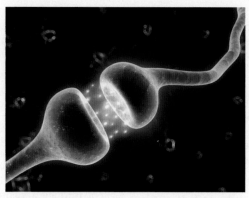

Neurotransmitters being sent from one neuron to another. This is how neurons communicate.

- Furthermore, the combination of DHA and phosphatidylserine powerfully supports energy production in brain cells. Scientists from the National Institutes of Health believe that phosphatidylserine, with attached DHA, is among the most critically important molecules for healthy brain function, and that phosphatidylserine works optimally in the presence of abundant levels of DHA.

- Research shows that supplementing with DMAE (another phospholipid) increases choline levels in the brain better than using choline itself. Having higher choline levels increases acetylcholine, a critical neurotransmitter involved in brain processes and muscle contraction. Boosting this neurotransmitter results in better mental function, better focus and drive in the gym, better muscle endurance and strength, improved mood and a greater sense of well being.

- DMAE provides numerous benefits, one being that is protects the integrity of cell membranes. This helps prevent premature aging. Other benefits of DMAE include its ability to elevate mood, counteract depression and boost memory and concentration.

- Unless you eat a lot of organ meats, like liver, kidney and brains (the richest sources of phospholipids), often prized in traditional cultures, you will need to supplement with phospholipids if you want to achieve optimum brain function.

- This is why I developed Super Brain Talk. Please do not think that I am trying to sell you this supplement (or any others mentioned in this book, at that). I developed these products so as I could regain my own health.

- You have more brain cells in your head than the number of trees in the Amazon rainforest. You have more connections between brain cells than the number of leaves on all the trees in the Amazon rainforest.

- The fact is, it's not the size of the brain that mostly determines intelligence, but the number of connections between neurons. The connections are physical entities, and can therefore be nurtured and stimulated with various measures.

- However, neurons differ from other cells in the body in some ways such as:

- Neurons have specialized projections called dendrites and axons. Dendrites bring information to the cell body and axons take information away from the cell body.

- Neurons communicate with each other through an electrochemical process.

- Neurons form specialized connections called "synapses" and produce special chemicals called "neurotransmitters" that are released at the synapse.

- There are approximately 1 quadrillion synapses in the human brain. That's 1,000,000,000,000,000 synapses! This is equal to about a half-billion synapses per cubic millimeter and DHA is required for them to function.

- Neurotransmitters are the runners that race to and from the brain, telling every organ inside of us of us what to do. Neurotransmitters touch the life of every cell.

- Amino acids are the precursors to neurotransmitters, and the production of these substances can be directly affected by your diet. So it is essential to eat quality protein with each meal

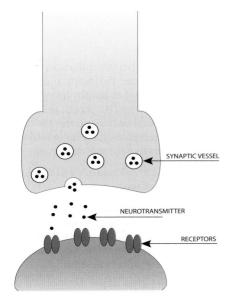

SYNAPTIC VESSEL

NEUROTRANSMITTER

RECEPTORS

Synaptic gaps are where signals jump from one cell to another to pass on the body's electrical messages. The more of these transmission centres or synapses on brain cells and the smoother the communication between them, the better the brain functions.

so that we have the substrates available to make our messenger molecules (neurotransmitters). There are many types of neurotransmitors, but our focus in this manual is on the importance of dopamine, acetylcholine, GABA (gamma-Aminobutyric acid) and serotonin:

- Dopamine is derived from the amino acids tyrosine and phenylalanine.
- Acetylcholine is derived from the B-vitamin choline.
- GABA is derived from the amino acids taurine, theanine and glutamine.
- Serotonin is derived from the amino acid tryptophan and 5 HTP.

- Neurotransmitters affect mood, sleep, concentration, weight, and can cause adverse symptoms when they are out of balance.

- So the key to what's going on in our skull are special brain chemicals called neurotransmitters. They are the messengers of mood.

- The body also produces its own uplifting chemicals, known as endorphins, by breaking down food, and it is therefore possible to raise the levels of these substances in the brain by eating foods containing a combination of nutrients which release endorphins. Low endorphin levels can be caused by certain vitamin and mineral deficiencies. Certainly, a lack of B vitamins (particularly B12) and vitamin C, or

of minerals such as iron, potassium and zinc, can cause you to feel low.

- The four key neurotransmitters that can help with mood , inhibit cravings and addiction can be subdivided into two major categories. Think of them as ON & OFF switches for your brain. Those that excite and activate you, and those that make you calm & happy.

- Both dopamine and acetylcholine are on switches that create our ability to focus and learn.

- Dopamine is often thought of as the pleasure, motivation, and reward neurotransmitter in the brain. Cocaine and stimulants like caffeine boost dopamine in the brain that's why these substances often become addictive and eventually dumb down your receptors to dopamine meaning you have to consume more each time to get a hit.

- Dopamine is built from the essential amino acids phenylalanine & tyrosine. Eating foods rich in protein, or supplementing your diet, with both these amino acids can help mood, energy, and attention.

- Dopamine levels are usually low in addicts, in people with low energy, depression and in ADHD.

- DHA shortages may result in low dopamine, serotonin and melatonin (our sleep hormone), leading to depression and sleep problems. Impaired serotonin function has been linked to long term aggression, violent behaviour and sleep disorders in humans.

- Omega 3 fatty acids naturally increase dopamine levels while lowering the AA:EPA ratio, as mentioned earlier. Animal and human studies show that fish oil raises dopamine levels in the brain. Dopamine has also been shown to stimulate the release of testosterone!

- If we add more omega-3, we can instantly raise dopamine by 40% Julia Ross, author of The Mood Cure

- It turns out that, among other things, omega-3 is an MAO (mono-amine oxidase) inhibitor, meaning it paralyzes the MAO enzymes that destroy mood-boosting brain neurotransmitters like dopamine.

- GABA and serotonin are our off switches and create a calming effect on the mind and body helping us sleep and relax. Because their functions are similar, similar symptoms may occur when either is deficient.

- One of the most reliable predictors of alcoholism is a chronic under secretion of GABA. People who don't have enough GABA almost invariably experience high levels of tension. They often self medicate with alcohol.

- Caffeine can exacerbate or even cause stress, anxiety, depression and insomnia because it interferes with a tranquillizing neurotransmitter chemical in the brain called adenosine.

- This is the chemical which turns down our anxiety levels - it's our body's version of a tranquilliser. Caffeine docks into a receptor for adenosine and regular use of caffeine is enough to produce anxiety and depression in susceptible individuals.

- New research published in the Journal of Alternative and Complementary Medicine shows that an hour of yoga raises levels of the inhibitory neurotransmitter GABA in the brain. Increased GABA levels reportedly help counteract anxiety and other neuropsychiatric disorders.

- The research, carried out at Boston University School of Medicine (BUSM) and McLean Hospital, used magnetic resonance spectroscopic imaging to examine two groups of people both before and after a one hour activity. One group practiced yoga, while the other read a book.

- Participants in the yoga group had a 27% increase in GABA levels, while those in the reading group remained unchanged. Co-authors Chris Streeter from BUSM and Domenic Ciraulo pointed out that this research shows a method of treating low GABA states.

- Green tea is also an ingredient that could help your GABA production. Naturally, green tea has L-theanine which when taken moderately can produce a calming effect to avoid drowsiness.

- For a solid dose of GABA, always include fresh citrus fruits in your diet. Foods that are high in glutamine can assist in GABA production. Some very helpful foods are beef liver, citrus, broccoli, halibut and lentils. As much as possible, include this in your daily diet with at least one to two servings every time you eat.

- Another good addition to your diet are nuts such as walnuts and almonds. Foods rich in L-theanine such as oats, spinach, whole grains can also assist in the production of GABA.

These foods can literally lower stress, while it provides other health benefits such as lowering the blood sugar.

- Gut bacteria significantly influences the communication between the brain and the gut. When the gut is full of healthy bacteria, it has the potential to regulate mood and positive feelings. Beneficial bacteria in the gut will increase GABA receptors in the brain to alleviate mood disorders like chronic depression.

- To produce GABA add taurine and theanine to your supplement stack.

- Serotonin plays a crucial role in maintaining our overall happy feeling. Serotonin deficiency or a decrease in the serotonin level is most likely to blame for depression, aggression, anxiousness, and elevated pain sensitivity.

- Serotonin can be the easiest deficiency of all to develop. The amino acid tryptophan is the only nutrient the body can use to make serotonin. According to the Lancet a 1997 study revealed that tryptophan is one of the first nutrients to be depleted by weight loss dieting. This could be another reason why dieting can cause anxiety and depression.

- Stress and high cortisol levels can decrease serotonin levels. Cortisol increases the activity of enzymes that break down tryptophan which leaves less substrate to make serotonin.

- High protein foods tend to lower brain tryptophan which in turn will lessen serotonin levels.

- Because carbohydrate consumption stimulates the uptake of tryptophan for the manufacture of serotonin. Carbohydrate cravings in many cases is really a craving for serotonin.

- In many species, its directly tied to appetite – deplete serotonin, and they act like they are starving.

- 90-95% of the human body's total serotonin is found in specialized cells in our guts.

- When the gut make too much serotonin, Irritable Bowel Syndrome could arise. Carbohydrates may be responsible for making too much serotonin. Excess carbohydrates are not only responsible for too much yeast growth in the guts causing those nasty holes in the gut lining but they are also responsible for too much serotonin production.

- If you want more information on nuerotransmittors for fat loss and mood, I highly recommend "The Mood Cure" by Julia Ross and "The Edge Effect" by Dr. Eric Braverman.

The Gut-Brain Connection

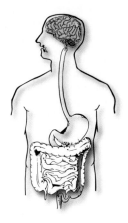

Our gut and our brain originate early in embryogenesis from the same clump of tissue which divides during fetal development. The health of your gut can have a huge influence on the health of your brain.

- For you to have a fully functioning well nourished brain you must first have a fully functional digestive system. After all if you can't digest the nutrients the brain needs to function you will suffer from brain drain no doubt about that. Remember the brain is totally dependent on what you eat and digest!

- Why do we get butterflies in our stomach before a performance? Why does indigestion produce nightmares? It turns out that both our gut and our brain originate early in embryo-genesis from the same clump of tissue which divides during foetal development.

- While one section turns into the central nervous system, another piece migrates to become the enteric nervous system. Later the two nervous systems connect via a cable called the vagus nerve - the longest of all the cranial nerves whose name is derived from Latin, meaning "wandering".

- The vagus nerve meanders from the brain stem through the neck and finally ends up in the abdomen. There's the brain-gut connection.

- Nearly every chemical that controls the brain in the head has been identified in the gut, including hormones and neurotransmitters

- According to Dr. Michael Gershon, M.D., author of `The Second Brain' and a neurobiologist at New York's Columbia-Presbyterian Medical

Center, the stomach is our second brain with an independent network of over 100 million nerve cells in the gut.

- If your gut has suffered a degree of damage perhaps through regular use of alcohol, coffee or painkillers, or through gut infections or antibiotics you are also more likely to react against the food you eat.

- The average person in the UK takes over 300 painkillers a year and are the guts worst enemies, because they damage it, making you more prone to allergy.

- I can recall one professional rugby player who, during his playing time, had taken an incredible amount of anti-inflammatories. He was still passing blood in his urine even many years after he retired.

- A leaky gut can lead to brain allergies which can dramatically impact your mood, attention, and behaviour. The most common and most serious undiagnosed immune or toxic reactions are to wheat and dairy.

- What is a leaky gut - The cells that line the intestinal wall are meant to act as a barrier to only allow fully digested nutrients through and into your blood stream to be utilized within your body.

- When leaky gut develops, these tightly packed cells begin to lose their structure and gaps form between them which allows undigested food particles, bacteria, yeast, toxins, and other harmful substances that exist within your gut enter into your blood stream. And once in your blood stream, these unwanted substances can travel freely anywhere within the body and account for countless chronic symptoms!

- The inflammation and toxic effects of gluten & casein (derived from wheat and dairy) are so powerful in derailing our brain function that they can lead to everything from brain fog, to depression, to ADHD, autism and dementia.

- University Western Ontario researchers investigated the "gut-brain" connection after many parents of autistic children reported significant improvements in the behaviour of their autistic children when they modified their diet, eliminating dairy and wheat products.

- I also want to make the very strong point that not everyone is allergic to wheat and dairy. You can easily get tested but ensure that you use a very reputable lab. If you are not allergic to these two proteins then, I have no doubt, that they offer some health benefits.

- Mercury is also known to inhibit the enzymes that digests gluten and casein, possibly increasing a person's susceptibility to wheat and milk allergy.

- Israeli doctors recently found that two women previously diagnosed with Alzheimer's actually had an inherited autoimmune diseases, an allergy to gluten. The women were put on a gluten free diet and miraculously their memories came back and the Alzheimer's disappeared. This obviously doesn't mean this would happen in every case but very interesting none the less.

- Gluten & caseine proteins are also known to exert opioid-like effects on the brain.

- These proteins attach to receptors in the brain. They are nearly identical in structure to natural opioid-binding peptides. (Can have morphine-like effects and become addictive)

- 57% of patients with neurological dysfunction (including Autism and ADD patients) were shown to have antibodies to gluten (a component of wheat and other grains.) Lahat E, et al. Prevalence of celiac antibodies in children with neurological disorders. Pediatr Neurol. 2000 May;22(5):393-6.

- A unique type of enterocolitis (infection of the colon) was found in 93% of individuals with developmental disorders. Wakefield AJ, et al. Enterocolitis in children with developmental disorders. Am J Gastroenterol. 2000 Sep;95(9):2285-95.

- Dr. Maios Hadjivassiliou of the United Kingdom, a recognized world authority on gluten sensitivity, has reported in the journal, The Lancet, that "gluten sensitivity can be primarily and at times, exclusively a neurological disease".

- That is, people can manifest gluten sensitivity by having issues with brain function without any gastrointestinal problems whatsoever. Dr. Hadjivassiliou indicates that the antibodies that a person has when they are gluten sensitive can be directly and uniquely toxic to the brain.

- 20% of children with coeliac disease have white matter lesions of the brain and the incidence is high enough that some authorities suggest that coeliac disease should be positively ruled out in all learning disabled children (J Ped, Dec 2001, Vol. 108).

- Cognitive decline and underachievement in post secondary education is 400% more likely in gluten sensitivity. Scandinavian Journal Of Gastroenterology, 2005.

Your Brain Thrives with the Right Exercise!

- Our ancestors were the ultimate athletes. Can you imagine the effort it took to hunt wild game, to gather fruits, nuts & plants etc. Their strength and endurance levels would be equivalent to any professional athlete today that I have absolutely no doubt about. Everything today is so easy for us in the Western world we piss moan and groan today if someone has moved our remote control for the T.V. and we have to get up and find it. We are designed to be physically active and this has an enormous effect on our brains as you are just about to find out.

Why Is Exercise Good For Mood?

1. Increased blood flow to the brain and more efficient oxygen and glucose metabolism.
2. Neuron response to stress is improved (especially in the hippocampus at least)
3. Increases serotonin to brain
4. Brain is protected against molecules that overexcite it, including free radicals, high glucose levels, and high glutamate levels

- Exercise produces BDNF which stands for "brain-derived neurotrophic factor. It's a protein actually, dubbed a master molecule and referred to as "Miracle-Gro for the brain".

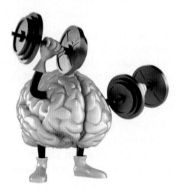

- BDNF is like miracle-grow for the brain!

- BDNF binds to receptors in the synapses between neurons, increasing voltage (yes your brain is electric!) and improving signal strength.

- BDNF Inside the cells, it activates genes that increase production of more BDNF and other important proteins as well as serotonin. Low levels of BDNF have been associated with depression and even suicide.

- Serotonin has a reciprocal relationship with BDNF, i.e. BDNF boosts serotonin production and serotonin signalling stimulates BDNF expression .

- One of the most exciting changes that exercise causes is neurogenesis, or the creation of new neurons. The new neurons are created in the hippocampus, the center of learning and memory in the brain.

- There also seems to be a role for neurogenesis in the treatment of depression. Studies show that the hippocampus of depressed women can be up to 15% smaller than normal.

- This damage may be reversed by BDNF-stimulated neurogenesis. BDNF as the key chemical underlying exercises impact on the hippocampus. Perhaps it is not exercise that has the curative power, but rather BDNF, and exercise is only the trigger.

- Humans start to lose nerve tissue beginning at age 30. Aerobic exercise reinforces neural connections by increasing the number of dendrite connections between neurons, creating a dens-

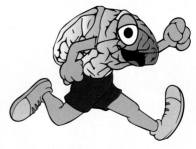

Exercise is great for our brain health and helps increase blood flow to the brain, increase serotonin levels and produces BDNF.

er network, which is then better able to process and store information.

- Norman Doidge, MD, author of "The Brain that Changes Itself", writes: The idea that the brain is like a muscle that grows with exercise, is not just a metaphor. Just like a muscle, the brain grows thicker as we use it.

- Endurance exercise appears to increase the brains capacity to concentrate. After rigorous exercise people are more attentive and ,because they can concentrate better, they have the ability to process and retain more information.

- In a recent German study volunteers who did two 3 minute sprints (separated by 2 minutes of lower intensity) during the course of a forty-minute treadmill session demonstrated higher increases in BDNF than non-sprinters.

- Not only that, the sprinters learned vocabulary words 20% faster than non-sprinting exercisers. It seems even a small amount of high-intensity exertion can have a profound effect on your brain.

What You Think About, You Bring About

- You and only you can program your brain/body to live in a world where you are kind, loving and happy this allows the body to be in a constant state of happiness which will have a positive effect on your fat burning hormones. Or you can choose to hate, have anger raging inside you and think the world owes you a living and be in a constant state of catabolism (when the body is breaking down tissue). The choice in how you think is yours and nobody's else.

- Body and mind are intertwined – every thought, feeling and intention you have sends

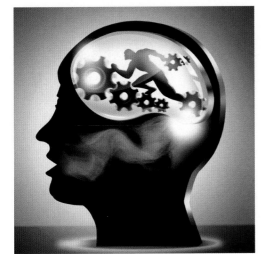

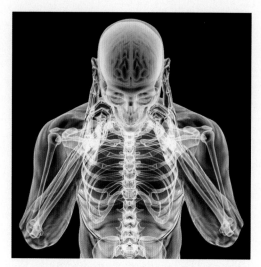

Do not let stress build up onto of you. It will have a negative impact on your search for fat loss and for health.

ripples throughout your body. They can be so powerful they can even effect your genes.

- We are all born with the potential to become living miracles. There are 3 factors involved in activating genes;
  - the genes themselves
  - the environment
  - the mind

- How you feel emotionally is without doubt the best possible indicator you have of whether you are heading towards HEALTH or DISEASE.

To detoxify our body we must also detoxify our mind, because our mind can sabotage even the most scientifically sound nutrition & exercise plan.

- Many of us are simply prisoners of our own thoughts, who create a life of self sabotage, keep repeating hurtful events that have happened in the past, hating the way we look and feel, envious of others, lost our passion and desire we once had as youngsters!

- You must never stop chasing you dreams! It is this purpose which will separate those people who live an ordinary live and those who live an extraordinary life. It has been estimated that we only activate 90-95% of our genes, meaning that we all have the scope to reach greater heights than could be imaginable.

- We all have the same number of genes within the human race. Those of which you look up to who have done incredible things; trust me you can achieve the same. You need to ensure that you have a purpose and are prepared to work to achieve it.

- I have been fortunate enough to have consulted for not only thousands of professional athletes, but also a lot of members of the general public. What I have always been amazed with is that, in the vast majority of people, many have accepted a mediocre life when, in reality, they could have lived an exceptional life.

Hatred paralyzes life; love releases it. Hatred confuses life; love harmonizes it. Hatred darkens life; love illumines it. Martin Luther King, Jr.

- From my years of training people from all walks of life, the first thing I look at is how much love and happiness they have presently. Why? The more love and happiness in their lives, the more stress I can apply as a Strength and Conditioning coach, and the better results they will have.

- When you have someone who is going through an extremely stressful event in their life, there is very little stress that they can cope with. You must remember that exercise is in itself stress. When you put stress on top of more stress, something has to give eventually.

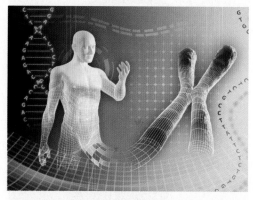

We have unlimited potential and can literally achieve miracles. You simply have to wake up all your genes for we only use 5 – 10% of our genes at any one time. Imagine if we used 100% of our genes?

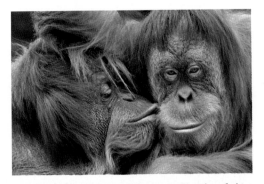

In one interesting experiment, monkeys were subjected to a flashing light, followed by an electric shock. Soon they began to react to the flashing light with a copious secretion of cortisol. If a monkey had one companion, however, the cortisol secretion was markedly lower. And if a monkey had five companions, no cortisol secretion at all occurred. This should magnify the fact that it is essential to keep a very good circle of friends and family around you who have a positve effect on you emtional health.

Even the most deadly snake bite doesn't kill you its the venom running through your bloodstream which will eventually paralyse your body, but what if the venom was stop by a tourniquet and the venom couldn't enter the bloodstream?

- This analogy is like the many stressful situations we face daily they can only do harm like the venom if allowed to run in our bloodstream where we release a chemical cascade of adrenaline and cortisol which can in excess cripple us. But thankfully you change the venom into positive juice within a split second by simply changing our thoughts from NEGATIVE TO POSITIVE.

- Former South African President Nelson Mandela, when asked how he survived years of imprisonment without growing bitter, replied, "Bitterness only hurts one's self. If you hate, you will give them your heart and mind. Don't give those two things away".

- The brain doesn't really distinguish, biochemically, whether a memory is short term or long term. Once the idea of a memory is released into biochemical code, the body responds to the chemicals. The body doesn't have a clue if the event is made up, currently happening or happened several years ago. Just thinking about previous deep emotional hurts can cause the body to respond as if those hurts are happening in that present moment.

- Every time we keep thinking about things that have hurt us emotionally in the past you release a cascade of stress hormones into the body and strengthen the connections in your brain for that hurt to hurt you more than it originally did.

*Do not dwell in the past,
do not dream of the future,
concentrate the mind
on the present moment.
Buddha*

- Depression and testosterone do not go together. If you want to increase your testosterone, you absolutely must get this under control: depression leads to lower testosterone levels.

- Men with abnormally low testosterone levels are almost three times more likely to be depressed than men with high testosterone.

- Let me remind you again of the study that found that the cortisol levels of the depressed individuals was 68% higher than those without depression. That same study found that testosterone were significantly lower in these individuals and were negatively correlated with cortisol levels. To put it directly: the higher the STRESS, the lower the TESTOSTERONE. Psychosomatic Med,1999, 61:292-296

- Studies have shown that when cortisol is released into the blood stream you become less sensitive to leptin, the hormone that tells your brain you are full. When this happens you tend to eat more, and crave more, sugar.

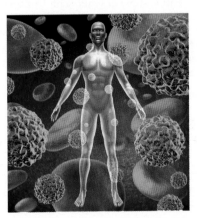

Dr. Steven Locke at Harvard University Medical School found that natural killer cell activity is diminished, not by severe changes or stressors in the life of healthy human volunteers, but by people's interpretatations of stress.

- It has also been demonstrated recently that the physical effects of stress can be greatly reduced if a person has a social support system of friends and family.

Stress makes you fat, no doubt about that. When your brain is chronically stressed your hormones get out of balance, when you are facing a stressful situation, whether real or made up in your head, you will release cortisol. Cortisol is responsible for setting off all the physiological responses associated with stress.

Love promotes growth & stress suppresses it!

- A study, published in 2005 in Archives of General Psychiatry and involving 42 married couples, showed that those who were most hostile to each other healed at only 60% of the rate of those who were least hostile to each other.

- I strongly believe with all my heart and from experience there is nothing more crippling to health than being with the wrong person. Choose your partner wisely and if it isn't right get out remember - one life, don't waste it with a twat:)

- It is so true that your perception of a situation can either be exceptionally positive or totally devastating. It all depends how you handle that stressor!

- A scientific study at Ohio State University Of Medicine was examining the effects of a high, fat high cholesterol diet on rabbits. Scientists were feeding them the diet for a period of time then examining them for evidence of atherosclerosis.

- The atherosclerosis level was expected to be very high in the vegan bunny but one group had 60% less of it than other groups. Eventually it was discovered that one of the technicians had taken this group out of their cages every day and stroked them. A repeat of the experiment confirmed this. The loving act of care and compassion had reduced levels of atherosclerosis by 60%! No drugs could do this!!!

- In 2005, scientists at the University of Miami School of Medicine found that when women were diagnosed with breast cancer were given three massage sessions per week for five weeks there was a significant increase in the number of natural killer cells and lymphocytes in their bodies, which are important components of the immune system. And, publishing in the International Journal of Neuroscience, they also reported these sessions reduced stress hormone levels by 31%, boosted serotonin by 28% and boosted dopamine by 31% - the latter two are essential for happiness & concentration.

- Laughter could be your best antidote to excess stress and absolutely no doubt help lose the fat off your gut. Dr. Lee Berk, of Loma Linda University Medical Center has written about the health benefits of laughter. He concluded that laughter boosts the immune system and reduces dangerous stress hormones in the body.

- In one remarkable study involving sixteen men who watched a funny video, levels of stress hormone cortisol fell by 39% after a good belly laugh. Adrenaline levels fell by 70%, while levels of the feel good hormones endorphins rose 27%. Not only that, but growth hormone levels sky-rocked by 87%. Now if that doesn't get you putting laughter in your fat loss program nothing will.

- Sigmund Freud identified the three parts of the emotional mind as the parent, adult and child. He noted that the child part of the mind is completely unconscious, while the parent part of the mind is completely conscious. The adult mind is partly unconscious, partly conscious. He concluded that too many people have locked away the child part of their emotional mind, sadly so, because when the parent or adult mind rules the emotions, life tends to be drained of joy, fun and adventure. Never lose the child in you; take very opportunity to laugh, be silly or mischievous.

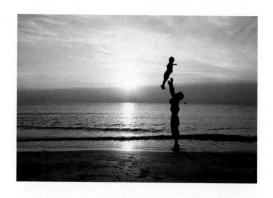

- I remember when my 6 year old son told me that, on the previous day, when no one was looking, him and a friend decided to lick a tree. I asked him why they had done this and what they got out of this. He looked me straight in the eye and said;

"It was fun Dad!"

- Tears are now rolling down my eyes with laughter. About 5 minutes later he announced to me that he wanted to go on holiday to Nigeria. Again, I asked him why? He replied, "everyone in my class has been to Nigeria Dad. And they all said it was fun"

- If you have forgotten how to have fun, may I suggest that you spend more time with children and you will soon learn how to reclaim the child that is within us all.

- I am very conscious of what I say to my 6 year old son Mansel as I want to program him with nothing but love, compassion for others and the belief that he can achieve everything in life that he sets out to do. Never forget that children, especially before the ages of 6, are like sponges - they believe everything whether true or false. I vividly remember my step grandfather telling my grandmother when I was very young that I was stupid and would come to nothing in this life. Encourage your children don't destroy them!

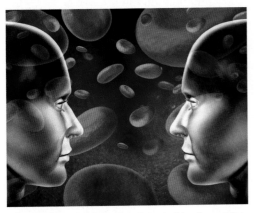

You can talk to your boby's cells and your body's cells can talk to you. You can talk to somebody elses body cells and, yes, they can reply to you.

A Rescuing Hug

An article that was publisheds some years ago detailed the first week of life of a set of twins. Apparently, each were in their respective incubators, and one was not expected to 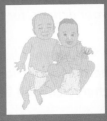 live. A hospital nurse fought against the hospital rules and placed the babies in one incubator. When they were placed together, the healthier of the two threw an arm over her sister in an endearing embrace. The smaller baby's heart rate stabilized and her temperature rose to normal.

Let us not forget to embrace those whom we love.

A Loving Touch

A groundbreaking and significant study on baby massage and premature babies was undertaken by Doctor Tiffany Field, the founder of the Touch Research Institute, which seeks to study the effects of positive touch and massage for individuals in society.

The study published in 1986 showed that;

 Premature babies that received gentle touch gained 47% more weight than a comparative group;

Their development and sensory awareness was enhancing enabling them to leave a medical setting 6 days earlier than a comparative group;

Further study of the babies who had received massage shown that eight months after birth they had increased motor and cognitive development.

Massage releases feel good hormones into the body, which increase appetite and enable restful sleep and relaxation. Massage helps to counteract stress and anxiety.

Watch your thoughts, for they will become words. Choose your words, for they become actions. Understand your actions, for they become habits.

Study your habits, for they will become your character. Develop your character, for it becomes your destiny

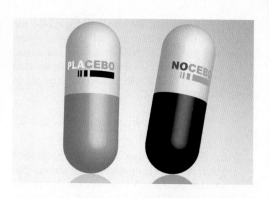

- We have a choice every day whether our thoughts create healing or disease it simply is our choice. Our thoughts are more important to our health than nutrition but when you combine good thoughts with good nourishment nothing is impossible, and I mean nothing!

Placebo = Healing Through Positive Thinking

- What if a scientist discovered a new drug that could cure or improve the symptoms of most known diseases with just one pill!

- Wouldn't it make headline news all around the world and become the greatest selling drug of all time? Such a drug already exists. Let me introduce you to the placebo effect.

- Research now shows that when we believe that we are taking a drug, but it is really a placebo, the brain lights up as if we really were taking the drug and produces its own natural chemicals.

- This has recently been shown with Parkinsons disease. The symptoms of Parkinsons disease arrive from impaired production of a substance called dopamine in part of the brain. This affects movement. Research has shown that Parkinsons patients, given a placebo, but told that it is an anti-Parkinsons drug, are able to move better.

- Brain scans have even shown that the brain is activated in the area that controls movements and dopamine is actually produced. The improved movement is not just a psychological thing, it is a physical release of dopamine in the brain.

- A serious skin disease called congenital ichthyosiform erythrodermia results in a hardening and blackening of the skin. A 16 yr old boy

was seen with this incurable skin condition by Hypnotist Dr. Mason who offered mental imagery to relax him and help him learn to see his skin normal. In 10 days the skin had returned to normal and the results were published in the British Medical Journal and were later verified by other medical researchers.

Never under-estimate the power of belief

Nocebo = Negative Beliefs That Can Make You Sick!

- The Nocebo Effect: Placebo's Evil Twin

- Ten years ago, researchers stumbled onto a striking finding: Women who believed that they were prone to heart disease were nearly four times as likely to die as women with similar risk factors who didn't hold such fatalistic views.

- The higher risk of death, in other words, had nothing to with the usual heart disease culprits -- age, blood pressure, cholesterol, weight. Instead, it tracked closely with belief. Think sick, be sick.

Health thrives in love and happiness. Disease thrives in hatred and anger

Wild Bill Cody's Story

This article was taken from the book 'Return from Tomorrow' by George G. Ritchie It is a true story of events in Dr. Ritchie's life while in the army during WWII, as recounted by himself.

"I was part of a group assigned to a concentration camp near Wuppertal, charged with getting medical help to the newly liberated prisoners, many of them Jews from Holland, France, and Eastern Europe. This was the most shattering experience I had yet had; I had been exposed many times by then to sudden death and injury, but to see the effects of slow starvation, to walk through those barracks where thousands of men had died a little bit at a time over a period of years, was a new kind of horror. For many it was an irreversible process: we lost scores each day in spite of all the medicine and food we could rush to them."

"Now I needed my new insight indeed. When the ugliness became too great a handle I did what I had learned to do. I went from one end to the other of that barbed wire enclosure looking into men's faces until I saw looking back at me the face of Christ. "

"And that's how I came to know Wild Bill Cody. That wasn't his real name. His real name was seven unpronounceable syllables in Polish, but he had long drooping handlebar mustaches like pictures of the old western hero, so the American soldiers called him Wild Bill. He was one the inmates of the concentration camp, but obviously he hadn't been there long: his posture was erect, his eyes bright, his energy indefatigable. Since he was fluent in English, French, German, and Russian, as well as Polish, he became a kind of unofficial camp translator."

"We came to him with all sorts of problems; the paper work alone was staggering in attempting to relocate people whose families, even whole hometowns, might have disappeared. But though Wild Bill worked fifteen and sixteen hours a day, he showed no signs of weariness. While the rest of us were drooping with fatigue, he seemed to gain strength. "We have time for this old fellow," he'd say. "He's been waiting to see us all day." His compassion for his fellow-prisoners glowed on his face, and it was to this glow that I came when my own spirits were low. "

"So I was astonished to learn when Wild Bill's own papers came before us one day, that he had been in Wuppertal since 1939! For six years he had lived on the same starvation diet, slept in the same airless and disease-ridden barracks as everyone else, but without the least physical or mental deterioration."

Perhaps even more amazing, every group in the camp looked on him as a friend. He was the one to whom quarrels between inmates were brought for arbitration. Only after I'd been at Wuppertal a number of weeks did I realize what a rarity this was in a compound where the different nationalities of prisoners hated each other almost as much as they did the Germans.

As for Germans, feeling against them ran so high that in some of the camps liberated earlier, former prisoners had seized guns, run into the nearest village and simply shot the first Germans they saw. Part of our instructions were to prevent this kind of thing and again Wild Bill Was our greatest asset, reasoning with the different groups, counseling forgiveness.

"It's not easy for some of them to forgive," I commented to him one day as we sat over mugs of tea in the processing center. "So many of them have lost members of their families." Wild Bill leaned back in the upright chair and sipped at his drink. "We lived in the Jewish section of Warsaw," he began slowly, the first words I had heard him speak about himself, "my wife, our two daughters, and our three little boys.

Dr Frankl's Story:

Dr. Victor Frankl was a psychiatrist and a jew. The Nazis imprisoned him in the death camps during World War 2 Germany, where he experience things so repugnant that he could scarcely reduce them to words. Frankl's parents, brother, and wife died in the camps or were murdered in the gas ovens. Of his immediate family, only his sister survived the camps. Frankl himself suffered torture and innumerable indignities, never knowing from one moment to the next if his captors would send him to the ovens or leave him among those who were left with the task of removing bodies or shoveling out the ashes of those who had been cremated while they were sill ALIVE.

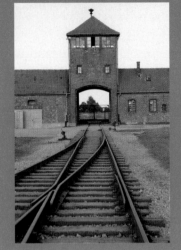

One day, naked and alone in a small room, Frankl began to become aware of what he later called the last of the human freedoms everything can be taken from a man but one thing: the last of human freedoms - to choose one's attitude in any given set of circumstances, to choose one's own way. Frankl openly acknowledged that the Nazi captors could control his entire environment and do what they wanted with his body. They could not however destroy his inner identity. Frankl came face to face with his reality that his own choices, not his circumstances, defined his identity. No matter how horrifying the environment in which he lived, and no matter how much humiliation and degradation others heaped on him, he was still in control of how he choose to respond. And the same is true for each one of us.

Conclusion

- From the information you have just read on the brain, I hope dearly that you nourish your brain with the correct nutrients to allow it to function at optimum efficiency. When the brain is well nourished, you must programme it with healing thoughts, positive thinking and not allow negative emotions effect your life.

- I highly recommend the books written by David R. Hamilton and "Deadly Emotions" written by Don Colbert. I also recommend;

  - "Change your thoughts change your life" - Dr Wayne Dyer
  - "Change your brain change your body" - Dr Daniel Amen
  - "Your miracle brain" - Jean Carper
  - "The Natural Way to Beat Depression" - Dr Basant Puri & Hilary Boyd
  - "Brain Longevity" - Dharma Singh Khalsa
  - "The UltraMind Solution" - Mark Hyman
  - "Spontaneous Evolution" - Bruce Lipton & Steve Bhaerman
  - "Molecules of Emotion" - Candace Pert
  - "The Biology of Belief" - Bruce Lipton
  - "The Omega Diet" - Artemis Simopoulos & jo Robinson

HABIT 4

HORMONES AND MITOCHONDRIA: THE KEYS TO FAT LOSS SUCCESS

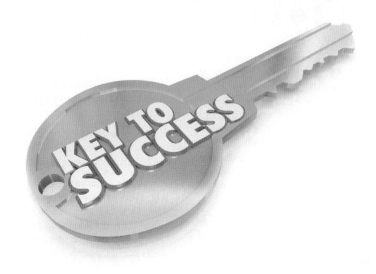

"When I was captain of Somerset County Cricket Club I went to see a well-known nutritionist (Phil Richards) in the UK. "You're very fit, aren't you?" he said, "but I can tell without even looking at your blood sample that you're not very healthy". I was a bit taken aback and asked what he meant. "I can see it in your face and your eyes. It happens to people who constantly train hard. They end up wearing their bodies out and become unhealthy. He (Phil Richards) went on to explain the importance of getting the balance right between training and recovery, and then showed me how nutrition plays a vital role in maintaining great health. His insights and strategies have had a profound impact on my life today."

Justin Langer (Australian Cricket Legend)

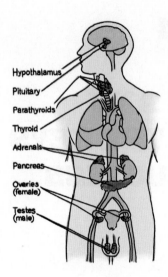

Hypothalamus
Pituitary
Parathyroids
Thyroid
Adrenals
Pancreas
Ovaries
(female)
Testes
(male)

- As this book talks a lot about hormones and mitochondria I thought it would be wise to dedicate a Habit to this fascinating subject so that you become familiar with the terminology of endocrinology (study of hormones) and our little energy factories (mitochondria). When you understand the fundamentals of hormones and mitochondria you will never look at fat loss the same, you will quickly realise for example counting calories is simply ineffective for fat loss.

- Remember from earlier in the book, there are two things which can either make us fat, tired and depressed or lean, energised and happy? Hormones and mitochondria.

- When these are not working efficiently it can make us fat, tired and depressed and on the flip side when they are functioning optimally you will be lean, energised and happy.

- Why is it that two people can eat the same amount of food and one gains weight while the other one does not? Its METABOLISM!

- What regulates metabolism? Your HORMONES & MITOCHONDRIA.

- However, be aware of the Metabolism Myth - because we equate thinness with health, you may think that because someone can eat what they want and not put on weight, they must have a healthy metabolism. However, this is not always true because the physiological definition of a healthy metabolism refers to all the processes of efficient regeneration, building up and using functional and structural proteins and fats and not just the ability to burn off sugar and stored fat as energy.

- Within the body there are various type of hormones which can have various effects;

  - We have anabolic hormones like testosterone and growth hormone which increase muscle mass and decrease our fat stores.
  - We have catabolic hormones like cortisol and glucagon which can break down muscle and convert to energy during times of calorie restriction and excess stress.
  - We have lipogenic hormones such as oestrogen with insulin being king here which stores fat. Insulin can also be anabolic; it can wear two hats, which I will get into later.
  - We have lipolytic hormones which help us burn fat such as glucagon, growth hormone, testosterone and the master blaster thyroid hormones.

- Hormones tell your body whether to burn fat or to store fat and they also tell your body either to build muscle or cannibalise muscle.

- Therefore understanding how to get hormones on your side is essential if losing fat and gaining lean muscle tissue is your goal.

- A study by a Harvard professor Dr. David Ludwig, studied three groups of overweight children, in which they fed each group a breakfast containing an identical number of calories. One group ate instant oatmeal, one group ate steel cut oats, and the third group had a vegetable omelette and fruit.

- Their blood was measured before they ate and every 30 minutes afterward for the next 5 hours. Then they ate a lunch that was identical to the meal they had eaten for breakfast. After finishing lunch, they were told to eat whenever they were very hungry for the rest of the afternoon. What happened was very interesting. The group that ate the instant oatmeal (the breakfast that entered the bloodstream and turned to sugar the fastest) ate 81% more food in the afternoon than the group that had the omelette. Not only were they hungrier, but their blood tests looked entirely different. The instant oatmeal group had higher levels of insulin, blood sugar, blood fats, and adrenaline even though they had consumed the same number of calories as the omelette group. The steel cut oats group also ate 51% more food in the afternoon than the children who ate the omelette.

- The conclusion here is that the kinds of calories you consume have a big impact on how much weight you gain, because different foods are metabolised in different ways. Also, the foods you eat will have an effect on which hormones are stimulated. This can have a profound effect on body fat composition. This is why any diet which bases it's philosophy on calories is one you should look at with extreme caution because in reality counting calories simply doesn't work long term.

- The outside of the body gives clues as to what's going on inside from a hormonal perspective and how/where you carry your fat. For example in the case of the adrenals if they are constantly bombarded with stress then as the result of excess cortisol you will tend to store fat around the abdominals (belly fat) and have skinny arms and legs.

- If there is an excess of oestrogen, you'll see excess fat accumulate around the hips and thighs, and if you are a man you get the added bonus of man boobs. When there is an weakness in the thyroid gland there will be an appearance of excess weight all over due to the effect of the thyroid on metabolism. The liver can also indicate a pot belly look alike symptom which could signal liver toxicity which will also affect your ability to lose excess weight. The liver can actually swell to the size of a football.

- For us to know how to optimize hormone & mitochondrial function, it is important for us first to know how hormones and mitochondria work at making our metabolisms work efficiently when they are healthy. You must always remember that for hormones & mitochondria to work at full efficiency they are both at the total reliance of the health of our cells. Look at cells like little people; keep them happy, feed them optimally and create the right environment and they will do an incredible job for you in return. Piss them off with negative thoughts, junk food and an hostile environment and you will have a rebellion on your hands and your metabolism will grind to a halt.

Men and Women have exactly the same hormones, only in different amounts.

- Hormones are secreted by the various cells, tissues and organs of the endocrine system. Natural hormones, the hormones our body makes, are usually short lived, staying in the blood stream for only a few minutes, or at most a few hours.

- This is just long enough to deliver their message. After the hormone has delivered its message, enzymes from the liver break up the hormones into pieces that are either flushed out as waste or re-used to build other molecules.

- Put simply, hormones are the body's chemical messengers that relay a signal from cell to cell.

- Two communication systems that operate within us:

  - The nervous system exerts point-to-point control through nerves, similar to sending messages by conventional telephone. Nervous control is electrical in nature and

LIVER   THYROID   CORTISOL   OESTROGEN

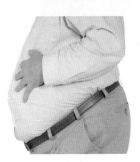 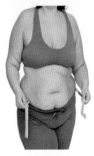 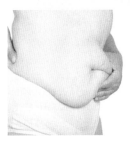 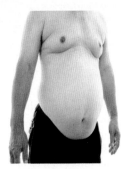

The outside of the body gives clues as to what's going on inside from a hormonal perspective and how/where you carry your fat. For example in the case of the adrenals if they are constantly bombarded with stress then as the result of excess cortisol you will tend to store fat around the abdominals (belly fat) and have skinny arms and legs. If there is an excess of estrogen you'll see excess fat accumulate around the hips and thighs and if you are a man you get the added bonus of moobs. When there is an weakness in the thyroid gland there will be an appearance of excess weight all over due to the effect of the thyroid on metabolism. The liver can also indicate a pot belly look alike symptom which could signal liver toxicity which will also affect your ability to lose excess weight.

fast.

- The endocrine system broadcasts its hormonal messages to essentially all cells by secretion into blood and extracellular fluid. Like a radio broadcast, it requires a receiver to get the message - in the case of endocrine messages, cells must bear a receptor for the hormone being broadcast in order to respond.

- As will be repeatedly demonstrated, the nervous and endocrine systems often act together to regulate physiology. Indeed, some neurons function as endocrine cells.

- As profound orchestrator's of all of life's processes, maintaining hormonal balance is imperative for optimum health. The entire hormonal system is interconnected. Therefore a change in one hormone equals a change in all hormones. This is why most hormone medications fail in the long run - when given singularly they knock other hormones out of balance.

- That is why endocrinologists, who are well experienced, will usually prescribe multiple hormones to solve a singular hormonal problem.

- Remember, natural hormones are so potent that they can produce very dramatic changes in cellular activity with very small amounts known as part-per-billion, or even parts-per-trillion, so minute that only extremely sensitive tests can measure them. Parts per trillion is equal to half a teaspoon of salt in 1000 Olympic sized swimming pool.

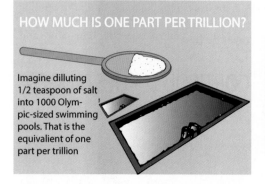

HOW MUCH IS ONE PART PER TRILLION?

Imagine dilluting 1/2 teaspoon of salt into 1000 Olympic-sized swimming pools. That is the equivalient of one part per trillion

- All endocrine glands are ultimately controlled by the hypothalamus located deep within the brain. The hypothalamus produces two types of regulating hormones, releasing ones and inhibiting ones, all of which act on the pituitary.

- The portal system within the stalk carries these command hormones from the hypothalamus to the front end of the pituitary, which is called

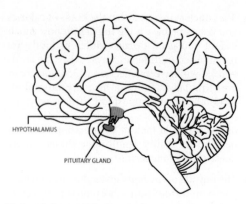

The hypothalamus and pituitary gland

the anterior pituitary. The back end the posterior pituitary is more of a storage area, particularly for vasopressin, which controls water balance, and oxytocin, the hormone of love and birth, both of which are manufactured in the hypothalamus.

- The pituitary and hypothalamus effectively function together as one unit, known as the hypothalamic – pituitary axis.

- The hypothalamus is in control because it is wired directly into its ultimate master, the brain. Everything you experience or perceive from running from an hairy arsed tiger, to a hot romance, to seeing no food in the fridge, where you thought there was a cream cake, the brain via the senses, gets to know first that it has to make decisions about what to do next and what hormones to release.

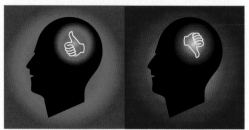

Our Thoughts Control Our Emotions And Our Emotions Control Our Hormones.

- Thinking negatively constantly will make you catabolic (breaking down), thinking positively will make you anabolic (building up). So it is very important from a hormonal, fat loss and health perspective that you think positive and be happy.

- Of course, there will be times when you are angry and want to scream your frustrations to the world. I suggest that you do this and get it out of your system. Do not hold any negative emotions within as this will eat you like a tumour.

- Hormones can be subdivided into groups based upon the dietary precursors from which they are derived. Polypeptide hormones are derived from amino acids, steroid hormones are derived from cholesterol and eicosanoids are generated from essential fatty acids. Therefore, you can see that your diet has a major impact on providing the building blocks for making these critical signalling agents.

- As well as our hormones being derived from food, food also has a massive influence on how our hormones behave. For example carbohydrates stimulate insulin, protein stimulates glucagon and fat is neutral but the building material for our steroid hormones.

- There are nine known groupings of endocrine hormone glands: three in the brain (pineal, pituitary and hypothalamus); three more in the throat (thyroid, parathyroids and thymus); two are in the abdominal region the adrenals and the pancreas; then the gonads testes for males, ovaries for females.

- Fat is the largest endocrine gland in the body. Being an important part of body composition, adipose (fat) tissue accepts a lot of hormonal signals and is able to produce and secrete hormones and hormone like substances, I cover this in habit 7.

How fat cells accumulate fat

- Adipocytes (fat cells) function to store calories in the body. When energy is needed, specific command signals mobilize adipocytes to release their stored fat.

- The adipocyte is the primary site for fat storage. Under the microscope, adipocytes appear

What types of hormones are there?

Hormones can be divided up on the basis of their chemical structure into 6 groups:

1. Those derived directly from the amino acid tyrosine, including:

  - thyroxine
  - triiodothyronine
  - adrenaline
  - noradrenaline

2. Those made up of short chains of amino acids, including:

  - adrenocorticotrophic hormone (ACTH)
  - corticotrophin releasing hormone (CRH)
  - thyrotrophin-releasing hormone (TRH)

3. Those made up of long chains of amino acids, including:

  - insulin
  - growth hormone (GH)
  - prolactin
  - parathyroid hormone (PTH)
  - cholecystokinin (CCK)
  - secretin

4. Those made up of proteins linked with glucose molecules forming glycoproteins, including:

  - thyroid stimulating hormone (TSH)
  - follicle stimulating hormone (FSH)
  - luteinising hormone (LH)

5. Those derived from cholesterol thus forming lipid soluble steroid hormones, including:

  - oestrogens
  - progesterones
  - testosterone
  - androstenedione
  - aldosterone
  - cortisol

6. The essential fatty acids omega-3 and omega-6 are transformed in the body into hormones called eicosanoids. They control other hormones and practically all important functions in the body.

bloated with triglycerides, which is the form which most fat exists in the body.

- Weight gain occurs when adipocytes (fat cells) accumulate a large amount of triglycerides and become enlarged. Obesity is characterized at the cellular level by an increase in the number and size of adipocytes in fat tissue.

- Adipocytes accumulate excess triglycerides due to overeating, insufficient physical activity, hormone imbalance and other causes. These factors, however, fail to address the reason why individuals seem to put on fat pounds despite making great efforts to eat less, taking dietary supplements and following other practices that should, in theory, lead to weight loss.

- But, as you saw in Habit 1, the role that toxicity, without calories, has in increasing adipocytes and so body fat.

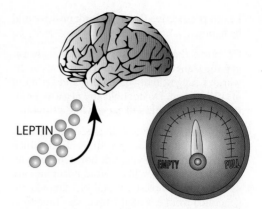

LEPTIN

EMPTY   FULL

The word leptin derives from the Greek word "leptos" meaning thin. It sends a signal to your brain about how much fuel you have within your body.

3 important adipocyte command signals for fat loss

- Adipocytes regulate their size and number by secreting command signals. One such signal is the hormone leptin, which is derived from the Greek term "leptos", meaning thin. Leptin is released by adipocytes to perform two critical functions. First it signals the brain that enough food has been ingested and shuts down appetite. It then seems to exert a process whereby triglycerides stored in adipocytes are broken down into fatty acids that can be used in energy production

- The second command signal released by adipocytes is a hormone called adiponectin. This hormone is an important modulator of insulin sensitivity. Adiponectin has been shown to have anti-atherosclerotic, anti-inflammatory and anti-diabetic roles. High circulating levels of adiponectin have been shown to protect against coronary artery disease, whereas low adiponectin levels are observed in overweight individuals. The insulin-sensitizing effects of adiponectin represent a novel treatment target for insulin resistance, Type 2 diabetes, and obesity.

- The third adipocyte command signal is glycerol-3-phosphate dehydrogenase. This enzyme is produced in adipocytes to help convert blood sugar into triglyceride stores in fat cells.

- Problems with leptin enforce "starvation metabolism" on an individual, even when there is plenty of food around. Eating in harmony with leptin is essential for healthy metabolism.

- When released by adipocytes, leptin performs two critical roles. First, it stimulates centres in our brain to give us the signal of satiety. This means, we "feel full", and stop eating. The other important job that leptin has is to help us access and utilize fat stores for fuel in our body. In other words, leptin helps us burn our stored fat.

- Leptin is actually a hormone – meaning that once it is released it will travel to another area of your body to make things happen. In the case of leptin, it is actually made in your white adipose tissue or stored fat. This finding alone has revolutionized the entire field of endocrinology – as previously stored fat was just thought to be a warehouse for extra calories. Our new understanding means that your stored fat is actually a metabolic organ, much like your thyroid gland or adrenal glands.

- Leptin is one of the most important hormones that regulates your body weight. It works with thyroid hormone, insulin, growth hormone, and adrenal hormones (like cortisol).

- Leptin is known as the fat hormone because it is made in you stored fat. Following a meal leptin is released from your fat, enters your blood, and travels to your brain. It delivers a message that you are full and also lets your brain know how much fuel you have on hand (like the petrol gauge in your car).

- It may seem illogical that leptin is much more abundant in the blood of obese individuals, but this is because obese people have more adipocytes that secrete leptin and C-reactive protein. C-reactive protein (CRP) is a marker of systemic inflammation and predictor of cardiac risk. As our abdominal girth increases, pro-oxidant cytokines, such as CRP, react with fat and create oxidized free radicals which can lead to atherosclerosis (hardened arteries), heart attack, stroke and cancer.

- In fact the hormone leptin actually reacts and binds with the pro-inflammatory marker, C-Reactive-Protein (CRP). CRP binds with leptin and blocks both the leptin transport across the blood-brain-barrier to signal satiety and also blocks the leptin signalling at a cellular level to break fatty acids down for energy expenditure. Hence, the release of C-reactive protein by adipocytes is a leptin-binding protein and neutralizes the natural adipocyte-controlling effects of leptin. The result is a vicious fat cycle, where more leptin accumulates in the blood of obese individuals because it is not able to be picked up by leptin receptor sites on cell membranes. This is leptin resistance. In habit 8 I there are effective protocols for lowering CRP levels.

How Do You Become Leptin Resistant?

- You become leptin-resistant by the same general mechanism that you become insulin-resistant (which we will cover in more detail later in the book) – by continuous overexposure to high levels of the hormone. If you eat a diet that is high in sugar (particularly fructose), grains, and processed foods – the same type of diet that will also increase inflammation in your body – as the sugar gets metabolised in your fat cells, the fat releases surges in leptin.

- Over time, if your body is exposed to too much leptin, it will become resistant, just as your body can become resistant to insulin.

- The only known way to re-establish proper leptin (and insulin) signalling is to prevent those surges, and the only known way to do that is via diet. As such, diet can have a more profound effect on your health than any other known modality or medical treatment.

- You must keep leptin in a state of healthy balance for your metabolism to work correctly and your appetite to be under control. This is not a situation where you take leptin hormone as a substance. This is a case wherein diet, exercise, lifestyle (stress management in particular), restful sleep, and various nutrients all help to optimize leptin function in your body.

- Allow 11-12 hours between dinner and breakfast. Never go to bed on a full stomach. Finish eating dinner at least three hours before bed. One of leptin's main rhythms follows a 24-hour pattern. Leptin levels are highest in the evening hours. This is because leptin, like the conductor in the orchestra, sets the timing for night time repair. It coordinates the timing and release of melatonin, thyroid hormone, growth hormone, sex hormones, and immune system function to carry out rejuvenating sleep. It does this while burning fat at the maximum rate compared to any other time of the day. And it does this only if you will allow it, by not eating after dinner.

- Allow 5-6 hours between meals. Do not snack.

- It is vital to create times during the day when triglycerides (fats) are cleared from your blood. If triglycerides build up during the day they physically clog leptin entry into your brain, causing leptin resistance – meaning that leptin cannot register properly in your brain to siganl satiety. Your metabolism is not designed to deal with constant eating and snacking. Doing so confuses your metabolism and results in you eating much more than you really need.

- Yes, you are supposed to get a snack between meals - but it is supposed to come from your liver.

- Snacking turns out to be one of the worst things you can do for fat loss. It doesn't matter how many calories you snack on, when you snack you throw powerful hormonal switches that cause leptin to malfunction and insulin will always remain high, which means you can

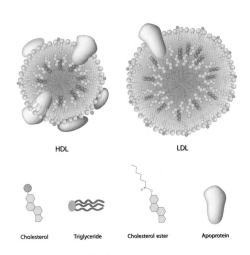

HDL   LDL

Cholesterol   Triglyceride   Cholesterol ester   Apoprotein

The lipoproteins of the blood

93

not burn fat. The fictitious idea that snacking is needed to stoke your metabolism or maintain your blood sugar is in no small part behind dietary advice that has helped cause an epidemic of obesity.

- Drink a green drink like goodness greens or green life in between meals this keeps hunger at bay and gives the body incredible nutrition without hormonal spikes. However, if you participate in intense physical exercise, then I can categorically say that you must snack in between meals. You will achieve outstanding body composition results whilst following such a regime.

- DO NOT EAT LARGE MEALS

- If you are overweight, always try to finish a meal when slightly less than full. The "full" signal will usually catch up in 10-20 minutes. Eating slowly is important. As you improve you will start getting full signals at your meals – listen to this internal cue and stop eating.

- Cortisol (our stress hormone) and leptin communicate in a reciprocal manner as one rises the other tends to fall. In non – stressed situations, both cortisol and leptin follow a 24 hour rhythm. The peak level of leptin is between midnight and two in the morning.

- Leptin is primarily an anabolic hormone (one that builds and repair); correct and properly communicating leptin levels during sleep are essential for repair and fat loss. The peak cortisol levels is six in the morning; it is the primary get up and go hormone, if you are dragging your ass out of bed most mornings still

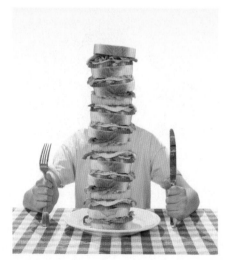

Do not overeat at meals!!!

exhausted, first look at repairing your adrenals by reducing stress in your life.

- When cortisol levels remain high due to constant stressors in your life (whether they are real or made up in your head), remember the body can't differentiate real stress or made up nonsense in your head. Under stress cortisol can influence the function of leptin and create a scenario where, if you are under constant stress, you can become resistant to leptin and this is a disaster for fat loss as well as our overall health.

- So you can now see it is very important getting leptin on your side in you ability to drop body fat. Properly working leptin permits fat burning to occur. It is the hormone that controls the rate of fat burning in the liver, muscles, pancreas, and heart.

- Once fat utilization is disturbed, carbohydrates also turn into fat. This means that insulin resistance can be a consequence of leptin resistance. If you are leptin resistant then there is a very strong likely hood that carbohydrates will be converted into fat, because of the body's inability to burn fat.

- Adipose tissue contains immune cells that in overweight people crank out inflammatory signals, TNFa and IL-6, twenty four hours a day, seven days a week. This is a relentless form of stress and not only do overweight people have to deal with the stress of life, they have to deal with the stress of highly inflammatory immune signals being generated by the extra pounds of fat they carry.

- Changing the type of fat in your diet can have a profound effect on these inflammatory signals dampening them down so you can overcome leptin resistance, reduce CRP & cortisol levels and this my friend makes losing body fat possible. Omega 3 fats, such as fish oil, can reduce TNFa and IL-6 (inflammatory signals) from the white adipose tissue.

- Individuals in inflammatory states such as rheumatoid arthritis can reduce their inflammation signals by a large percentage using pharmaceutical grade fish oil. Always choose high quality fish oil, like PRP Ultimate Fish Oil. This can help you also overcome leptin resistance which will help facilitate fat loss.

- Fish oils are also proven to reduce insulin resistance and have a direct bearing on glucose utilization, including the ability of muscles to use and store glucose. In order to overcome

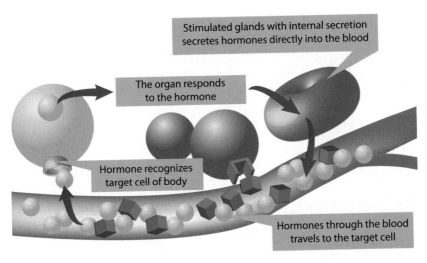

Stimulated glands with internal secretion secretes hormones directly into the blood

The organ responds to the hormone

Hormone recognizes target cell of body

Hormones through the blood travels to the target cell

leptin resistance, glucose metabolism must work properly. This is why extremely low or zero carbohydrate diets do not work in the long run. Fish oils with their unique ability to enhance glucose utilization can have a significant effect on increasing leptin and insulin sensitivity, which are two major players in fat loss.

- In a recent study fish oil and a GLA (Gamma Linolenic Acid) demonstrated the ability to reduce pro-inflammatory immune cell activity by up to 65% percent within four weeks (PRP's Ultimate Fish Oil also contains high dose GLA).

- Adiponectin, like leptin, is a hormone secreted from your adipose tissue. It is a powerful hormone that regulates insulin function and reduces inflammation in your circulatory system. As the amount of fat tissue increases, the level of adiponectin decreases. Larger fat cells naturally produce less adiponectin. Levels of adiponectin also appear to be directly related to abdominal fat.

- While a variety of nutrients have been shown to support healthy levels of adiponectin, a new study points out that the basics of increased fibre, fish oil intake, and regular exercise all help raise your adiponectin levels.

- A review of the scientific literature regarding the influence of diet and adiponectin levels showed that Daily intake of fish or omega-3 supplementation increased adiponectin levels by 14-60%. A 60-115% increase in adiponectin levels was obtained with fibre supplementation.

- Ghrelin is another hormone which is important in decreasing body fat. Put simply, ghrelin is the hormone that tells us to eat, and leptin is the hormone that tells we've had enough and it's time to stop eating. Ghrelin is secreted by the stomach and seems to function as a meal-initiation signal, apparently changes in response to low calorie dieting in order to help maintain body weight. I discuss ghrelin in more detail in habit 7. I must credit Byron Richards on his book "Mastering Leptin", which allowed me to understand the real truth about leptin and its role in fat loss and health.

- For the endocrine gland hormones to send their message efficiently to the target cells you need a very healthy cardiovascular system. This is because it is the blood that is the transportation mechanism for the hormones. I devote habit 9 to this very important subject titled "Nutritional Cardiology".

How Hormones Effect Cells

- On the surface of cells are receptors that hormones joins with. These receptors and the hormones are created so specifically for one another that the hormone dispatched never adheres to the wrong receptor.

There are three distinct classes of hormone communication:

1. Endocrine - glands produce and release these hormones into the bloodstream, where they will travel and bind with a specific receptor. (Like the diagram at the start of the chapter)

2. Paracrine - these hormones don't travel randomly in the bloodstream. They are cell-to-cell regulators that have very defined constraints on how far they can travel. Examples of paracrine hormones are histamines which are released as local responses to stress and injury.

3. Autocrine - These hormones are sent out from the cell to test the immediate environment and then come back to report to that cell what lies just outside its perimeter. The most important autocrine hormones are the eicosanoids which are derived from EFA's.

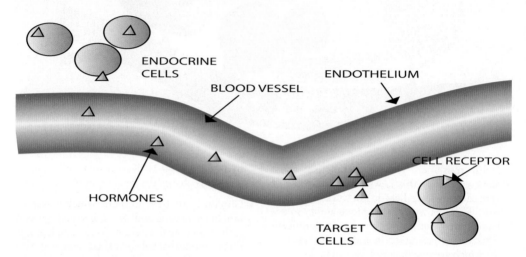

PARACRINE

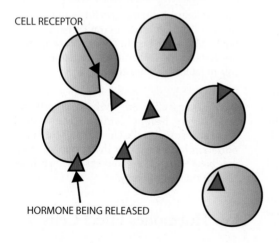

AUTOCRINE

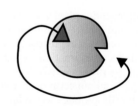

- Every hormone thus resembles a key, and the receptor affected by it resembles a special lock that only that key can open.

- Virtually every cell in the body is studded with thousands of tiny structures called receptors. Think of receptors like our eyes, ears, nose, smell and sense of touch. Their job is to pick up

signals coming at them from the surrounding space. They are so important that, 40% of our DNA is devoted to making sure that they're perfectly reproduced from generation to generation.

- Once the receptors receive a signal, the information is transferred deep within the cell's interior. The information coming in directs things like cell division, cell migration for attacking enemies, making repairs and cell metabolism, to name but a few of the myriad of activities that are going on in our incredible cells.

- The signal comes from other cells and is carried by our hormones, neurotransmitters and peptides referred to as ligands. The term ligand comes from the Latin word "to bind", and is used because of the way the substances latch so tightly to the cell's surface receptors.

- Information carrying ligands are responsible for 98 % of all data transfer in our body and brain. The remaining 2% of communication takes place in the synapse, between brain cells firing and releasing neurotransmitters across a gap to attach to receptors and unload their information.

- Dr. Candace Pert, in her book, Molecules of Emotion, talks about the brain as a "bag of hormones". Of course, given the role of the brain in regulating hormones and itself being affected by hormones. 98% of the brain communicates by hormones & 2% by synapses.

- Upon reaching the cell the hormone often activates a gene within a cell to make another necessary compound.

- Getting to a target cell is no easy task for a hormone since most cells (muscles, heart tissue, lungs, and especially the brain) are protected from the blood stream by the endothelial cells that line the blood vessel walls.

- These cells act as a potent barrier to prevent many things (based primarily on size) passing from the bloodstream into the space known as the interstitial space between the endothelial cells and the actual target tissues of the hormones.

- If the endothelial cell barrier is functioning well, hormones are not impeded from reaching target cells. Any dysfunction to the endothelial cells will cause dysfunction of your hormonal system by decreasing the concentration of the active hormone in the interstitial space. We will discuss the health of the endothelium in greater detail in Habit 8.

- If the hormone can't get to its target site, it's as if it weren't there in the first place, even though there may be higher than normal levels of the hormone in the blood stream. This is why a lot of blood tests for hormones today simply don't tell you what's happening at the cellular level where it matters!

- Steroid hormones cause changes within a cell by first passing through the cell membrane of the target cell. Steroid hormones, unlike non-steroid hormones, can do this because they are fat-soluble. Cell membranes are composed of a phospholipid bilayer which prevents fat-insoluble molecules from diffusing into the cell.

- Improving cellular membrane health is absolutely critical for hormones to function efficiently; what membranes love are essential fatty acids in balance (omega 3 & 6), phospholipids and antioxidant protection.

Fat-soluble vitamin E and co-enzyme Q-10 protect the fatty cell membrane and the mitochondria, while water-based vitamin C and glutathione protect the cell interior. R-Lipoic acid has the unique ability to go anywhere.

- What cells hate are free radicals in excess, hydrogenated fat (trans fats), toxins and hormone disruptors this combined deafens the cell receptors to the talkative hormones. And this creates multiple health problems.

Peptide Hormones

- Peptide hormones are composed of amino acids.

- A peptide hormone binds to a cell-surface receptor, it does not enter the cell. The resulting complex activates an enzyme that catalyses the synthesis of cyclic AMP from ATP. Cyclic AMP activates other enzymes that are inactive.

- Cyclic AMP is a second messenger; the hormone is the first messenger.

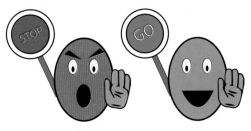

There are molecules within cells which give the green or red light to different reactions

- These are the ultimate key to hormonal action and act through the following sequence of events:

  1. A hormone like insulin docks on a cell receptor
  2. The receptor which spans the membrane of the cell undergoes a change that is transmitted to the interior of the cell.
  3. Depending on the receptor and the hormone that has activated it, another molecule is synthesized within the cell that completes the message.

- These new molecules are called second messengers of which there are two primary kind: Cyclic AMP, which is considered the "green light" for cells. "Good" eicosanoids interact with receptors that produce this second messenger.

- Inositol triphosphate which is equivalent to the "red light" for the cell and usually has a physiological action opposite to that of cyclic AMP. Bad eicosanoids use this pathway.

- If the green light and red lights are balanced and working smoothly the result is wellness. If you have excess of red lights, then your traffic signals are out of balance, the result is the development of chronic disease.

- The great complexity of your biological Internet comes down to maintaining the appropriate balance of green and red lights in each of the trillions of cells throughout the body.

Nonsteroid Hormone Action

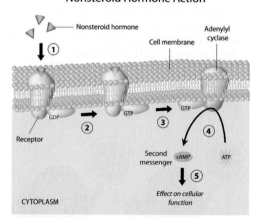

How non-steroid hormones work. Second messengers are the molecules that relay signals from receptors on the cell surface to target molecules inside the cell, in the cytoplasm or nucleus. They relay the signals of hormones like epinephrine (adrenaline), growth factors, and others, and cause some kind of change in the activity of the cell. They greatly amplify the strength of the signal

- Cyclic AMP levels are chronically diminished by elevated insulin levels! Growth hormone release and release of thyroid stimulating hormone need cyclic AMP before they can be released from the pituitary gland. Thyroid hormone will not be released into the blood stream without cyclic AMP and the sleep inducing melatonin hormone will not be produced from serotonin without cyclic AMP.

- Back in 1982, John Vane won a knighthood, a Nobel prize for his work on eicosanoids, hormones that last but a few seconds and are produced by cell in your body.

- Since eicosanoids are produced in every cell, not one specific one, it is as if you had 100 trillion separate eicosanoid glands capable of making these exceptionally powerful hormones.

- We know that all forms of inflammation are ultimately controlled by Eicosanoids. It is the balance of eicosanoids in your body that is so important to your health. Simply stated good eicosanoids promote cellular health and bad eicosanoids produce cellular destruction.

- Remember that anything that causes inflammation will, in turn, cause insulin resistance and increase body fat!

- All eicosanoids are derived from dietary fat, in particular the polyunsaturated essential fatty acids that must be supplied by the diet. There are only three such essential fatty acids that can be made into eicosanoids: dihomo gamma linolenic acid (DGLA), arachadonic acid (AA), and eicosapentaenoic acid (EPA).

- DGLA and AA are omega 6 fatty acids, and EPA is an omega 3 fatty acid. The really good eicosanoids that accelerate cellular rejuvenation come from DGLA, the really bad eicosanoids that accelerate cellular destruction come from AA and EPA helps maintain a dynamic balance between DGLA and AA as well as diluting out any excess of AA in the cell.

- Omega-6 fats in excess are readily converted to arachadonic acid, a precursor to pro-inflammatory prostaglandin E2 (PGE2).

- As powerful as eicosanoids are, they are ultimately controlled by the diet. All pro inflammatory eicosanoids are derived from the long chain omega 6 fatty acid, called arachadonic acid (AA).

- What's interesting to understand the more the ratio favours high AA from omega 6 then the more inflammation that will occur which increases cortisol levels & decreases testosterone!

- Gamma linolenic acid (GLA) is found in plant sources like evening primrose & borage oil. Its functions and benefits are very similar to DHA and EPA. Like DHA, GLA maintains the permeability and flexibility of cell membranes, creating cells that can obtain the needed nutrients for proper functioning.

GLA improves cell sensitivity to insulin, reducing our chance of developing diabetes, heart disease and excess body fat. This is why I added GLA to my Ultimate Fish Oils, so that it works synergistically with EPA & DHA to help dampen down inflammation within our bodies.

- GLA goes to DGLA (dihomogammalinolenic acid) almost automatically. Once at DGLA, there are two biochemical paths available. One path leads to good eicosanoids and the other leads to the bad eicosanoids.

- To go down the bad road, DGLA is converted by the delta 5 Desaturase (D5) enzyme to arachadonic acid, which is the precursor to bad eicosanoids. So we see D5 is key.

- If we can inhibit this enzyme, the less arachadonic acid, the less bad eicosanoids and thus the less problem with our health, i.e. the less pain, inflammation heart disease, stroke, obesity, etc.

- High levels of insulin activate enzymes that actually cause the body to produce more Arachadonic Acid (AA).

- What controls D5? It is activated by insulin. So you can see controlling your blood sugar is also very important in controlling your eicosanoids and your inflammation levels.

- High levels of insulin activate enzymes that actually cause the body to produce more Arachadonic Acid (AA).

- Another key to the puzzle is an Eicosapentaenoic Acid (EPA). EPA is a key inhibitor of D5. This shows that fish oils have many remarkable benefits to our health

- So I hope you have a basic understanding of hormones and how they communicate with the cells as the more efficient the messages from the hormones can be heard by the cell, the easier it will be to lose fat and gain lean muscle tissue. It was the work of Dr Barry Sears which educated me on the improtance of eicosonoids and I must give him huge credit for sharing this information in his books.

- In the upcoming habits we go into hormones in more depth but at least you know the basics. Now we look at the other part of the equation for enhancing our metabolism so we can stay lean & healthy and please enter the mitochondria.

Mitochondria

- The primary role of mitochondria is to extract energy from nutrients to produce adenosine triphosphate, or ATP, which our body uses to create energy for a whole host of cellular processes. We are constantly using ATP, whether we're running, walking, thinking, breathing, pumping blood through our cardiovascular system, or singing a song. Think of a physiological process, and ATP is involved. Without mitochondria, then, we wouldn't be able to get much of anything done. We simply wouldn't be alive.

- The role of your metabolism is to take the oxygen you breathe and the food you eat and process it to make energy, the fuel of life. This energy is made in tiny little factories in our cells called mitochondria.

Mitochondria are responsible for approximately 90% of all energy produced within the human body.

- Mitochondria are the only places inside your muscle cells where carbohydrate, fat, and protein can be broken down in the presence of oxygen to create the energy you need to exercise.

- When the mitochondria are not working to full capacity, you suffer all the symptoms of low energy, fatigue, slow metabolism, weight gain, memory loss, inability to put muscle on and the list goes on. It comes down to a simple numbers game: the more mitochondria you have, and the more efficient they work, the more fat you will burn as well as building more muscle.

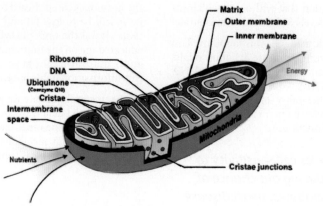

The anantomy of our mitochondria

- For example, one study found reduced mitochondrial function associated with low testosterone.   Diabetes Care, 2005, 28:1636-1642

What causes mitochondria to be less efficient

- At the moment our understanding is that the causes fall into two main groups: either nutritional deficiencies or toxins.

- When toxins enter the body and move throughout the tissues, they come into contact with the mitochondria and damage them. The toxins can prevent ATP production and in one study 48% of the mercury that was found inside the individual cells were found in the mitochondria themselves.

- Mitochondrial damage caused by toxicity, ageing, or lack of essential nutrients and antioxidants can lead to lower mitochondrial capacity, which may result in steroid hormone decline, loss of muscle, gain in fat, general weakness and metabolic decline.

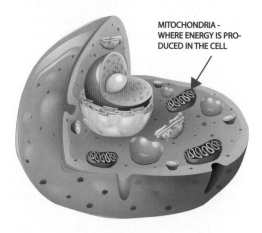

MITOCHONDRIA - WHERE ENERGY IS PRODUCED IN THE CELL

- A published paper (co-authored by the UCSD Statin Study director) suggests that statin-induced damage to the body's mitochondria is the true cause of the commonly-reported side effects of statin use.

- Mitochondria are essential to energy. CoQ10 in the mitochondria help produce energy and fight free radicals. Unfortunately for statin-users, CoQ10 travels along the same pathway as some types of cholesterol. Following its scorched-earth policy to a tee, statins block that pathway, meaning CoQ10 can't get through to help mitochondria destroy free radicals. More free radicals running rampant means more inflammation– which is the true cause of heart disease.

- It is clear that obese people have fewer and more poorly functioning mitochondria than leaner people do. Perhaps that is why lean people stay lean and obese people stay obese. So you can see increasing and enhancing mitochondria is far more important than counting calories.

- The major factors that damage the mitochondria are oxidative stress, or free radicals, too many calories and not enough nutrients in your diet. Toxins, such as mercury, as we have just seen, also contribute to the damage. Anything that causes inflammation causes damage to the mitochondria and certain medicines such as statins will also effect the efficiency of mitochondria, this will be discussed more in Habit 8.

- We have our own anti-oxidant systems to protect us but these are easily overwhelmed by a toxic, low nutrient, high calorie diet.

- The endogenous anti-oxidants we make, called superoxide-dismutase, catalase and glutathione peroxidase are dependent on essential dietary nutrients to help them work well including; zinc, copper, manganese, vitamin c and selenium which are often deficient in our processed food diets of today.

According to Professor Enzo Nisoli the average adult possess approximately 10 million billion mitochondria, which corresponds to approximately 10% of our body weight. That is some serious energy generating capacity.

- The more mitochondria you have, and the more efficiently they consume oxygen, the faster your metabolic rate, the easier it is for your body to burn calories and the more energy you have.

Important substrates for the mitochondria to function efficiently

- CoQ10
- L-Carnitine
- D-Ribose
- Magnesium

- CoQ10, L-carnitine, D-ribose, and magnesium, individually and collectively help increase energy, or ATP, production in your body by supporting mitochondria within cells. D – Ribose helps fill the body's energy tank while L-Carnitine and CoQ10 help the body convert fuel to energy. Magnesium is a vital mineral used by the enzymes that make energy synthesis and recycling possible

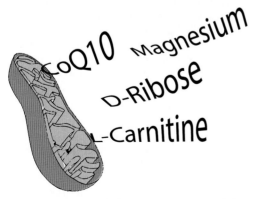

Fuel your mitochondria with The Fantastic 4 - magnesium, CoQ10, D-ribose and L-carnitine. I gained this informatin from the excellent work of Dr Stephen Sinatra and his book "Metabolic Cardiology"

- CoQ10, L-carnitine, D-ribose, and magnesium are covered in great depth in Habit 8 on nutritional cardiology. This habit will help you get your heart, blood vessels & blood in tip top condition which enhances our hormones and increases our oxygen levels.

- CoQ10 supplementation also improve performance. Dr J. Van Fraechem give a group of healthy young men 60 mg of CoQ10 per day for 8 weeks. They did not change their usual level of daily exercise or diet yet increased their maximum exercise capacity by 28%!

- High intensity exercise has been shown to lower CoQ10 most probably due to the consequence of an excess of free radicals caused by increased metabolic demands of chronically exercising muscles.

- Carnitine is the gatekeeper for fat burning, it picks up fat and transports it into the mitochondria for burning to create ATP. The more Carnitine present the more fat burnt and this is essential for effective fat loss.

- Most fat utilization occurs in the cell's mitochondria. The greater the number of mitochondria, the more efficient fat utilization will be. Because muscle is the largest mitochondria containing tissue, muscle composition directly affects fat utilization. Any intelligent fat loss program should include a strength training program to increase muscle and improve our anabolic hormones.

- This is why slimming programs that do not take into account the essential role that muscle plays in increasing our metabolic rates often fail in the quest for fat loss.

- Why? These programs are mostly based on calorie deficits which cause the body to become highly catabolic, meaning that we loss a shit load of muscle and end up becoming a smaller, fatter version of ourselves from when we started.

- During long endurance training fats become a major energy source. You will not run out of fats to burn but you might run out of L-Carnitine, which is essential for fats to be used as energy. Endurance exercise rapidly depletes the pool of L-Carnitine in muscle, so the amount of carnitine available is a limiting factor on the energy supply of endurance athletes.

- Carnitine also increases maximum use of oxygen in athletes. This effect was first observed by Dr. Brian Liebovitz at the University of Cal-

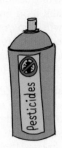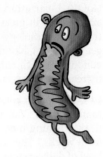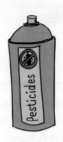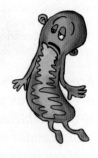

Pesticides, just like toxic metals, can have devastating effects on our mitochondria. Many pesticides are developed to target the mitochondria specifically.

ifornia. It has been confirmed by two Italian studies. Both give athletes 4 grams of L-carnitine daily and V02 max increased significantly.

- D-ribose is essential as a building block of ATP (adenosine triphosphate), it rapidly restores depleted energy by providing substrate for ATP production.

- Strenuously exercised muscle may have lowered levels of ATP by 20%. It may take 3-4 days to replenish these ATP levels. Supplementing with ribose can increase the replenishment of ATP by up to 4 times

- Supplemental D-ribose absorbs easily and quickly through the gut and into the bloodstream. About 97% gets through.

- Dosages between 5–15 grams depending on activity and heart problems.

- Since all enzymatic reactions involving ATP have an absolute requirement for magnesium, it makes perfect sense to include magnesium to any program which wants to enhance ATP production within the mitochondria.

- As you can now see you need a cocktail of micro-nutrients for the mitochondria to produce ATP efficiently they are magnesium, co-enzyme Q10, L-carnitine and D-ribose. This is why I developed Cardio Fuel to boost mitochondria function.

- I will cover this in great depth in the habit on nutritional cardiology.

Enhancing Mitochondria

- In 2006, Harvard researchers found that the red pigment in grapes called resveratrol could extend life in mice by protecting their mitochondria. These mice actually lived 15% longer than average, even while eating a bad diet. In fact, they even became fitter and lost weight.

- So how could they eat poorly and not exercise, but become fitter and live longer? One word: mitochondria. It turns out that the resveratrol protected and improved the function of the mitochondria through its effects on special master aging genes.

- Intense scientific interest into the function of mitochondria during exercise dates back to the early 1950s, when physiologists noticed that the breast and wing muscles of chickens had few mitochondria, while those of pigeons and mallards contained high densities of the little structures. Of course, chickens can't fly, while mallards and pigeons are the endurance athletes of the bird world, leading researchers to believe that mitochondrial concentrations were closely related to exercise capacity.

- We don't make new mitochondria or improve our existing ones just for kicks, just like we don't build lean muscle mass by sitting around. We have to give our bodies a reason to do it. We have to challenge our cells through purposeful aerobic and anaerobic conditioning. Make sure that your training is very challenging.

- Scientists were somewhat surprised to learn that mitochondria contain their own genetic material - and that all the mitochondria in an individual's body are inherited from one's mother, not father (this is because the egg contains mitochondria, while sperm cells are mitochondria-free). This may seem strange, since the egg is rather immobile and the sperm are distance swimmers, but the bottom line is that sperm are so tiny that mitochondria would weigh them down excessively on their harrowing passage toward the egg. The consequence of this, of course, is that you tend to inherit your exercise capacity from your mother, not your dad.

- Of course, scientists began experimenting with ways to increase mitochondrial densities. At first, it was believed that the mitochondria might be under hormonal control and early research efforts were indeed able to show that mitochondrial numbers were increased when levels of a key hormone produced by the thyroid gland - thyroxine - increased. In laboratory rats, the simple addition of desiccated thyroid to normal rat food caused an explosive increase in mitochondrial size and density in both the heart and liver. This clearly shows how important a fully functional thyroid is in energy metabolism and habit 5 is all on the thyroid and how to get it healthy.

- Exercise physiologist John Holloszy, of the Washington University School of Medicine in St. Louis, showed that chronic exercise could put mitochondrial numbers on the upswing. Holloszy simply had one group of lab rats to run on treadmills for up to 120 minutes per day at intensities of about 50-75% of VO2 max for a period of 12 weeks, while a second group lolled in their cages. At the end of the 12-week period, Holloszy found that the running rats had increased their mitochondrial densities by approximately 50-60% and had also doubled their concentrations of 'cytochrome c,' a key compound found inside mitochondria which is crucially important in aerobic energy production

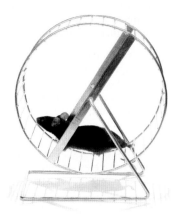

Studies in humans, and animals, have shown that aerobic exercise and increase mitochondrial number and function

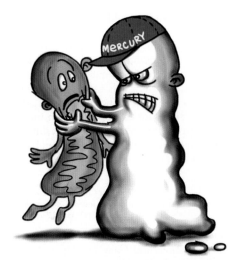

Mercury in our body has the ability to strangle our mitochondria and making them less efficient

('Effects of Exercise on Mitochondrial Oxygen Uptake and Respiratory Enzyme Activity in Skeletal Muscle,' The Journal of Biological Chemistry, vol. 242(9), pp. 2278-2282, 1967).

- Of course, exercise physiologists then began wondering which type of training was best for perking up mitochondrial numbers. Should one train fast? Long and slow? Mix fast efforts with slow ones? How long should one exercise (how many miles per workout and week) in order to optimise mitochondrial density?

- Holloszy and his co-workers at Washington University were the first to really tackle this question.

- In a fairly simple piece of experimental work, Holloszy et al had one group of rats running 10 minutes per day, another running for 30 minutes, a third group exercising for 60 minutes, and a fourth working for 120 minutes per day. Training took place five days a week for 13 weeks, and training intensity was fixed at about 1.2 mph (or about 32 metres per minute and 313 minutes for the 10K, which is an intensity of around 50-60% VO2max for a healthy lab rat).

- Not too surprisingly, the two-hour per day runners turned out to have the best mitochondrial set-ups. For example, compared to sedentary rats, the 10-minute per day exercisers had about 16-per cent more cytochrome c, while the 30-minute workers boosted cytochrome c by 31%. However, rats who ran for an hour expanded cytochrome c by 38%, and the two-hour rats increased it by 92%!

- Holloszy's study provided nice support for the specificity of training principle, too, for during a rugged endurance test staged at the end of the research period, the 10-minute rats lasted 22 minutes, the 30-minute ones for 41 minutes, the hour-long rats ran strenuously for 50 minutes, and the two-hour trainees stayed on the treadmills for a whopping 111 minutes! Of course, run time to exhaustion was directly related to cytochrome c concentration; the more c a rat had, the longer it could run at a tough pace

    (*'Skeletal Muscle Respiratory Capacity, Endurance, and Glycogen Utilization,' American Journal of Physiology, vol. 228(4), pp. 1029-1033, 1975*).

- Other researchers wanted to explore the intensity question, and Gary Dudley and his colleagues at the State University of New York at Syracuse did just that. Like Holloszy, Dudley had his rats training five times a week and used a variety of different workout durations, from five minutes up to 90 minutes per day. However, unlike Holloszy, Dudley restricted his study to only eight weeks and used a range of different training intensities - 100% VO2max, 85% VO2max, 70% VO2max, 50% VO2max, and 40% VO2max. Dudley also looked at how different intensities and durations influenced different muscle fibre types (fast twitch, aerobic fast twitch or 'intermediate', and slow twitch), which no one had ever done before

    (*'Influence of Exercise Intensity and Duration on Biochemical Adaptations in Skeletal Muscle,' Journal of Applied Physiology, vol. 53(4), pp. 844-850, 1982*).

- In contrast to what Holloszy had found, Dudley was able to show that training beyond about 60 minutes per workout was without benefit in terms of increasing cytochrome. In other words, a rat training at about 70-75% VO2max could upgrade cytochrome c by expanding workout duration from 30 to 60 minutes - but not by increasing workouts from 60 to 90 minutes. This was true at all intensities studied by Dudley - and also with all three muscle fibre types. Progressing beyond about 60 minutes per workout simply didn't have much value when it came to the mitochondria.

The faster you train, the better

- However, Dudley's most interesting findings were those related to intensity of training. He was able to show that in fast-twitch muscle fibres, just 10 minutes of fast running (at close to 100% VO2max) per day was enough to rough-

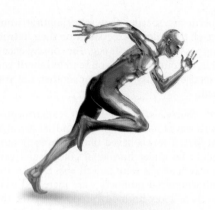

Walking or jogging may not be enough, as some research shows. However, sprinting or interval running is not suitable for everyone, as I will explain in Habit 10

ly triple cytochrome c concentrations over an eight-week period. In contrast, running for 27 minutes at 85% VO2max daily only hoisted cytochrome c by 80%, while 60 to 90 minutes at 70-75% VO2max nudged cytochrome c upward by just 74%. So much for the theory that intense exercise can hurt mitochondria.

- So what's the bottom line? As Dudley and his colleagues put it, "an increase in the intensity of training brings about the greatest adaptive response in the mitochondria".

- You must remember that, you can only train intensely when you have an excellent base of health and fitness

- Expressing the crucial importance of intensity another way, Dudley and co-workers said, 'For the same adaptive response, the length of daily exercise necessary to bring about the change becomes less as the intensity of exercise is increased.' In other words, 10 to 15 minutes of running at close to 100% VO2 max in a workout can do much more for you than running for 60 to 90 minutes at slower intensities.

- Although this research is very impressive and show us that high intensity training is an effective way to increase mitochondrial efficiency, from my own experience, I have found that, I get much better gains, form a fat loss perspective by doing lots of endurance training. I had virtually no gains from high intensity interval training. My observations, after training 1000s of professional athletes, is quite simple; the more fast twitch fibre the athlete, the more he will gain from high intensity training. The opposite is then true for the slow/mixed -twitch fibre athlete, like myself, who will get better results from endurance type training.

- World class endurance athletes might have up to 10% of their cells composed of mitochondria instead of 2% for sedentary person. So essentially they have five times as many little energy factories as the average person and this is why they can run so fast for so long.

- Muscle biopsy studies have shown that there are two major changes associated with mitochondrial energy production following endurance training: an increase in the number and the size of the mitochondria.

- Endurance training also increases the number of red blood cells that deliver oxygen to muscle cells with more efficiency.

- When you exercise correctly, you increase your muscle mass and increase your oxygen intake. These are both important factors in positively effecting your mitochondria. By increasing your muscle mass, you increase the number of cells in your body that contain large numbers of mitochondria. Your muscles have one of the highest concentrations of mitochondria.

- When you increase your oxygen intake, your direct your mitochondria to process more oxygen more quickly. The more oxygen the body consumes the more fat it will burn. When you workout, your mitochondria work out. That means they get better and better at consuming oxygen so, in short, exercise increases your metabolic power.

- Loss of muscle is actually one of the reasons yo-yo dieters can not seem to lose weight. They lose and gain over and over again but the big problem is that when they lose weight, they also lose muscle. Since muscle is much more metabolically active and burns 70x as many calories as fat cells, losing muscle slows down their metabolism, making it easier to gain weight and harder to lose it. You must gain muscle to lose fat

- The loss of muscle has a tremendous impact on your ability to lose weight. This is why it is absolutely paramount that a well designed strength training plan is at the core of your fat lose plan.

- For enhanced fat loss mixed weights, endurance, speed, power and bingo you are in the exercise fat loss game. I give you all the information you need in Habit 9 to design your own exercise plan to gain lean muscle and improve cardiovascular fitness. So when you train next make sure you give your mitochondria a workout so they become more efficient at burning fat 24/7.

Conclusion:

- I hope you can now see the importance of understanding hormonal health, cellular health and enhancing mitochondrial function in your quest for a lean and healthy body. The rest of the habits will cover hormones and mitochondria, as well as cellular health, so you know how to manipulate these factors to optimize metabolism and become a fat burning machine instead of a fat storing machine.

- If you want to learn even more about this topic then I suggest that you start with such books as "The Hormone Cure" by Sara Gottfried, "The Hormone Solution" by Thierry Hertoghe, "Sexy Hormones" by Lorna Vanderhaeghe & Alvin Pettle, "The Truth About Hormones" by Vivienne Perry" and "Natural Hormonal Enhancement" by Rob Faigin.

HABIT 5

THYROID: MASTER OF METABOLISM

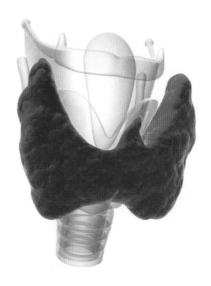

"Phil's knowledge of healthy living and nutrition is limitless. With his dietary advice and training techniques Phil transformed a squad of 40 professional rugby players into one of the most physical and dynamic outfits in the premiership. A very driven individual he strives to be the best and get the most out of whomever he works with."

Will Skinner (Professional Rugby Player, Harlequins & England)

Thyroid: Master Of Metabolism

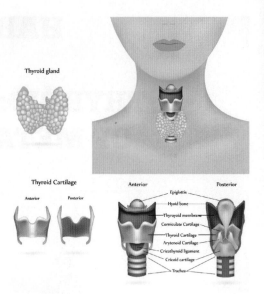

Thyroid gland

Thyroid Cartilage

Anterior   Posterior   Anterior   Posterior

Epiglottis
Hyoid bone
Thyrohyoid membrane
Corniculate Cartilage
Thyroid Cartilage
Arytenoid Cartilage
Cricothyroid ligament
Cricoid cartilage
Trachea

- Sitting at the base of the throat, the thyroid gland produces hormones that regulate basal metabolic rate, the speed at which our bodies burn food for energy. The thyroid gets its directions from the hypothalamus, at the base of the brain, by way of the pituitary gland. On a signal from the hypothalamus, the pituitary sends thyroid-stimulating hormone (TSH) into the bloodstream. It travels to the thyroid gland and causes the release of thyroxine (T4), which is partly converted into triiodothyronine (T3). Through a feedback mechanism, the hypothalamus determines when levels of T4 and T3 are low and alerts the pituitary to supply more TSH.

- The thyroid gland is under the control of the pituitary gland, a small gland the size of a peanut at the base of the brain.

- The thyroid's main role in the endocrine system is to regulate your metabolism, your body's ability to break down food and convert it to energy. Food essentially fuels our bodies, and our bodies each "burn" that fuel at different rates. This is why you often hear about some people having "fast" metabolism and others having "slow" metabolism.

- The thyroid produces several hormones, of which two are key: triiodothyronine (T3) and thyroxine (T4). These hormones help oxygen get into cells, and regulate metabolism.

- How do thyroid hormones get to the cells? In order for the thyroid hormones to travel through the blood to reach the cells, a transport protein is needed. The three transport proteins are thyroxine-blinding globulin, albumin and transthyretin (thyroxine-binding pre-albumin). All these transport proteins are produced by the liver, though transthyretin is also produced in the choroid plexus and thus is the main thyroxine-binding protein in the brain and spinal cord. In the rest of the body, transthyretin carries about 10% of the hormone while albumin binds around 15-20% and

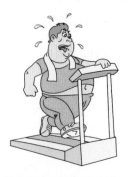

No matter how much you exercise, you will struggle to lose weight if your thyroid is not functioning properly.

thyroxine-binding globulin carries about 70% of the thyroid hormones. Protein malnutrition, alcoholism and liver disease can impair the production of these carrier proteins. T3 binds more weakly (is more easily released into cells) than T4. Thyroid hormones are thought to easily penetrate cell membranes.

- How does T4 become metabolically active in the cell? The active form of thyroid hormone is T3 but the thyroid gland releases 14 times more T4 than T3. Thus in the cell, the T4 must be converted to T3 by type l 5"-deiodinase, a selenium-dependent enzyme. (Selenium deficiency in rats decreased enzyme activity by 90%). Type ll 5"-deiodinase is most active in the anterior pituitary, the central nervous system, placenta and brown (high mitochondrial content) fat. T4 can also be converted to reverse T3 (rT3) by the enzyme, 5" deiodinase (especially type l 5' deiodinase in the liver). Reverse T3 is an inactive form of the molecule. The production of rT3 is thought to be a way the body prevents the accumulation of excess T3. Both T3 and rT3 are further reduced to T2 (two iodine molecules), T1 (a single iodine molecule) and T0 (thyronine without any iodine). The half-life of T3 is one day while the half-life of T4 is about a week. The released iodine and thyronine return to the thyroid gland for re-assembly into T4 and T3.

- Every cell in the body has receptors for thyroid hormone. These hormones are responsible for the most basic aspects of body function, impacting all major systems of the body. For example, the activity of the Krebs cycle within the mitochondria is very thyroid dependent.

- Just as importantly, thyroid hormones increases the metabolic rate of almost every tissue in the body. Its effects on metabolism are astonishing. For example, a person whose thyroid gland reduces the production of T4 can experience as much as a 40% drop in metabolism, or basal metabolic rate (the rate at which the body spends energy for maintenance activities).

- It is believed that T3 can increase the mitochondria's ability to burn calories and thus raise the basal metabolic rate (BMR). In addition, T3 will also cause an increase in the number and size of the mitochondria, which will further serve to increase BMR.

- One can imagine the thyroid gland as a furnace and the pituitary gland as the thermostat. Thyroid hormones are like heat. When the heat gets back to the thermostat, it turns the thermostat off.

- The production and release of thyroid hormone in the thyroid gland is regulated by a feedback system in your brain—the hypothalamus and pituitary glands—which make TRH (thyroid-releasing hormone) and TSH (thyroid- stimulating hormone), respectively. If everything works as designed, you will make what you need and the T4 will be converted to T3. The hormones work in a synchronous feedback loop, creating a state of dynamic balance. There really is no start-and-stop place in the system; however, you may understand it better in this way: the brain's central command centre, the hypothalamus, detects a need for more

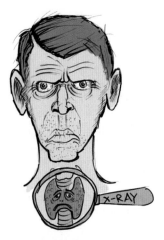

There are many things which can have a negative impact on your thyroid gland. A tired thyroid gland will make you sick, tired and, more than likely, overwieght.

thyroid hormone and releases TRH, which sends a signal to the pituitary (the second in command in the brain) to release more TSH, which is then released into the bloodstream, goes to the thyroid gland, and stimulates the production of T4 and small amounts of T3.

- The function of the thyroid gland is to take iodine, found in foods, and convert it into thyroid hormones: thyroxine (T4) and triiodothyronine (T3). T3 and T4 are then released into the blood stream and are transported throughout the body where they control metabolism (conversion of oxygen and nutrients to energy).

- The thyroid gland needs iodine and the amino acid L-tyrosine to make T4 and T3. A diet deficient in iodine and poor protein sources can limit how much T4 & T3 the thyroid gland can produce and lead to hypothyroidism. PRP Iodine Forte contains iodine, tyrosine & selenium.

Iodine Deficiency and the Thyroid

- Since iodine is needed for the production of thyroid hormone, and the body does not make iodine, we have to get it through what we eat. It is commonly found in foods such as salt-water fish, seaweed, sea vegetables, shellfish and iodine-containing multivitamins.

- Worldwide, the number one cause of hypothyroidism is iodine deficiency, which remains a public health problem in 47 countries; about 2.2 billion people (around 38% of the world's

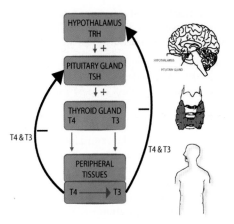

The thyroid hormone feedback loop. The hypothalamis and pituitary gland have create the signal to prodcue more T4 & T3. As this occurs, there is a negative feedback loop to signal a reduction in TRH and TSH release from the hypothalamus and pituitary

population) live in areas with iodine deficiency. An article in The Lancet in 2008 stated that, "According to WHO, in 2007, nearly 2 billion individuals had insufficient iodine intake, a third being of school age. Thus iodine deficiency, as the single greatest preventable cause of mental retardation, is an important public health problem."

- Thyroid cells are the only cells in the body which can absorb iodine. These cells combine iodine and the amino acid tyrosine to make T3 and T4.

- T3 is critically important because it acts on special receptors on the nucleus of the cells that send messages to your DNA to turn up your metabolism, to increase the fat burning in your mitochondria, and to generally make every system in your body work at the right speed. This is why T3 lowers your cholesterol, improves your memory, keeps you thin, promotes regrowth in cases of hair loss, relieves muscle aches, relieves constipation etc.

- If you produce too little T3, or if the T4 you produce is not being properly converted into this active thyroid hormone (which can happen when any step in the process is inhibited), your whole system goes haywire: your metabolism and mitochondria don't get the proper signals, you gain weight and you suffer from the symptoms of hypothyroidism.

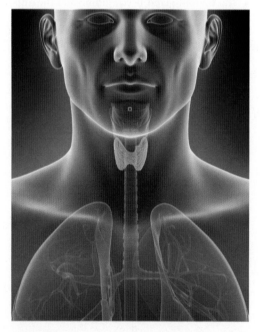

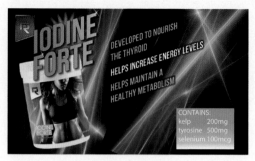

In order to produce thyroid hormones, you need an adequate supply of iodine, tyrosine and selenium. That is why I developed this product. It contains all of the ingredients you need to nourish your thyroid

- Thyroid peroxidase (TPO) is the enzyme responsible for making thyroid hormones. It liberates iodine to be added to tyrosine for T4 & T3 production. This process involves many cofactors, including selenium, copper, magnesium, niacin, riboflavin, vitamin B6 & zinc. Therefore, a deficiency in any of these vitamins and minerals could lead to thyroid problems.

What Else Can Effect the Thyroid?

- The enzyme thyroid peroxidase is also blocked by mercury in the body, primarily from dental mercury amalgam fillings and thimerosol, a mercury preservative found in vaccinations and other medicines.

- Vitamin A is another critical nutrient for thyroid activity. Vitamin A appears to influence how well the thyroid hormone receptors in the nucleus function.

- The normal thyroid gland produces about 93% T4 and about 7% T3. However, T3 possesses about four times the hormone "strength" as T4.

- Hopefully you are starting to see that even a mild thyroid problem can make it difficult to lose weight, regardless of how much exercise you do or what food you are eating.

- Thyroid hormone also increases the utilization of carbohydrates and fat from food, along with the rate of protein synthesis. It stimulates the appetite and the movement of food through the digestive tract. Thyroid hormone increases the uptake of oxygen into the cells, which speeds aerobic respiration.

- Nothing escapes the influence of T3, since it can also stimulate almost all aspects of carbohydrate metabolism. It can increase the absorption of glucose by the intestinal tract, increase the uptake of glucose by the cells, and increase glycolysis(breakdown of glycogen). In glycolysis, the excess glucose that is not needed for glycogen production is broken down and burned by the mitochondria to produce even more ATP.

Signs of Hypothyroidism

- Do you feel fatigued, lethargic, and sluggish, especially when you wake in the morning? Do you have poor-quality, cracked nails? Are you cold all the time? Do you have dry skin, coarse hair, or hair loss? Are you depressed? Are you constipated? Do you have muscle and joint pains? Have you lost the outer third of your eyebrows? Do you have trouble losing weight no matter what you do?

- If you answer yes to any of these questions, you may be suffering from hypothyroidism, a potentially dangerous health condition that occurs when the production, conversion, or action of the thyroid hormones in your body is inhibited, resulting in too little active thyroid hormone in your blood.

Common symptoms of hypothyroidism (producing too little thyroid or thyroid hormones not working efficiently)

- Physical Symptoms:
- Fatigue
- Weight Gain
- Aches and pains in joints and muscles
- Constipation
- Dry and itchy skin
- Brittle hair
- Hair loss, including loss of eyebrow hair
- Feeling cold even in warm temperatures
- Milky discharge from breasts
- Infertility
- Heavy Menstrual Periods
- The outside of your eyebrows are much thinner than normal and vitiligo can be a sign of hypothyroidism .

Symptoms of Untreated Hyperthyroidism in Adults (producing too much thyroid hormone)

- Cardiovascular System (increased heart rate, increased diastolic blood pressure, heart flutter - atrial fibrillation)
- Central Nervous System (difficulty sleeping, difficulty concentrating, nervousness, irritability, changes in vision)
- Gastrointestinal Tract (increased frequency of bowel movements, increased appetite, weight loss)
- Musculoskeletal System (fatigue and muscle weakness)
- Kidneys (leg oedema)
- Reproductive System (decreased menstrual flow, reduced fertility

Thyroid Blood Tests

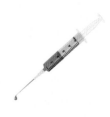

- The diagnosis of hypothyroidism by laboratory methods is primarily based on the results of total T4, free T4, T3, and TSH levels. The typical blood tests measure thyroxine (T4), which accounts for approximately 93% of the hormone secretion by the thyroid. However, the form that affects the cells the most is T3 (triiodothyronine) which cells make from T4.

- If the cells are not able to convert T4 to the four-times more active T3, a person can have normal levels of thyroid hormone in the blood, yet be thyroid-deficient. This is why blood tests can be inaccurate and you need to look at symptoms as much as the blood tests! If you're taking prescription thyroxine (T4) but are not feeling any better, it's likely that the T4 is not converting to active T3 hormone.

- Selenium is a component that helps convert T4 to T3, so deficiencies of selenium can impair thyroid function and worsen hypothyroidism. So if you are on thyroid medication and you still do not feel any better then it could be due to the fact that you have a selenium deficiency, which would be very common today with our nutrient deficient soils. I also want to point out that mercury, either from amalgam fillings, food or environmental exposure, can also deplete selenium levels. But it could also due to many other factors as well. The conversion to T3 can also be hampered by nutritional deficiencies such as inadequate omega-3 fatty acids, low zinc, chemicals from the environment, or by stress. So often, taking T4 alone will result in only partial improvement.

Your Numbers, Your Doctor, and You

- Here's an important point to remember if you do get tested and your numbers are not "normal." Hypothyroidism has a huge range, from very mild to quite severe. Not only that, one person whose TSH tests result in a reading of 2.5 may feel perfectly fine, while another person with the same reading may be suffering a battery of symptoms. The numbers and the symptoms don't always correlate. Most of the time, taking thyroid medication will cure your symptoms and you will feel better within a matter of days; by six weeks on the medication you'll have a very good idea of how it's working. Unless you tell your doctor how you're feeling, he or she has nothing to go on but your test results. You need to share with your doctor if your symptoms are getting better (or worse),

and you need to be consistently retested to see how your medication is working. Your numbers may go back to normal, but if you're still not feeling well it's your responsibility to tell your doctor so that more tests can be taken or your medication can be tweaked until you find what works best for you

- It is possible, however, to go overboard with thyroid medication. Too much thyroid medication can stress out the adrenal glands, which will then overproduce cortisol as well as deregulate (impair) the ratio of cortisol and DHEA and epinephrine and norepinephrine. This will leave you more fatigued than you were in the first place, because the rest of your body's systems will not be able to produce the energy needed to keep up with your now revved-up thyroid.

- It is possible for individuals to be hypothyroid and have elevated levels of T4. This is sometimes seen in liver disease. The liver utilizes large amounts of thyroid. If liver cells are not able to use all the thyroid brought to them by the blood stream, the thyroid backs up and the blood levels of thyroid hormone rise, similar to when a stream is dammed.

- The most important single test for thyroid function is basal temperature. The reason for this is that thyroid hormone increases the conversion of ATP to ADP to power all the metabolic functions of the cell. In that conversion, 50% of the energy is released as heat. That heat is needed to maintain bodily functions by maintaining the proper temperature range for enzymatic activities necessary for life. Body temperature is a good measure of basal metabolic rate and is cheaper and simpler to per-

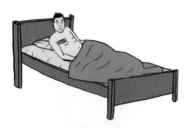

You can use a thermometer to check your waking temperature. This will help you assess whether you have an under active thyroid.

form than measuring the rate of conversion of oxygen to carbon dioxide, which is the "gold standard" measure of metabolic activity.

Thyroid Self-Test:

- The basal temperature in menstruating women is most accurately measured on the 1st, 2nd, 3rd or 4th day of the menstrual cycle (preferably beginning on the 2nd day). Males, pre-pubertal girls, and post-menopausal or non-menstruating women may take basal temperatures any day of the month. You should take your temperature 3 days in a row.

- To test yourself for an under active thyroid, keep an electronic thermometer by your bed at night. When you wake up in the morning, place the thermometer in your armpit and hold it there for about 10 minutes. According to Broda Barnes, MD (a pioneer in thyroid metabolism), if the average temperature is below 97.8 Fahrenheit, then the diagnosis of a low functioning thyroid system is likely. An average temperature between 97.8 and 98.2 is considered normal.

An average temperature above 98.2 is considered high and might reflect an infection or a hyperthyroid condition. At least three days of measurement are necessary for an average.

- Dr. Broda Barnes also shown that cold hands and feet of the hypothyroid patient signify poor circulation to the skin, which results in a susceptibility to skin infections. There are very few people with skin diseases of any kind who would not benefit by thyroid.

- Cortisol is a key factor in setting the temperature of the body, so with high cortisol levels the body temperature in the morning will also be low. Why? High cortisol levels reduce the

thyroid hormone T3. When T3 is low, metabolism slows and body temperature dips, hence the connection between thyroid and adrenals.

- High cortisol also inhibits the messenger hormone thyroid stimulating hormone (TSH) – which is sent from the pituitary gland to the thyroid gland to release T4 – T3.

- Low adrenal function often leads to low thyroid function, classically evidenced by high levels of thyroid binding globulin (TBG), low free T4, low free T3, high TSH, slow ankle reflex and low body temperature.

- The adrenal glands main purpose is to produce and release certain regulatory hormones and chemical messengers, and the connection between thyroid and adrenal gland is a very important clinical consideration.

- Cortisol produced by your adrenal glands helps enable thyroid hormones pass from your blood into your cells. Cortisol raises your cellular level of glucose which works with your cell receptors to receive T3 from the blood to the cells.

Cortisol affects the thyroid gland in three ways:

1. Cortisol is required to facilitate release of TSH from the pituitary gland.

2. Cortisol facilitates conversion of the inactive T4 hormone to the active T3 form.

3. Cortisol allows each T3 cell receptor to more readily accept T3.

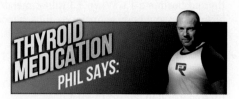

I have witnessed my mother prescribed an incredibly high amount of thyroxine and the effect that it had on her was terrible. She could not even get out of a chair, she was that exhausted, and her lips were purple. I thought she was going to die, and that is no exaggeration. After a few days of going from doctor-to-doctor, thankfully one switched on doctor looked at the dosage she was taking and said, "I believe that the amount of thyroid medication you are taking is too high". He reduced it immediately and, as if by magic, her symptoms disappeared. It was after this experience that I decided to investigae thyroid health, function and metabolism so that I could help people who have thyroid problems. By the way, the thyroxine that my mother takes has had no effect on her energy levels, unless she takes my Iodine Forte. But, please remember, do not take any supplements with prescription medication without advice from a medical professional.

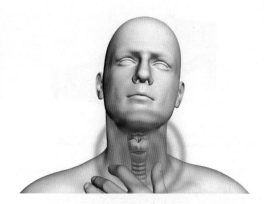

Stress and Your Thyroid

- Stress is one of the worst thyroid offenders. Your thyroid function is intimately tied to your adrenal function, which in turn is intimately affected by how you handle stress.

- Many of us are under chronic stress, which results in increased adrenaline and cortisol levels, and elevated cortisol has a negative impact on thyroid function. Thyroid hormone levels drop during stress.

- When stress becomes chronic, the flood of stress chemicals (adrenalin and cortisol) produced by your adrenal glands interferes with thyroid hormones and can contribute to obesity, high blood pressure, high cholesterol, unstable blood sugar, and more. A prolonged stress response can lead to adrenal exhaustion (also known as adrenal fatigue), which is often found alongside thyroid disease

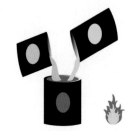

- Administering thyroid medication in cases of advanced adrenal fatigue without concurrent attention to adrenal recovery will often fail. In many cases, it is analogous to pouring oil onto a fire. An already weak adrenal system, in a low energy state, may not be able to carry the burden of extra energy output that the thyroid hormones are demanding. What the adrenals need is rest, not extra work.

- Cortisol is necessary to produce thyroid hormones, and also necessary for your body to convert T4 to the active T3 (as we have seen), as well as thyroid receptor function. When your thyroid hormone receptors aren't working properly, any thyroid hormones you do make can't get into your cells. Without enough cortisol, the thyroid receptors can eventually even disappear, until you correct the deficiency. This is why a lot of people on thyroid medication don't see any benefits; because the doctor doesn't address adrenal function as part of the treatment.

- Hypocortilism, or low cortisol, occurs when the adrenal glands are unable to make a normal amount of the main stress hormone, cortisol. Often those with hypothyroidism are suffering from low cortisol levels. If the hypocortisolism is undiagnosed, or inadequately treated, thyroid medication may work only temporally or completely fail to help with symptoms or even make the problems worse.

- Too much cortisol, on the other hand, causes thyroid resistance, where your tissues no longer respond to thyroid hormones as they should. Your levels of T3 and T4 will look normal on a blood test but they are not working at a cellular level, where all the action takes place - another reason why blood tests can give you the wrong answer when it comes to thyroid function.

- Your adrenals rely heavily on your thyroid to function correctly. None of the adrenals vital activities can be accomplished without adequate thyroid support. In fact, virtually every cell in your body has receptors for both cortisol and thyroid hormones. You must have adequate levels of both in your cells for your body to do its job and be healthy. If you have hypothyroidism (reduced thyroid function), production of cortisol drops. And conversely if you have hyperthyroidism (elevated thyroid function), you produce higher levels of cortisol.

- Hypothyroidism slows your adrenal glands and also stresses your body; increasing adrenaline output and further taxing the adrenals. In addition, hypothyroidism leads to an increase in cortisol binding globulin, a protein that binds cortisol and makes it unavailable to the body. This then becomes a vicious cycle, with low thyroid function leading to low adrenal function, which leads to even lower thyroid function. Get your adrenals and thyroid working in harmony together which will give you vibrant health and optimum body fat levels.

- In order for thyroid hormone to become effective (as already mentioned) it first must be converted from T4 into its more active T3. When you're dieting, or under a lot of stress and making high levels of cortisol in response to the situation, your body converts T4 to reverse T3 instead of the dynamo T3. Reverse T3 ties up your thyroid receptors and prevents you from using the active T3 which enhances metabolism and fat burning. This results in symptoms of hypothyroidism no matter what your actual levels of thyroid hormones are. That's why its so hard to lose weight by extreme dieting or when you are under extreme stress or both. Your body goes into survival mode and drops metabolism and that's why rT3 increases at the expense of it's fat burning brother T3.

- Hypothyroidism can be primary or secondary. If hypothyroid symptoms, such as low body temperature, fatigue, dry skin and weight gain persist despite thyroid replacement therapy regardless of laboratory values, one must look elsewhere for the cause of the low thyroid function

- Secondary hypothyroidism is low thyroid function caused by malfunction of another organ system. One of the most frequently overlooked causes is adrenal fatigue, as we have just discussed.

- Thyroid binding sites can also be taken up by oestrogen and heavy metals like mercury cre-

ating hypothyroidism even though your body is producing thyroid hormones.

Oestrogen Dominance & Thyroid Function

- Oestrogen causes food calories to be stored as fat. Thyroid Hormone causes fat calories to be turned into usable energy. Thyroid Hormone and Oestrogen therefore have opposing actions.

- High oestrogen levels lead to excessive production of thyroid-binding globulin (TBG) by the liver. If the TBG levels are high it will bind more thyroid hormones, thus reducing the free thyroid hormones available in the blood. Therefore, thyroid hormones cannot be used by the cells that require them for maintaining the body's metabolism.

- Although there are enough thyroid hormones in the blood, they are not taken up by the body's cells, as they are inactivated by TBG. Oestrogen dominance therefore often leads to thyroid problems.

- This is one of the reasons why blood tests reveal 'normal' levels of thyroid hormones in such situations, but some women still show classical symptoms of thyroid problems.

- Oestrogen has also been found to bind to thyroid binding sites within the cell. So excess oestrogen thus also decreases thyroid function by tying up its binding site with ease.

- Thyroid hormone is essential and influential in regulating appetite and metabolism as leptin and ghrelin. Without an optimum balance of leptin and ghrelin in your brain, you simply

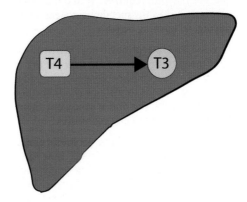

60% of the conversion of T4 into T3 takes place in the liver, provided that the liver is health

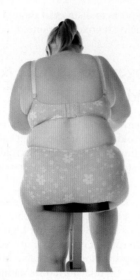

Oestrogen dominance is often associated with high levels of fat around the thighs and buttocks.

cannot achieve or maintain a normal weight. The intimate relationship between leptin and thyroid hormones is amazing. First, leptin promotes thyroid growth and thyroid hormone production. Leptin signals the hypothalamus to send the message to the pituitary to tell your thyroid to produce the right amount of hormone needed for metabolism.

- Without leptin, or when leptin is inefficient, the communication between your hypothalamus, pituitary and thyroid gland fails to produce the right amount of hormones. Leptin also tells the cells in your body to convert enough T4 to T3. When leptin signalling is not at its best, thyroid hormones become less efficient in your cells and your body burns even less energy and fat.

- Just as leptin influences the thyroid, thyroid hormone itself effects leptin levels and leptin efficiency. Leptin requires thyroid hormone to carry out its healthy metabolising, energy producing, fat burning benefits.

- If your T3 is low, leptin will not efficiently spark your metabolism. So you can now see that you can not just take one hormone like thyroid and expect the pounds to melt away; all hormones work synergistically and if you want them to function efficiently - just get healthy.

- Thyroid hormone also has a profound effect on hunger hormone, ghrelin, levels. Low thyroid causes ghrelin to rise, making you hungrier and slowing metabolism even further. Restoring thyroid hormones to normal levels causes ghrelin to drop.

- Amazingly, thyroid hormone has the ability to convert fat cells into calorie burning, heat producing cells. Even leptin cannot produce this effect without thyroid hormone. The hormones leptin, ghrelin and thyroid hormone work on the mitochondria to either enhance calorie burning and heat production (leptin and thyroid hormone) or slow heat production, which slows metabolism (ghrelin).

- It is worth noting again, that if you are trying to lose weight by cutting calories, thyroid hormone will work against you, slowing your metabolism. Starvation and calorie restriction lower both thyroid hormone and leptin, causing your mitochondria to burn fewer calories and generate less heat. After all, your body is trying to preserve your life. Why would it burn up your energy stores?

- The amount of glucose in liver cells regulates the enzyme that converts T4 to T3. This means that hypoglycaemia or diabetes (in which glucose doesn't enter cells efficiently) will cause hypothyroidism, when T4 can't be converted into T3.

- When a person is fasting, at first the liver's glycogen stores will provide glucose to maintain T3 production. When the glycogen is depleted, the body resorts to the dissolution of tissue to provide energy. Eating carbohydrate can allow the liver to resume its production of T3.

- Low carb diets disrupt thyroid hormone; researchers have found that during the low carbohydrate diet Reverse t3 increased and T3 decreased, but they remained unchanged dur-

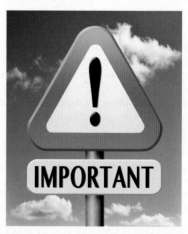

Lack of glucose in the cell is the most important factor in decreasing T3 production. Iodine attaches to insulin receptors and improves glucose metabolism, which is good news for people with insulin resistance & diabetes.

ing the carbohydrate – rich diet. Rt3 blocks T3 from entering the cells to increase metabolism.

- The thyroid gland assists the pancreas and liver in maintaining stable blood sugar. A hormone released by the thyroid, thyroxine, increases insulin response. Hypothyroidism threatens the supportive role and contributes to hyperglycaemia and poor insulin response.

- The exact effects of thyroid hormone on insulin secretion remains poorly understood. However, a clinical trial demonstrated that a hypothyroid state resulted in a reduction in both insulin binding and a number of insulin receptors in the livers of experimental rats.

Other benefits of Iodine

- Japanese women, who are eating lots of seaweed, have the highest iodine intake (13.8 mg. daily) of women anywhere in the world. They also have the lowest incidence of breast cancer in the world.

- "Iodine deficiency may lead to an under-active thyroid and ultimately to a goitre, and goitres have been clearly associated with an increased risk of breast cancer."

Breast Cancer: A Nutritional Approach by Carlton Fredericks, Ph.D.

- "At iodine sufficiency, the largest amounts of iodine are found in fat tissue and muscle (striated) tissue. If obesity is present, the body's need for iodine increases, as the fat cells of the body would require more iodine. Women's breasts are major sites for iodine storage. Maintaining adequate iodine levels is necessary to ensure an adequately functioning thyroid gland and normal breast architecture. I believe it will also lower the incidence of breast cancer and help women overcome breast cancer."

Iodine: Why You Need It, Why You Can't Live Without It by David Brownstein, M.D.

- The thyroid contains more selenium by weight than any other organ. As we have already discussed, selenium is a necessary component of the enzymes that remove iodine molecules from T4 converting it into T3; without selenium there would be no activation of thyroid hormone.

- Selenium also plays a role in protecting the thyroid gland itself. The cells of the thyroid generate hydrogen peroxide and use it to make thyroid hormone. Selenium protects the thyroid gland from the oxidative damage caused by these reactions. Without adequate selenium, high iodine levels lead to destruction of the thyroid gland cells.

The liver-thyroid connection

- T4, as we now know, is not the active thyroid hormone; it must be converted into T3 in your body in order to exert its effects. The majority of this conversion does not occur in your thyroid gland. Most T4 to T3 conversion happens in your liver, kidneys and muscles.

- In fact, 60% of T4 is converted into T3 in the liver providing it is functioning at full effectiveness. Now you can see why a dysfunctional liver can lead to a cascade of hormonal problems.

- If you are taking thyroid hormone medication in the form of thyroxine, it too must be converted into the active form in your body. Therefore if you are taking thyroid medication but still not feeling much better, your liver could be to blame! It is vital that you work on improving the health of your liver if you want healthy thyroid hormone levels.

- Thyroid hormones affect the liver cells responsible for detoxification most of all. When thyroid function is low, due to hypothyroidism, the enzymes that carry out detoxifying tasks simply can't do their job efficiently.

- If you have a fatty liver or a sluggish liver, this conversion will not be effective. This can leave you feeling tired, depressed, puffy, overweight and with dry skin and thinning scalp hair. Indeed, you would have a thyroid problem caused by a faulty liver.

The gut-bacteria-thyroid connection

- One little known role of the gut bacteria is to assist in converting inactive T4 into the active form of thyroid hormone, T3. About 20% of T4 is converted to T3 in the GI tract, in the forms of T3 sulphate (T3S) and triidothyroacetic acid (T3AC). The conversion of T3S and T3AC into active T3 requires an enzyme called intestinal sulfatase. For this to happen you need lots of healthy bacteria.

Autoimmune Thyroid Disorders

- Studies show that 90% of people with hypothyroidism are producing antibodies to thyroid tissue. This causes the immune system to attack and destroy the thyroid, which over time causes a decline in thyroid hormone levels.

- What the vast majority of hypothyroidism patients need to understand is that they may not have a problem with their thyroid, they have a problem with their immune system attacking the thyroid.

- An Italian study found that those with a significant allergy to gluten also developed a significant allergy to their own thyroids, which disappeared when the gluten was removed for three to six months.

- Several studies show a strong link between autoimmune thyroid disease (AITD), both Hashimoto's (hypothyroidism) and Graves (hyperthyroidism), and gluten intolerance. The link is so well-established that researchers suggest all people with Auto Immune Thyroid Disorder be screened for gluten intolerance.

- What explains the connection? It's a case of mistaken identity. The molecular structure of gliadin, the protein portion of gluten, closely resembles that of the thyroid gland. When gliadin breaches the protective barrier of the gut, and enters the bloodstream, the immune system tags it for destruction. These antibodies to gliadin also cause the body to attack thyroid tissue. This means if you have AITD and you eat foods containing gluten, your immune system will attack your thyroid.

- Even worse, the immune response to gluten can last up to 6 months each time you eat it.

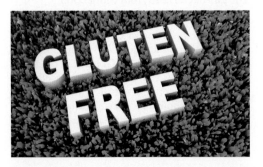

There's no "80/20' rule when it comes to gluten. Being "mostly" gluten-free isn't going to cut it. If you're gluten intolerant, you have to be 100% gluten-free to prevent immune destruction of your thyroid.

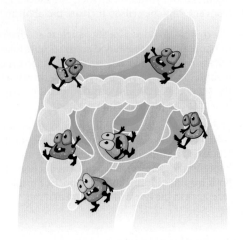

Gut bacteria plays a role in converting T4 into T3

This explains why it is critical to eliminate gluten completely from your diet if you have AITD.

Environmental Chemicals

- Perfluorooctanoic acid (PFOA) studies have shown that people with the highest 25% of PFOA concentrations (above 5.7ng/ml) were more than twice as likely to have thyroid disease than those with the lowest 50% of PFOA concentrations (below 4.0ng/ml). PFOA is found in non-stick cookware, stain-resistant clothing and carpeting, food packaging and other consumer goods.

- Scientists generally agree that Polychlorinated biphenyls (PCBs) alter thyroid hormones in the human body. PCBs have a shape very similar to thyroid hormones, which allows them to interfere or compete with normal hormones.

- Food can be a major source of human PCB exposure, usually from fish and animal fat. Bottom feeders and other aquatic organisms ingest and accumulate PCBs, resulting in bio-concentration upward in the food chain.

- Mercury also has significant effects on the thyroid. There is ample evidence that mercury leaching from dental amalgam fillings contributes to thyroid disease and anaemia. Mercury from dental fillings can migrate to the thyroid gland and can sit on the thyroid's iodine receptors, blocking iodine from reaching the receptors and thereby preventing full activation of the thyroid.

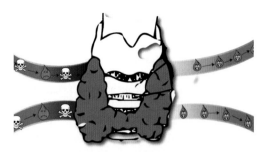

All of your blood passes through the thyroid every 17 minutes as it secretes iodine to kill germs

- Another serious problem toxins create is a reduction in thyroid hormone levels and an increase in the excretion of thyroid hormones by the liver. Toxins induce a liver enzyme (Hepatic UDPGT), which promotes T4 excretion in the bile. This leaves you with less around to do the job of boosting your metabolism.

- In addition to all this, toxins compete with thyroid hormones by blocking your receptors and vying for thyroid transport proteins (the proteins which carry thyroid hormones around the body), making it even more difficult for your thyroid hormones to do their job.

- Your thyroid hormones are very vulnerable to chlorine, fluorine and bromine (which are halides like iodine). This means that they compete for your iodine receptors. If you are exposed to a lot of these halides, you will not hold on to the iodine you need.

- Bromine is present in many places in your everyday world - plastics, pesticides, hot tub treatments, fire retardants, some flours and bakery goods, and even some soft drinks.

- Bromine binds to the body's receptors and block the absorption of iodine receptors primarily in the thyroid and stomach. The list of bromine is long, varied and frightening:

  - Used in most grains
  - Used in bleached and enriched flour
  - Used as a retardant in furniture, carpets and clothing
  - Used as a preservative in nuts and oils
  - Sprayed on strawberries and vegetables
  - Used as a fumigant for termites
  - Used as an antibacterial agent along with chlorine in hot tubs and pools
  - Used in Paxil and Prozak
  - Used in carbonated drinks

- Used in computers and automobiles

- Chlorine also blocks iodine in the body, so chlorinated water (both drinking and bathing) should best be avoided when possible to maintain a healthy thyroid.

- Fluoride, a common additive to your water supply, and an ingredient in the toothpaste you and your children use, may be contributing to the increased rates of hypothyroidism - and other health concerns - in the UK without improving dental health. Dr. John Yiamouyiannis examined the raw data from a large study that was conducted by the National Institute for Dental Research (NIDR). He concluded that fluoride did not appear to have any decay preventing success, as there was little difference in the DMFT values (the mean number of decayed, missing or filled teeth) for approximately 40,000 children. It did not matter whether they grew up in fluoridated, non-fluoridated or partially fluoridated communities.

(Yiamouyiannis, J.A. "Water Fluoridation and Tooth Decay: Results from the 1986-87 National Survey of U.S. Schoolchildren", Fluoride, 23, 55-67, 1990).

- A larger study has been conducted in New Zealand. There, the New Zealand National Health Service plan examines the teeth of every child in key age groups, and have found that the teeth of children in non-fluoridated cities were slightly better than those in the fluoridated cities.

(Colquhoun, J. "Child Dental Health Differences in New Zealand", Community Healthy Services, XI 85-90, 1987).

- In a study published online in Environmental Health Perspectives, a US National Institute of Environmental Health Sciences' journal, the researchers found, amongst other things that: "The children in high fluoride areas had signif-

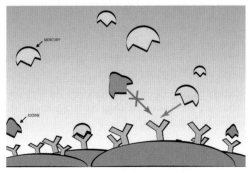

Mercury is just one of many foreign elements that compete with iodine at thyroid receptors

icantly lower IQ than those who lived in low fluoride areas".

- Another key quote from the Reuters article on the subject: "It's senseless to keep subjecting our children to this on going fluoridation experiment to satisfy the political agenda of special-interest groups," says attorney Paul Beeber, NYSCOF President. "Even if fluoridation reduced cavities, is tooth health more important than brain health? It's time to put politics aside and stop artificial fluoridation everywhere, says Beeber."

- Up until the 1950s, European doctors used fluoride to reduce the activity of the thyroid gland for people suffering from over-active thyroid (hyperthyroidism).

- Up to half of those drinking fluoridated water also suffer 'dental fluorosis' - a mottling of the teeth thought to be caused by its effects.

- In my humble opinion, fluoridation is mass medication and dumbs society down by decreasing thyroid function, it has absolutely nothing to do with protecting your teeth.

- In 1991 Robert Carton, former president of the Union of Government Scientists at the US Environmental Protection Agency – the body that oversees drinking water quality in the US – has described fluoridation as "the greatest case of scientific fraud of this century, if not of all time."

- Iodine intake immediately increases the excretion of bromide, fluoride, and some heavy metals including mercury and lead. Bromide and fluoride are not removed by any other chelator or detoxifying technique other than iodine.

- Genistein is particularly harmful for people who have pre-existing low or marginally low thyroid function. Genistein is one of several known isoflavones. Isoflavones, such as genistein and daidzein, are found in a number of plants, with soy beans and soy products like tofu and textured vegetable protein (such as margarines) being the primary food source. A daily dose of genistein as low as 30mg can affect normal thyroid function.

- Mega consumption of isoflavones such as soy burgers can bring the total daily genistein intake to over 200mg.

Thyroid and Mental Function

- There is an old medical saying that just a few grains of thyroid hormone can make the difference between an idiot and an Einstein. It aptly characterizes the thyroid as a quickener of the tempo of life.

- Dr. Barry Durant-Peatfield, in his book "Your Thyroid and How to Keep It Healthy", states; "Brain cells have more T3 receptors than any other tissues, which means that a proper uptake of thyroid hormone is essential for the brain cells to work properly."

- Thyroid hormones are one of the major "players" in brain chemistry disorders. And, as with any brain chemical disorder, until treated correctly, thyroid hormone imbalance has serious effects on the patient's emotions and behaviour.

- Furthermore, because the brain requires sufficient thyroid hormones to function optimally, a low thyroid hormone status can contribute to overall loss of function and degeneration in the brain, including the areas of the brain that govern mood (Davis 2007).

- Overt hypothyroidism has been shown to disturb serotonin signalling in the brain, which can contribute to depression (Stipcevic 2009).

- Findings that T3 is very highly concentrated near the junctions between brain cells strongly support the concept of T3 as a brain chemical transmitter that is essential for maintaining normal mood and behaviour.

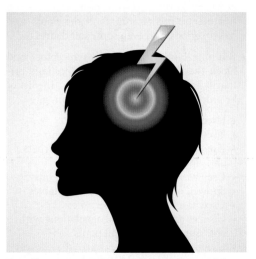

Thyroid hormones are essential for a functioning brain and the prevention of mood disorders

- Extensive human research has led scientists to conclude that serotonin levels in the brain decrease if T3 is not delivered in the right amount. Thyroid hormone in the brain has the ability to enhance the production of serotonin in brain cells.

- The potent thyroid hormone T3 is found in greater quantities in the limbic system, a region of the brain that regulates mood, emotions, and perception of happy and sad events.

- Hashimoto's (an autoimmune disease of the thyroid) can cause a person's metabolism to swing between overly active to overly depressed. These swings can mimic the symptoms of bipolar disorder and cause misdiagnosis and inappropriate treatment

    (Chang 1998; Kupka 2002; Cole 2002; Frye 1999).

- Any patient suffering from depression should be routinely assessed for hypothyroidism. There should be no exceptions; between 30-50% will be found to be hypothyroid, and as a result of treatment, their depression will begin to lift in weeks

- Conventional medicine will turn with little thought to psychotropic antidepressants. The problem with these is that they are sometimes difficult to stop taking and is not targeting the problem, especially if it related to thyroid problems.

- Here is a frightening thought: patients have been diagnosed with dementia and Alzheimer's disease, when in reality what they had was a thyroid disorder. A 2008 study, published in the Archives of Internal Medicine, found that older women who had levels of TSH that were either too high or too low had more than twice the risk of Alzheimer's disease than those with more moderate levels (the same was not true of men). This is another reason that testing your thyroid become part of your standard testing routine as you get older!

- In terms of immunology, the thyroid gland acts as a gatekeeper: every 17 minutes all the blood in the body passes through the thyroid, where this gland's secretion of iodine kills germs that have come into the body (through absorption of food in the digestive tract, skin injury, respiratory intake, etc.)

- Pathogenic micro-organisms, the primary causative agent for disease in the body, are made weaker during their passage through the thyroid gland. With each "17 minute passage" they are made still weaker until most are killed, provided the thyroid has its normal supply of iodine.

Benefits of Coconut Oil

Lauric Acid a Key Component to Health

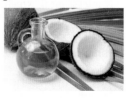

- Lauric acid is a medium chain fatty acid which is abundant in coconut oil, and considered responsible for many of its health benefits. Coconut oil is about 50% lauric acid. The only other abundant source found in nature is in human breast milk. Dr. Jon J. Kabara, Ph.D. and Professor Emeritus of Michigan State University says, "Never before in the history of man is it so important to emphasize the value of Lauric Oils. The medium-chain fats in coconut oil are similar to fats in mother's milk and have similar nutriceutical effects."

- In the body Lauric acid, which accounts for 55% of the total fatty acids in extra virgin coconut oil, converts to monolaurin.

- Research by lipid biochemists has shown monolaurin to inactivate fungi such as Candida albicans, and such bacteria as Listeria, Staphylococcus, and Streptococcus.

- Dr. Mary Enig, a Ph.D. nutritionist/biochemist and one of the world's leading authorities on fats and oils, goes on to say, "Approximately 50% of the fatty acids in coconut fat are lauric acid. Lauric acid is a medium chain fatty acid, which has the additional beneficial function of being formed into monolaurin in the human or animal body.

- Monolaurin is the antiviral, antibacterial, and antiprotozoal monoglyceride used by the human or animal to destroy lipid coated viruses such as HIV, herpes, cytomegalovirus, influenza, various pathogenic bacteria including listeria monocytogenes and heliobacter pylori, and protozoa such as giardia lamblia. Some studies have also shown some antimicrobial effects of the free lauric acid."

- Coconut oil can also protect against diabetes. Long chain fatty acids found in most vegetable oils are likely to be deposited in blood vessels or stored near the internal organs as fat. Excess fat storage around the internal organs promotes insulin resistance and ultimately diabetes. Long chain fatty acids also hinder glucose absorption, which keeps the glucose levels in the bloodstream dangerously elevated. The medium-chain fatty acids in coconut oil, on the other hand, are used immediately for energy after consumed. Coconut oil also helps to stabilize blood sugar levels immediately after a meal, which prevents glucose spikes and hypoglycaemia risk.

- Coconut oil is also a wonderful food to help stimulate the metabolism and aid with weight loss efforts. The mechanism of coconut oil's effects is by stimulating the thyroid gland and by reducing the appetite. The medium-chain fatty acids in coconut oil are instantly burned when consumed, which results in a boost in thyroid levels for hours. Furthermore, coconut oil helps you feel full and satisfied earlier in a meal and helps with satiety for hours afterwards. This combination makes it a perfect supplement to the diet in those wishing to lose weight.

- One of the most outstanding benefits of consuming MCFA's is that they do not require the liver and gallbladder to digest and emulsify them. This means instant energy and increased thermogenesis (increased metabolic rate in the body) which leads to more heat production as well as improved circulation. For anyone with impaired fat digestion or a removed gallbladder, coconut oil is the only oil to consume as it is very easily digested.

Conclusion:

- Well now you can see how important the thyroid is for health and fat lost and, the huge number of factors which can inhibit the thyroid from working efficiently, leaving you often piling on the pounds and feel extremely tired and negatively effecting your mood.

- Hopefully from this chapter you are know more knowledgeable on maintaining a healthy thyroid and, remember all hormones work in synergy.

- If you want to know more about your thyroid gland and thyroid hormones then the books that I suggest that you read are;

- "Ultra Metabolism" - Mark Hyman
- "The Anti-Ageing Zone" - Barry Sears
- "Master Your Metabolism" - Jillian Michaels
- "Hormonal Balance" - Scott Isaacs
- "Thyroid - Guardian of Health" - Philip Young
- "Why Do I Still Habe Thyroid Symptoms?" - Datis Kharrazian
- "The Thyroid Solution Diet" - Ridha Arem
- "Hypothroidism - the unsuspecting illness" - Broda Barnes & Lawrence Galton

HABIT 6

ANABOLISM VS CATABOLISM

ANABOLISM   **CATABOLISM**

GET THE HORMONE BALANCE RIGHT FOR OPTIMUM FAT LOSS AND HEALTH

I have known Phil now for a number of years. I can confidently say that he is now at the forefront of conditioning and nutrition practices both in professional sport and respective to general health of the public. I had the pleasure of working closely with Phil during the 2006-7 season as Leicester Tigers almost became the first club to win every available trophy, narrowly missing this goal by losing the final game of the season. Phil's contribution that season was invaluable."

Craig White (High Performance Coach Leicester, Wales & British Lions)

- A steroid is a chemical substance with four carbon ring structures attached to each other in a very specific and unique fashion. Cortisol, DHEA, testosterone, pregnenolone, progesterone, and oestrogen are all steroid-based hormones that chemically look very similar to each other in terms of their basic molecular structures. They are all made in the adrenals with cholesterol being the raw material. However, their actions differ markedly, with enormous differences in how they function and in the roles they play in the various chemical factories of our bodies.

- All of our steroid hormones are made from cholesterol. Steroid hormones have pregnenolone and progesterone as basic precursors. The diagram at the bottom of the page shows how steroid hormones are all made from cholesterol. Some of the hormones in this pathway in the diagram can be converted into others, and some can convert back, while others cannot as you can see below.

- In this habit we will look at the connection between pregnenolone, cortisol, testosterone, DHEA, oestrogen & progesterone in helping to decrease body fat composition and improve our overall health.

The Cholesterol Myth

- Are you still under the impression that cholesterol is a dietary villain and a primary cause of heart disease? And do you avoid eating healthy

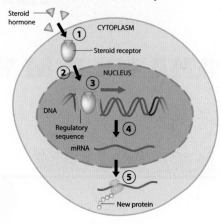

Steroid Hormone Response

How a steroid hormone effects a cell

animal foods like eggs, butter and grass-fed beef because of "high-cholesterol" fears?

- The pharmaceutical industry and the food industry have developed a trillion pound business based on the nonesense that cholesterol is the main cause of heart disease. Let me tell you in simple terms; inflammation is the cause of heart disease - not cholesterol - as you will see in habit 8.

- Cholesterol is the precursor to steroid hormones and 80-90% of cholesterol is made by the liver. So the health of your liver is essential for steroid production. If you eat a low-fat diet to drop your cholesterol, your body simply makes more cholesterol to compensate. If you

HOW STEROID HORMONES ARE MADE IN YOUR BODY

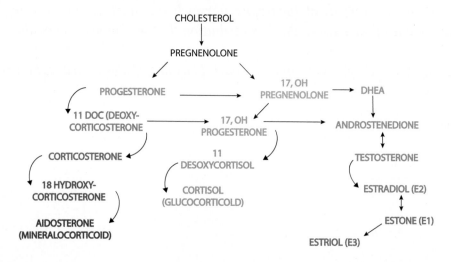

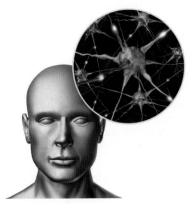

Cholesterol plays an essential role in your brain, which contains about 25% of cholesterol. It is critical for synapse formation, i.e. the connections between your neurons, which allow you to think, learn new things, and form memories.

eat a diet high in cholesterol, your body will simply make less.

- Cholesterol has many health benefits. Many research studies have revealed, for instance, that cholesterol plays a key role in regulating protein pathways involved in cell signalling and may also regulate other cellular processes. It's already known that cholesterol plays a critical role within your cell membranes, but research suggests cholesterol also interacts with proteins inside your cells, adding even more importance.

- Your body is composed of trillions of cells that need to interact with each other. Cholesterol is one of the molecules that allow for these interactions to take place. Also, cholesterol is the precursor to bile acids, so without sufficient amounts of cholesterol, your digestive system can also be adversely affected.

- Low cholesterol levels have been linked to violent behaviour, and changes in brain chemistry, particularly a reduction in serotonin activity. Furthermore, you need cholesterol to produce steroid hormones, including your sex hormones, as already discussed.

- All statin drugs block the biosynthesis of both cholesterol and CoQ10, which explains statins' common side effects such as fatigue, muscle pain and muscle weakness.

- So for those of you who think cholesterol is the enemy, you would be dead without it; far from being the enemy it is critical for life.

- Research on statins found powerful evidence that statins induce injury to mitochondria.

With injured mitochondria, the body produces less energy and more "free radicals".

- As statins block the production of cholesterol in the body, they also block the production of much of the body's Co-Q10, which is also important in preventing free radical damage. In addition, statins reduce the very blood cholesterol that is needed to carry Co-Q10 and other fat-soluble antioxidants throughout the body. I talk more about statins throughout the book and how the evidence clearly shows that cholesterol is not the cause of heart disease.

Let's look at Pregnenolone?

- Pregnenolone is a natural hormone, produced primarily by the adrenal glands, but also in the brain, liver, skin, testicles and ovaries. In the body, pregnenolone is used either as pregnenolone itself, or it is converted to DHEA (dehydroepian- drosterone), which in turn is converted into androgens (e.g. testosterone), oestrogens and other steroids, and through another pathway, it is converted into progesterone.

- There are over 150 different steroid hormones which are made from pregnenolone in the body in total – it generates a whole symphony of hormones – in short it is "The Symphony of Life".

- It is interesting to note that there is a clear difference in the metabolism of pregnenolone in human males and females – in males the metabolic pathway seems to favour conversion into testosterone and in females the conversion into oestrogens.

- Pregnenolone is called the mother of all steroid hormones for a good reason. It is a steroid hormone at the top of the hormonal production cascade. It is also the precursor in the synthesis of female hormones such as oestrogen and progesterone, mineralocorticoids such as aldosterone that is responsible for sodium regulation, glucocorticoids such as cortisol that suppresses inflammation and helps to reduce stress, and androgens such as testosterone. Pregnenolone is therefore aptly called a pro-hormone. During periods of stress, the output of adrenal steroids such as cortisol will increase, which will put a great demand on pregnenolone production. This may lead to pregnenolone deficiency, which in turn may lead to reduction of both glucocorticosteroids and mineralocorticoids such as cortisol and aldosterone respectively.

- Numerous studies have shown the effects of pregnenolone on the body and brain. In normal people, pregnenolone will boost energy, elevate mood and improve memory and mental performance. Pregnenolone will also create a sense of well being while improving the ability to tolerate stress. Furthermore, pregnenolone has a host of other benefits, which include the ability to influence cerebral function, the female reproductive cycle, immune defences, inflammation, mood, skin health, sleep patterns, stress tolerance, and wound healing.

- Production of pregnenolone decreases with stress, aging, depression, hypothyroidism and exposure to toxins. It can also be depleted when levels of other hormones, such as cortisol, are low, as it is used to replenish those supplies.

Cortisol: the steroid hormone for stressful times

- Cortisol is a steroid and one of the primary stress hormones. Production is stimulated within the endocrine system's hypothalamic-pituitary-adrenal (HPA) axis. Secretion comes from the adrenal glands.

- Ironically named the master "stress" hormone, cortisol regulates the way your body uses various fuel sources and is essential for recouping energy following stress. When your adrenals are healthy, you will produce 35–40 mg of cortisol per day.

- Normal cortisol hormone levels tend to follow a 24-hour circadian rhythm; the lowest level being at night during sleep that gradually increase to when you need to wake up and get moving. The high cortisol levels present in early morning rapidly drop off and then continue to decline for the remainder of the day. You can see a diagram of the daily rhythm on the next page. Under ideal conditions, your cortisol levels should be neither consistently high nor low, but fluctuate in a fairly rhythmic pattern

The primary role of cortisol is to help mobilise energy for fuel.

- Excess cortisol impedes the entry of amino acids into muscle cells for protein synthesis, and instead transports them to the liver to be used as energy.

- This is why individuals involved in strength training may experience a decrease in muscle mass and increases in body fat if they do not take the necessary steps to reduce/control cortisol levels. Cortisol is one of the main reasons athletes at all levels take one step forward & two back, unless they know how to play the anabolic v catabolic game.

- If there is a true anti–muscularity drug, it is chronic stress. This was demonstrated in one experiment with young soldiers undergoing Army Training. At the peak of training, their testosterone levels dropped by 30%.

- Within weeks after the course ended, thus removing the psychological and physical stress, their testosterone levels returned to their pre–training levels. Stress is one of the most serious threats to testosterone production, and chronic

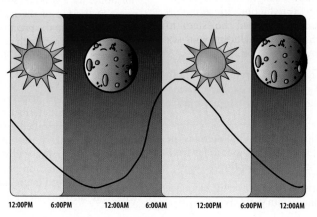

A diagram of "normal" daily cortisol rhythm

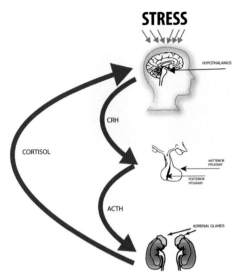

STRESS

The HPA response begins when the hypothalamus secretes corticotropin releasing hormone (CRH) which directs the pituitary gland to release the hormone adrenocorticotropic hormone (ACTH). ACTH then directs the adrenal glands to secrete more hormones, including epinephrine, norepinephrine, and cortisol

stress is epidemic in our 21st century way of life.

- Remember the study from habit 1 where researchers found that the cortisol levels of depressed individuals were 68% higher than those without depression? That same study found that testosterone, both night time and 24-hour, were significantly lower in these individuals and were negatively correlated with cortisol levels. To put it directly: the higher the cortisol, the lower the testosterone.

Controlling Stress Is The Key To Your Fat Loss Success.

- Remember this very important point: the less stress in your life, the more material you have for growth and repair. The more stress in your life, the less material you will have for growth and repair. It is exceptionally difficult to be lean and healthy when you can't control stress.

- Whether they signal attack, retreat or surrender, every cell responds accordingly, and you feel the results. It is through the actions of the adrenal hormones that your body is able to mobilize its resources to escape or fight off danger (stress) and survive. In a more primitive society that would mean being able to run away quickly, fight or pursue an enemy or game, endure long periods of physical challenge and depriva-

tion, and store up physical reserves when they are available.

- Short, intermittent bursts of cortisol helped our ancestors survive in the wilderness and still come to our aid today. But unlike our ancestors, we face chronically stressful situations such as job loss and financial insecurity. Additionally, there are new biological stressors such as obesity and environmental toxins.

- The biological stress response is designed to be short term so, if it is aroused too often or lasts too long, it can potentially affect your overall health and well being.

- If you are constantly bombarded by stressors your cortisol and adrenaline will remain elevated; this is a disaster if trying to lose body fat! If your adrenals remain in a state of heightened alert and continue to produce adrenaline and cortisol, you're exposed to chronically elevated blood sugar, which raises insulin levels and can result in insulin resistance and type II diabetes.

- The effects of chronic, over-exposure to cortisol can be devastating. Prolonged cortisol elevation causes the immune system to go on red alert and inflammatory activity becomes chronic and also causing insulin resistance. As well as this, excess cortisol breaks muscle tissue down, to be used as fuel, and this then lowers metabolism.

- Stresses can be physical, emotional, nutritional, chemical, physiological or hormonal. Your body responds identically to all of these stressors, because it cannot distinguish the differences between them – stress is stress no matter what the source is. If you want to have a lean, healthy body then you must control stress. If you don't control stress, then stress will con-

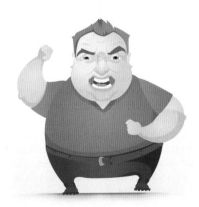

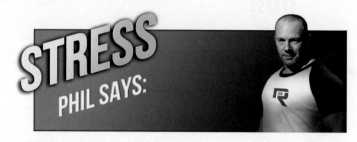

STRESS
PHIL SAYS:

No matter what you may have been through, even unspeakable pain, you are still in control of your identity. No event can change you on the inside unless you allow it to do so. No person can cause you to respond in a particular way on the inside unless you choose to do react that way. The freedom to forge your own opinions, ideas, attitudes, and choices rests solely and uniquely with you. When I personally learnt this my life changed immediately. I, like most people, have had my share of stressful situations in life, and for decades I would stew in my negative emotions going over events until I felt the same anger the event caused me when it happened. If you are locked into dragging up past events it is impossible to move forwards with any hope. Learn to live with hope, joy and happiness and your life can change in an instant.

trol you - which usually means becoming sick, tired and obese.

Stress and abdominal fat

- The link between cortisol and abdominal fat comes from the signal the hormone sends for fat storage to your abdominal fat cells. The fat cells in your abdominal area have four times more cortisol receptors than fat located elsewhere in the body, making them more sensitive to cortisol and causing them to respond more strongly to fat storage.

- Elevated cortisol causes your body to store more of our calories as fat, especially around your stomach and the sides of your face and this increases the breakdown or catabolism of muscles. The physical profile associated with chronic high cortisol is a bit like Humpty Dumpty - you have a rounded moon face, large belly and skinny arms and legs.

- Excessive cortisol can also stimulate your appetite, causing overeating, and cravings for sugary and high calorie fatty foods that are too strong to fight. Another key issue in weight gain is the relationship between insulin, a hormone made in your pancreas, and cortisol. When your body is stressed, cortisol is released to raise levels of fat and glucose (blood sugar) in your bloodstream and thereby increase energy and muscle strength. The increased blood sugar stimulates increased insulin, which has the job of keeping blood sugar levels within a very narrow range.

- When insulin is released continually, your cells eventually become desensitized to it, and high levels of blood sugar and insulin build up in the blood. This can cause insulin resistance and eventually type 2 diabetes .

- The reason fat accumulates around your middle is because it is close to the liver, where it can be quickly converted back into energy if needed.

- The connection between stress and obesity cannot be overlooked. Cortisol signals a metabolic shut down that makes losing weight almost impossible.

- It's as if the body feels it is under an attack, such that it must hoard all its resources, including

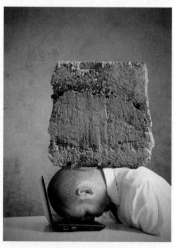

Stress can have a huge impact on your hormones, turning you into a fat storing machine

fat stores, and won't let go of them under any inducement.

If a person has excess body fat, they will make an enzyme called aromatase which will convert testosterone into oestrogen, increasing oestrogen levels.

- Stress makes you burn fewer calories and cortisol can actually reduce the body's ability to release fat from its fat stores to use for energy! Stress hormones cause increased body fat in the abdominal region, exactly where we don't need or want it.

HSD: The Body's "Fat Storage" Enzyme

- So how does stress lower testosterone? Most of the research in this area was done through Population Council endocrinologist Matthew Hardy and his work on rats. He and his teams found out how stress lowers your testosterone: through a tricky little enzyme called 11ßHSD-1

- In males, the body produces most of its testosterone in the Leydig Cells of the testes and this enzyme keeps cortisol from pushing down your testosterone. It literally puts the brakes on cortisol from destroying your testosterone. However, in times of stress, there is simply too much cortisol compared to 11ßHSD-1 and this leads to a decrease in your testosterone production.

- One of the complicating factors in the stress/cortisol/fat relationship is an enzyme deep within fat cells called HSD - short for 11-beta-hydroxysteroid-dehydrogenase-1.

- HSD functions to convert inactive cortisol (called cortisone) back into active cortisol, which then functions as a potent fat-storage signal within fat cells, especially abdominal fat cells.

- Recent research tells us that HSD activity is higher in abdominal fat cells than it is in fat cells in other parts of the body - which may be the reason why cortisol exposure is associated with higher levels of fat in the abdominal region, as compared to fat levels in other parts of the body, such as the thighs or buttocks.

- Researchers in Berlin, Germany, have suggested that the regulation of cortisol levels within cells by HSD is just as important as cortisol lev-

els in the plasma. This means that the adrenal glands are not the only place in the body for "production" of cortisol; fat cells can produce their own fat-storing cortisol via reactivation of inactive cortisol by the HSD enzyme.

- This leads to higher cortisol levels within fat cells and a further increase in fat storage and the size of fat cells. Overall, according to the German scientists, it is this mechanism of "self-production" of cortisol within individual fat cells that may represent the most important pathogenic signal for central (abdominal) obesity.

- Researchers from the University of Birmingham, in England, have some especially de-

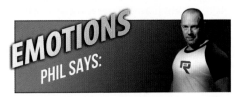

Our deadly emotions play havoc with our cortisol levels for example I get bombarded everyday with messages on what are the best supplements to reduce cortisol and I reply, "Be happy and have a positive attitude towards life is the quickest way to drop cortisol, and put yourself in an anabolic state. You and only you can choose how you will think and feel in any circumstance, event, relationship in your life. When you react with hostility, hatred, jealousy, anger and aggression this just sends your cortisol levels through the roof and you have to decide is it worth having such feelings every time you are faced with a stressful situation. Yes, of course, there will be times when situations agitate you but learn to control the situation instead of the situation controlling you. Life is often said to be 10% what happens to us and 90% how we respond to it."

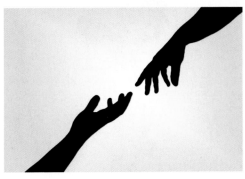

When you are on your knees from life's stressful events, those who help you in these situations, are your true friends.

pressing news for people trying to lose weight by extreme dieting. Studying the metabolic effects of a very low calorie diet (eight hundred calories per day) for ten weeks, they found that the stress of the diet significantly increased cortisol levels throughout the body, but also increased HSD activity within fat cells by 3.4 times.

- In a series of experiments conducted by researchers from Harvard University, the British Heart Foundation, Merck pharmaceuticals, and a Swedish biotechnology firm, not only has HSD over-activity been identified as a cause of obesity and diabetes, but reducing its activity has been shown to reduce belly fat - despite a high-fat and high-calorie diet!

- Danish scientists have found that higher levels of growth hormone are associated with reduced HSD activity, a finding that may explain some of the primary effects of growth hormone in reducing body fat (especially abdominal fat) and increasing muscle mass.

- Flavonoids have been found to help balance HSD activity. The most potent of the flavonoids for balancing HSD activity are found in the form of substances known as polymethoxylated flavonoids (PMFs) found in oranges (nobiletin and tangeretin), which can be up to three to five times stronger than other flavonoids. However, PMFs come from citrus peels, which you're probably not eating very many of.

Limit alcohol if you want to get your cortisol levels back to a healthy level as alcohol raises cortisol, and the effect persists for twenty four hours in men and probably longer in women.

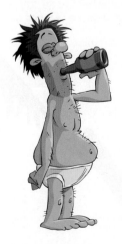

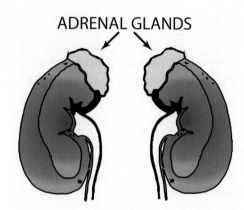

ADRENAL GLANDS

The adrenal glands sit on top of the two kidneys. The make and release steroid hormones

- Drinking too much alcohol is a forced chemical stressor; your body secretes cortisol to overcome the toxic effects of alcohol just as it would a lethal poison. Too much alcohol blocks your liver from breaking down glycogen into sugar for brain energy, and cortisol helps your body bypass this blockage by breaking down your muscles to turn into glucose to make new sugar a process called gluconeogenesis. So, not a situation you want if you are after a leaner body. There is no easy way to say this drop the booze if you want to drop the fat its that simple.

- Eliminate caffeine from your diet; it's the quickest way to reduce cortisol production and elevate the production of DHEA, the leading anabolic youth hormone. 200 mg of caffeine (one 12 oz mug of coffee) can increase blood cortisol levels by 30% in one hour! Cortisol can remain elevated for up to 18 hours in the blood. This is the easiest step to decrease your catabolic metabolism and increase your anabolic metabolism.

Adrenal Fatigue

- No bigger than a walnut and weighing less than a grape, each of your two adrenal glands sits like a tiny pyramid on top of each kidney ("ad" "renal" means "over" the "kidneys"). But don't let their size fool you; these powerful little endocrine glands manufacture and secrete steroid hormones such as cortisol, oestrogen and testosterone that are essential for life, health and vitality. They modulate the functioning of every tissue, organ and gland in the body to maintain homoeostasis (a constant internal environment) during stress and keep you alive.

- The main purpose of the adrenals is to enable the body to deal with stress from every possible source, ranging from injury and disease, to work and relationship problems. They largely determine the energy of your body's responses to every change in your internal and external environment.

- In adrenal fatigue, more cortisol is secreted during the early stages. In the later stages of Adrenal Fatigue (when the adrenal glands become exhausted), cortisol output is reduced.

- Normally after many years on the roller coaster of stress when initially the adrenals are spewing out cortisol to help counteract the stress response they then become exhausted like all things in life when you keep pushing them into the ground. Then you are faced with low cortisol which is an issue you won't hear your main stream doctor unless you are flat on your back, in adrenal crisis, with blood pressure so low that you can't send oxygen to your brain and wanting to faint all the time.

1. Do you have a hard time falling asleep at night?
2. Do you wake up frequently during the night?
3. Do you have a hard time waking up in the morning early, or feeling refreshed?
4. Do bright lights bother you more than they should?
5. Do you startle easily due to noise?
6. When standing from sitting or from lying down, do you feel light-headed or dizzy?
7. Do you take things too seriously, and are easily defensive?
8. Do you feel you don't cope well with certain people or events in your life?

- Any of the above sound familiar? If so time to heal those adrenal glands.

Testing Adrenal Function

- Take and compare two blood pressure readings—one while lying down and one while standing. Rest for five minutes in recumbent position (lying down) before taking the reading. Stand up and immediately take the blood pressure again

- If the blood pressure is lower after standing, suspect reduced adrenal gland function the de-

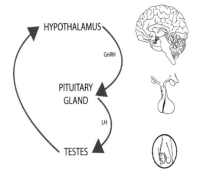

In males, the hypothalamus secretes gonadotropin-releasing hormone (GnRH) which then stimulates the release of leutenizing hormone (LH) secretion from the pituitary gland. LH then stimulates cells in the testes to create testosterone

gree to which the blood pressure drops while standing is often proportionate to the degree of hypoadrenalism.

- An interesting study showed that light exposure in the early morning has a strong impact on the morning cortisol peak. For those who awoke to bright light, cortisol levels about half an hour after waking were 35% higher than for those who awoke during darkness (Frank, Scheer, and Buijs 1999). One easy way to help normalise your production pattern if your cortisol levels are low is to increase your exposure to light during the day, especially in the early morning.

Nutrients that help decrease excess cortisol

- For many years, studies have shown that phosphatidylserine is able to cut elevated cortisol levels induced by mental and physical stress. In one early study, 800 mg per day given to healthy men significantly blunted the rise in cortisol caused by physical stress. That's why I prescribe PRP's Super Brain Talk as it is an incredible anti anxiety product in my eyes.

Ginkgo biloba

- For the last 5,000 years, leaves of the ginkgo tree have been used to treat various medical conditions. While ginkgo is currently used to help combat the debilitating effects of memory decline and dementia, emerging evidence suggests that it may be useful in treating the impact of stress and elevated cortisol levels. A recent double-blind, placebo-controlled study, published in the Journal of Physiology and Pharmacology, examined ginkgo's effects in modulating cortisol and blood pressure levels in 70 healthy male and female subjects. When subjected to physical and mental stressors, subjects who were given 120 mg per day of a standardized ginkgo extract saw smaller increases in their cortisol levels and blood pressure than did their counterparts who were given a placebo.

- When you are faced with a stressful situation, your vitamin C is rapidly used up in the production of cortisol and related stress-response hormones.

- In two separate studies about vitamin C supplementation (1,000–1,500 mg per day for one week), ultra-marathon runners showed a 30% lower cortisol level in their blood when compared to runners receiving a placebo.

Vitamin C is utilized by the adrenal glands in the production of all the adrenal hormones, most notably cortisol.

- It is interesting to note that, humans do not produce vitamin C. There are 3 other species that don't either; guinea pigs, fruit bats, and other primates. Those animals who do produce vitamin C, do so whilst under extreme stress; under times of stress they release a large amount of vitamin C. When a goat is under extreme stress, it has been estimated to produce 100 000mg of vitamin C, in 24 hours.

- In those animals who can produce vitamin C, glucose is one of the main substances used. From my research, it is best to take vitamin C at least 2 hours away from carbohydrate sources. This is because glucose competes with vitamin C at the same cell receptor sites. It you have just eaten a meal containing 100g of carbs that is made equals 100 000mg of glucose and you take 1000mg of vitamin C with the same meal, you have 1000 molecules vs 100 000 at the same receptor sites.

- I recommend that you take a minimum of 3000mg of vitamin C a day, in divided dosages throughout the day. The more stress that you have in your life (physical, mental, chemical or emotional), the more I would increase the dosage. A good rule of thumb is that, you will know if you are taking too much vitamin C because you will be shitting through the eye of a needle!

- Another study, published in the journal Psycho-pharmacology, reviewed evidence showing that vitamin C can reduce high cortisol levels brought about by psychologically induced stress. In a randomized, double-blind, placebo-controlled trial, researchers gave 3000 mg per day of vitamin C or a placebo to 120 volunteers who were subjected to psychological stress through the Trier Social Stress Test (TSST), which consists of 15 minutes of psychological stress induced via a mock job interview, followed by a mental arithmetic challenge. Subjects who took vitamin C had lower blood pressure, subjective stress, and cortisol measures compared to those who were given placebo.

Testosterone: required for men and women

- Often referred to as the "hormone of desire," testosterone is involved in maintaining muscle mass, mood, sex drive, and energy levels in both men and women.

- Testosterone is actually produced by an intricate chain of events beginning in the hypothalamus. The hypothalamus secretes gonadotropin-releasing hormone (GnRH) to the pituitary gland in controlled pulses or bursts, which in turn causes the release of leutenizing hormone (LH) from the pituitary gland.

- And it is leutenizing hormone that stimulates the Leydig cells of the testes to create testosterone. Why the science lesson? Because it is important to know that disease or damage to anything in this physiological chain, i.e. the hypothalamus, pituitary or testes, can cause hypogonadism, or low testosterone and will make it very difficult for you to significantly increase your testosterone.

- If you've sustained a blow to the head or a traumatic brain injury, caused by a stroke, heart attack, or loss of oxygen for long periods of time, low testosterone may result.

How Testosterone is Stored in the Body

- On average, a man's body produces about 6-8 mg of testosterone a day, but not all of that testosterone floating in our bloodstream can be used by our bodies. Our total testosterone can be broken down into the following three subtypes:

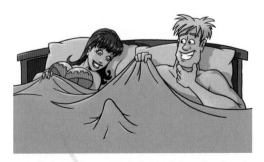

Normally testosterone is 30% higher in the morning than the evening. This may explain why men are more interested in sex in the morning and is part of the reason for spontaneous morning erections. In fact, the loss of morning erections is a sure sign that testosterone is declining and heart disease could be taking a grip, or your mrs has grown a lot of facial hair and you no longer find her attractive.

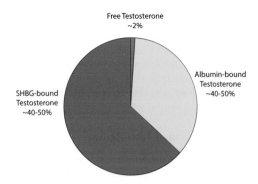

Only around 2% of the testosterone in the body is free. The rest is bound to either albumin or SHBG

1. Free Testosterone.

- This is testosterone in its purest form. The reason it's called "free" is because there aren't any proteins attached to it. Unbound to other molecules, free T can enter cells and activate receptors in order to work its virile magic on your body and mind. Despite free testosterone's benefits, it makes up only 2-3% of our total testosterone levels. To maximize the benefits of T, we want to do what we can to increase the amount of free testosterone in our bloodstream.

2. SHBG-bound Testosterone.

- About 40-50% of our total testosterone is bound to a protein called sex hormone binding globulin (SHBG). SHBG is produced in our livers and plays an important role in regulating the amount of free testosterone in our bodies. The downside to SHBG-bound T is that it's biologically inactive, meaning our bodies can't use this type of testosterone to help build muscles or boost our mood. SHBG isn't bad, but too much of it is. Excess SHBG is why it's possible to have high total testosterone levels, but still suffer symptoms of testosterone deficiency — the SHBG binds itself to too much testosterone and doesn't leave enough of the pure stuff. Research suggests that diet and lifestyle changes can help reduce the amount of SHBG in our system, making more free T available.

- Fish oil has been shown to lower SHBG. Again, this is anti-andropause because andropause is known for slowly raising SHBG levels with age, which means that more SHBG is bound to your testosterone leaving you less free testosterone.. The net effect of taking fish oil, then, is the opposite and will leave you with more free testosterone.

- Fish Oil has also been shown in one study to increase Leutenizing Hormone (LH). Leutenizing Hormone (LH), is the hormone that triggers or signals testosterone production.

3. Albumin-bound Testosterone.

- The rest of our testosterone is bound to a protein called albumin. Albumin is a protein produced in the liver, and its job is to stabilize extra-cellular fluid volumes. Like SHBG-bound testosterone, albumin-bound testosterone is biologically inactive. However, unlike SHBG-bound T, the bind between albumin and testosterone is weak and can be easily broken in order to create free testosterone when needed. Because albumin-bound testosterone is easily converted to free T, some labs lump it together with free testosterone whenever you get tested.

- Studies have found that after age 30, testosterone levels in men may decline an average of 2% a year.

Average Testosterone Levels by Age in Men	
AGE	AVERAGE
15-24	750NG/DL
25-34	700NG/DL
35-44	650NG/DL
45-54	600NG/DL
55-64	550NG/DL
65-74	500NG/DL
75-84	450NG/DL
85-89	400NG/DL

- There are 5 reasons as to why free testosterone levels may be low:

1. Too much testosterone is being converted to oestrogen through the activity of aromatase.
2. Too much free testosterone is being bound by SHBG. This would be especially apparent if a male's total testosterone levels are high but free testosterone levels are low.
3. The pituitary gland is not secreting enough LH to stimulate gonadal production of testosterone. In this case, total testosterone would be low.
4. The gonads have lost their ability to produce testosterone, despite adequate amounts of LH. In this case, the level of LH would be high despite a low testosterone level.
5. DHEA is abnormally low.

Testosterone - just for men? Hardly!

- Although women produce only about one-tenth the testosterone of men, women produce 300 micrograms per day, whilst men produce 6 – 8 milligrams per day. You can see how little testosterone a women produces, this is a major reason as to why a woman should never fear putting on large amounts of muscle whilst doing strength training. Let me make it clear - for a woman to carry large amounts of muscle on her frame, she would either need to have a severe hormonal problem or be taking performance enhancing drugs.

- A woman's levels of testosterone drop by about 50% by the age of forty-five compared to the amount she produced at age twenty.

- In a scientific review by the North American Menopause Society, nine out of ten studies on testosterone in women showed increasing testosterone levels to be effective in improving sexual desire, energy levels, body composition changes, and overall emotional outlook.

- One study, published in 1996 in the Journal of Clinical Endocrinology and Metabolism, showed that obese women who boosted their testosterone levels lost significantly more abdominal fat and gained more muscle mass compared to women who were given a placebo and whose testosterone levels remained suppressed.

- Researchers at the University of Washington, in Seattle, have shown that among women who lose weight using dietary restriction alone, each 2% loss of body weight is associated with a fall in testosterone levels of 10-12%. This is another reason which shows that raise loss diets who focus on calorie restrictions are not only stupid, but, in the long term, will have a negative effect on your hormones and increase your body fat.

- Most testosterone production in women comes from the ovaries and in men from the testes, but in both genders a substantial amount of testosterone also comes from the adrenal glands—the same gland responsible for cortisol production.

Male Hormone Restoration

- Recent studies have demonstrated that low testosterone in men is strongly associated with metabolic syndrome, type 2 diabetes, cardiovascular disease (Miner and Seftel 2007), and an almost 50% increase in mortality over a seven year period (Malkin et al 2010). Restoring testosterone to youthful ranges in middle-aged, obese men resulted in an increase in insulin sensitivity as well as a reduction in total cholesterol, fat mass, waist circumference and pro-inflammatory cytokines associated with atherosclerosis, diabetes, and the metabolic syndrome (Kapoor et al 2006, Malkin et al 2004, Heufelder et al 2009). Testosterone therapy also significantly improved erectile function (Fukui 2007) and improved functional capacity, or the ability to perform physical activity without severe duress, in men with heart failure (Malkin et al 2007).

- Fat cells convert testosterone into oestrogen. Furthermore, low testosterone is correlated to being overweight. Fat cells are loaded with aromatase, the enzyme that converts testosterone to oestrogen. The higher your percentage of body fat, the more oestrogen you can produce and the fatter you will become, unless you control your diet and use supplements plus exercise to lower oestrogen production.

- To increase your testosterone levels, you must, I repeat you MUST, decrease your stress levels. The reason for this is that testosterone and cortisol are both made from cholesterol. The more stress in your life, the more cortisol that is required (using up this substrate) and so the less substrates you have to make testosterone. Remember, excess stress, whether you are a male or female, will make you tired, dumb and flabby.

Sunshine Increases Testosterone

- Vitamin D, a steroid hormone, is essential for the healthy development of the nucleus of the sperm cell, and helps maintain semen quality and sperm count. Vitamin D also increases levels of testosterone, which may boost libido. In one study, overweight men who were given vitamin D supplements had a significant increase in testosterone levels after one year. Vitamin D deficiency is currently at epidemic proportions in the UK, and many other regions around the world, largely because people do not spend enough time in the sun to facilitate this important process of vitamin D production.

- So the first step to ensuring you are receiving all the benefits of vitamin D is to find out what your levels are using a 25(OH)D test, also called 25-hydroxyvitamin D. This test should be available by asking your doctor to perform a routine blood sample. Or you can find a lab that will also do this test for you.

- A few years back, the recommended level was between 40 to 60 nano-grams per millilitre (ng/ml), but more recently the optimal vitamin D level has been raised to 50-70 ng/ml.

- To get your levels into the healthy range, sun exposure is the BEST way to optimize your vitamin D levels; exposing a large amount of your skin until it turns the lightest shade of pink, as near to solar noon as possible, is typically necessary to achieve adequate vitamin D production. If sun exposure is not an option, a safe tanning bed can be used (Always read the instructions). I personally use a UVB sun bed three times per week for 2 minutes, skin colouring will determine exposure. I only use

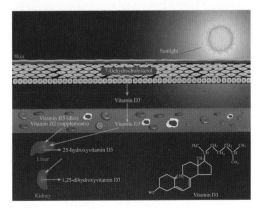

Vitamin D metabolism from sunlight

the UVB sun bed during the winter months, or days in the summer where there is no sun exposure. Otherwise, if it is a nice sunny day (which is extremely rare in the UK) I will bare my body and get my free vitamin D. Remember, you only get the maximum exposure of UVB rays between 12-3pm. The darker the skin colour, the more time needed require sun exposure. I am whiter than white, so, after 10-15 minutes of sunshine, I put my t-shirt and cap on, I'm done.

- A vitamin D3 supplement can be taken orally, but research suggests the average adult needs to take 8,000 IU's of vitamin D per day in order to elevate their levels above 40 ng/ml, which is the absolute minimum for disease prevention. Research has also shown the close connection between vitamin A and vitamin D. They work synergistically. If you take too much of one then you will deplete the other. This is why I advise that you do your own research before consuming any high dose supplements. This is why I have added vitamin A to my Ultimate Fish Oil supplements; vitamin D protects omega-3 fats, but I was conscious of the fact that excess vitamin D can deplete vitamin A.

Remember Stress Kills Testosterone

- When you're under a lot of stress, your body releases high levels of the stress hormone cortisol. This hormone actually blocks the effects of testosterone, presumably because, from a biological standpoint, testosterone-associated

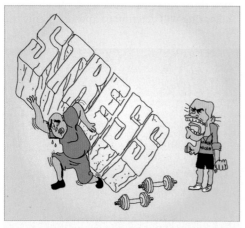

Exercise is just another form of stress. Too much or the worng type can wreak havoc with our hormones. Beasting yourself or others may not always be the most appropriate way to train for fat loss.

behaviours (mating, competing, aggression) may have lowered your chances of survival in an emergency (hence, the "fight or flight" response is dominant, courtesy of cortisol).

You must do everything in your power to be happy and focus on what's good in your life and ignore the negatives. This will have a big impact on increasing testosterone levels

- Excess intake of carbohydrates especially those that raise blood sugar rapidly create chronically elevated levels of the hormone insulin and cortisol. These two hormones oppose the action of testosterone and can diminish it's production by up to 25%, according to some research

- Men with low levels of testosterone could be at greater risk of developing diabetes, a study has suggested. Edinburgh University researchers found low testosterone levels are linked to a resistance to insulin.

- If you don't consume enough carbohydrates though your body takes this as a sign of stress and lowers your testosterone levels. So dose-response is the key, meaning lots of exercise = lots of carbs very little exercise = very little carbs.

- Cholesterol is the building block of testosterone as we now know, so it would make sense that a meat-eating, cholesterol-consuming diet would yield more of the big T than a vegetarian diet would.

- And indeed, that's what a 1985 study found when it looked at a large cross-section of omnivores and vegetarians. What was surprising was how significant the difference was: The meat-eaters actually had 36% more T than the guys who stuck to rabbit food....

- A 1989 study found pretty much the same thing: The meat-eaters ate more fat, more cholesterol, more saturated fat, and less fibre than the vegetarians and had 31% more testosterone.

- A Dutch study published in 1992 looked at changes in T levels on these two diets. A group of young male endurance athletes ate and trained on each diet for 6 weeks. (Half started on the meat-rich diet, half on the vegetarian diet; then they switched). Total testosterone declined 35% when the athletes used the vegetarian diet.

- Dutch research shows that athletes had higher testosterone levels when eating meat-based protein, compared with other sources, such as dairy and eggs. So even an ovo-lacto-vegetarian diet would not be good for T levels.

- And this shows that it is not just the fat and cholesterol in meat that raises T levels as these are found in dairy and eggs. It has something to do with meat itself.

- I can relate to this as I was a vegan for 3 years after becoming a cellular microscopist. The research that I followed, which I now realise was flawed was based on a vegan diet promoting healthy blood and an alkaline body. I followed this diet and, I can honestly say, that I had the strength levels of a pregnant goldfish and I also became fatter. Many years on, after extensive research on how to build healthy blood, I realise that you must have quality meat in your diet. Also, when you understand the hormonal system, especially steroid hormones, you realise how you need cholesterol in your diet as the precursor to all of our steroid hormones. You will find zero cholesterol in a plant based diet. This may explain why I had the sexual drive of a castrated bull.

- A study done at Penn State University showed high protein consumption to have a higher negative correlation with testosterone than any other macro-nutrient. A high protein diet stimulates enzymes in the liver to break testosterone down and eliminate it from the body, so stick to around 30–50 grams of protein per serving for optimum absorption.

Factors that can inhibit testosterone

- Zinc inhibits levels of aromatase, the testosterone to oestrogen converter and declining levels of zinc are extremely common in the western diet. Zinc is also necessary for normal pituitary function, without which the proper hormonal signals will not be sent to the testicles to stimulate the production of testosterone.

- One recent study shows that cell phone usage may lower male fertility levels. Researchers have not yet isolated an underlying cause, but a likely culprit is alterations in the brain's pituitary output, since the men had lowered levels of Leutenizing Hormone which is required for testosterone production. ScienceDaily, 19 May 2011. Web. 23 May 2011, Queen's University, "Cell phone use may reduce male fertility, Austrian-Canadian study suggests

- An Italian study analysed 3,484 Italian men who were already being treated for erectile dysfunction. They found that those who were taking statins for their cholesterol had signifi-

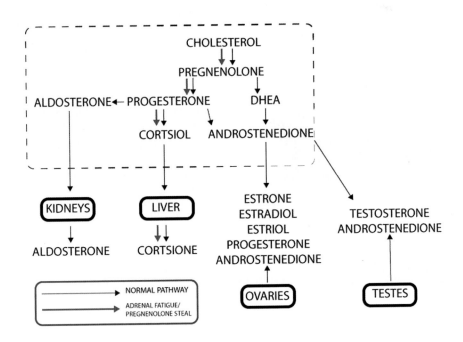

cantly lower testosterone levels than men who weren't on statins. The researchers also found an increased incidence of hypogonadism in those taking statins. Hypogonadism is a condition in which the body doesn't produce enough testosterone, which may lead to erectile dysfunction, as well as a decrease in muscle mass and body-hair growth.

- If you take statins, this isn't a reason to stop, but it is something you should be aware of. (Going cold turkey on any prescription medication without consulting with your physician is a bad idea, by the way).

- Testosterone builds and keeps heart muscle strong. In fact, there are more testosterone receptors in the heart than in any other muscle of the body! This is why low testosterone levels can be fatal to both sexes. This is another reason why you have to question all of those middle-aged men and women who are taking statins. Is it the wisest thing to do for heart health? In my opinion, it is medicine gone mad, all based on monetary gain, and not based on scientist.

- Researchers from the University of Connecticut have shown that over-trained athletes have elevated levels of sex hormone–binding globulin (SHBG, which binds testosterone, making it unavailable to the body) and reduced testosterone levels—both of which could be prevented by a well planned nutrition, training and recovery program.

Don't Over Train

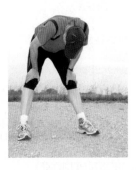

- A low testosterone person needs to be careful about their training program: study after study has shown that over-training significantly reduces testosterone levels for 1-4 days afterward! And, by the way, it doesn't matter whether it's endurance or weight training – the downward effect on testosterone levels is the same.

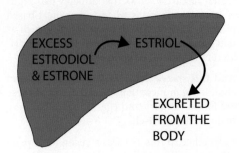

The liver converts ertodiol and estrone into estriol to be excreted from the body

- Rest and regeneration will help you increase your testosterone. If you don't, your circulating testosterone levels can plunge by as much as 40%, as was discovered by studies performed at the University of North Carolina.

- One short term study of 8 young men with an average age of 17 showed significant increases in baselines testosterone (7.5%) in only 11 weeks. This is a nice increase in testosterone when you consider that it occurred in less than three months! What did these young pups do to increase their already abundant testosterone? They simply engaged in "explosive strength training" for these 11 weeks. Eur J of Applied Physio, 2004, 91(5-6):698-707

- Are there any studies showing that this extrapolates to longer time frames? Yes! One study of nine elite weight lifters over a two year period showed significant increases in testosterone, leutenizing hormone and the ratio of testosterone to SHBG. The authors concluded that "the present results suggest that prolonged intensive strength training in elite athletes may influence the pituitary and possibly hypothalamic levels, leading to increased serum levels of testosterone". J Appl Physiol, 1988, 65:2406-2412

- Yet another study showed that elite weight lifters had significantly higher testosterone levels than elite cyclists. In other words, the body seems to adapt to the kind of exercise placed before it. In everyday language that means that weight lifting and weigh training very likely lead to increases in testosterone over time. J of Sports Sciences, 2004, 22(5):465-478

- Sports scientists often use the ratio between cortisol and testosterone as an indicator of how easily the body builds up muscle. That's why some sports scientists advise athletes to do power training early in the evening: testosterone levels may well be somewhat lower than earlier in the day, but cortisol levels are radically lower at this time of the day.

- Strength training is really a kind of hormone therapy, write researchers at the Spanish University of Extramadura in the European Journal of Applied Physiology. According to the researchers, regular weight training raises testosterone levels by forty percent.

- I will show you the best exercises for hormonal benefits and weight loss in habit 10.

DHEA: The fountain of youth

- DHEA (dehydroepiandrosterone) is one of the critical hormones that scientists are calling the "fountain of youth". This hormone is made from cholesterol by the adrenal glands and is a precursor to 18 steroid hormones including oestrogen and testosterone. Healthy DHEA production is critical for lean muscle development, fat burning, bone growth, skin health, and immunity.

- DHEA, dehydroepiandrosterone, is a naturally produced pro-hormone and is the most abundant basic building block for hormones in the human body.

- From birth men and women alike gradually produce more and more DHEA until about age 25. After age 25 we produce about 2% less per year each year. So by age 35 we make about 20% less than we did at age 25, and by age 50 we are making half as much. By age 70 most people make minimal amounts of DHEA.

- In 2009, scientists confirmed that low DHEA levels in men were linked to diabetes and coronary heart disease. DHEA powerfully modulates gene expression to shift the metabolic balance in favour of energy utilization and away from storage as fat.

- Many researchers believe that DHEA's anti obesity effects are due to its ability to block a specific enzyme called glucose-6-phosphate-dehydrogenase (G6PD). Scientists believe that DHEA, by inhibiting G6PD, actually blocks the body's ability to store and produce fat.

- High stress and poor sleeping habits also cause increased cortisol levels. When these issues become chronic they cause a phenomenon called 'pregnenolone steal. Pregnenolone is a by product of cholesterol metabolism that is

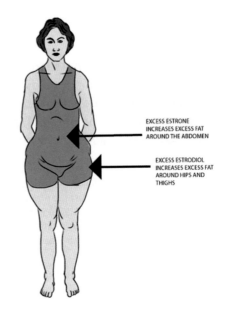

EXCESS ESTRONE INCREASES EXCESS FAT AROUND THE ABDOMEN

EXCESS ESTRODIOL INCREASES EXCESS FAT AROUND HIPS AND THIGHS

necessary to produce both cortisol and DHEA. High stress causes this process to shift towards cortisol production. This shift essentially 'steals' the necessary pregnenolone from the DHEA production pathway to produce more cortisol. This process depletes DHEA levels. This is known as the pregnenolone steal.

- When our cortisol levels are managed through stress reduction the raw materials from which our bodies manufacture our DHEA are freed up to manufacture this essential fat busting hormone. So one of the most effective ways to increase DHEA is to manage stress, I have learnt to do this after being a stress head all my life and I've seen my body fat literally dropping off once I reduced all of the stress in my life, no amount of exercise or healthy eating did that for me.

- High sugar and carbohydrate consumption increases blood sugar and insulin levels. Elevated insulin causes a decreased production of DHEA in the adrenals. Blood sugar imbalances also create critical vitamin and mineral imbalances that stress the adrenals and reduce DHEA production. Alcohol and caffeine consumption also decrease DHEA levels.

- Many people rush out and look for DHEA boosting supplements; however, lifestyle factors that deplete DHEA levels should be addressed first. The most important factor includes reducing/eliminating adrenal stressors such as stress, leaky gut syndrome, parasites and other infectious agents, chronic inflammation, physical stress, nutrient deficiencies, poor sleep, & blood sugar imbalances.

Eliminate/reduce caffeine from your diet. It's the quickest way to reduce cortisol production and elevate the production of DHEA, the leading anabolic youth hormone.

- 200 mg of caffeine (one 12 oz mug of coffee) has been shown to increase blood cortisol levels by up to 30% in one hour! Cortisol can remain elevated for up to 18 hours in the blood. This is the easiest step to decrease your catabolic metabolism and increase your anabolic metabolism.

- If you do need coffee in your life, I suggest that, you either go for a brisk walk after or some form of exercise as this will help reduce the subsequent increase in stress hormones.

- When I was head of S&C at numerous rugby clubs, I banned all of the players from coffee/caffeine products before games. Why? Because my research had led me to believe that excess caffeine over-excites the brain and, during crucial decision-making moments, you are more likely to make mistakes. Another observation was that, when you are consuming too much caffeine, you are of the false belief that you are doing more work than you really are.

- Trust me, for a number of years before this, I had used a number of drinks that contained caffeine, and other stimulants. I found that it always affected the players' ability to sleep that night after the game. Over a long season, this led to huge problems with poor sleep and so inadequate rest.

- An anti-inflammatory diet is a critical part to de-stressing the body and boosting DHEA levels. This diet should be very low in sugar and very rich in phytonutrients (chemical compounds found mostly in coloured fruits and vegetables) and trace minerals from fresh, raw or lightly steamed vegetables. Powerful anti-inflammatory herbs such as tumeric, ginger, rosemary, thyme, oregano, & cinnamon should be generously consumed on a regular basis.

- Healthy fat consumption is an essential part of creating cholesterol which is needed to produce DHEA. Healthy fat sources include coconut products, avocados, olive oil, nuts, seeds, & purified omega-3 fish oil supplements. Healthy protein sources to boost DHEA production include wild-caught fish, grass-fed red meat, liver and free range chicken, turkey, and organic eggs.

- Other lifestyle factors that are critical for healthy DHEA levels include regular sun exposure and/or supplementation to maintain vitamin D (25-OH) levels between 70-100 ng/ml.

- Meditation is often used as an antidote to stress and has been found to increase DHEA levels. In fact, in a meditation study, a group of 45 year old males who regularly meditated were found to have 23% more DHEA than a smaller group who didn't meditate. In women, the meditators had 47% more DHEA. Another scientific study found that for every 20% increase in DHEA, there was a 48% drop in heart disease and a 36% drop in death from any cause.

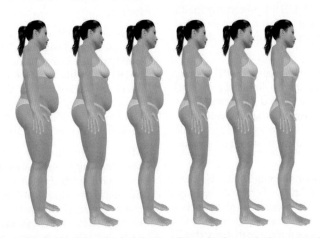

Female hormones play a huge role in female's ability to lose body fat. You will struggle to lose weight if you cannot play the hormone game!

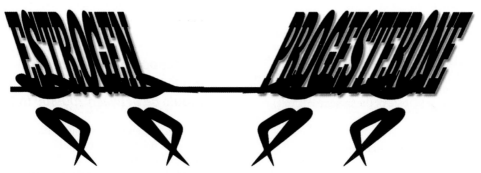

Estrogen and progesterone are antagonistic in many of their actions

Female Hormones

- The two primary female hormones secreted by the ovaries are oestrogen and progesterone. The properties of one offsets the other and together they are maintained in optimal balance in our body at all times. Too much of one hormone or the other can lead to significant medical problems.

- Oestrogen is produced in the ovaries. It regulates the menstrual cycle, promotes cell division and is largely responsible for the development of secondary female characteristics during puberty, including the growth and development of the breast and pubic hair.

- Men produce some level of oestrogen, though on a much smaller scale than women. In men, small levels of oestrogen are produced in the testes, but can also be produced in the liver, adrenal glands and fat cells. It has been shown that excess fat can lead to raised oestrogen levels in men.

- When oestrogen levels start to get high in men, health problems start to arise. Elevated oestrogen levels in men have been shown to contribute to prostate cancer, heart disease, and gynecomastia (man boobs). Since high levels of oestrogen are typically accompanied by lower levels of testosterone levels in men, other changes also occur including; loss of muscle mass, fatigue, depression, low libido and erectile dysfunction.

- Excessive oestrogen in men raises body fat and can contribute to a host of other problems.

- Aromatase is the enzyme that is responsible for converting testosterone into oestrogen and is found most prominently in fat cells. This is the link; the more body fat a man (and a woman)

has, the more aromatase, and therefore oestrogen, they are likely to have.

- What Exactly is Oestrogen?

- Oestrogen is a naturally occurring human hormone. In fact, it is not a single hormone, but a collective name for several variants. Estrodiol is the most potent, with estrone and estriol, its much weaker sisters. In healthy young women, the typical mix approximates 15/15/70% respectively. This is the combination worked out by Mother Nature as optimum for human females.

- Estradiol is produced by the ovaries, and promotes fat storage around the hips and the thighs.

- Estrone is produced by fat cells from the conversion of male hormones (androgens). This type of oestrogen promotes the storage of fat around the middle.

- Estriol is a weak form of oestrogen, the liver converts estradiol and estrone into estriol to be excreted from the body.

- Oestrogen and progesterone work in synchronization with each other as checks and balances to achieve hormonal harmony in both sexes.

- Oestrogen is a pro-growth hormone. Since too much of anything is generally not good, the body has another hormone to offset and counterbalance the effects of oestrogen. It is called progesterone.

- Progesterone, as its name implies, is a pro-gestation hormone. In other words, it favours the growth and well-being of the foetus. Without a proper amount of progesterone, there can be no successful pregnancy. It protects us against the "growth effect" of oestrogen.

- Progesterone is made from pregnenolone, which in turn comes from cholesterol. Production occurs at several places. In women, it is primarily made in the ovaries, just before ovulation, and increasing rapidly after ovulation. It is also made in the adrenal glands in both sexes and in the testes in males. In women, its level is highest during the luteal period (especially from day 19 to 22 of the menstrual cycle).

Functions of Progesterone

- Progesterone acts primarily as an antagonist (opposite) to oestrogen in our body. For example, oestrogen can cause breast cysts while progesterone protects against breast cysts.

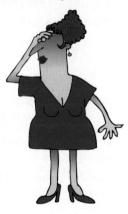

- When the hormonal balance between oestrogen and progesterone is off, the following symptoms of such imbalance include: hot flashes, vaginal dryness, water retention, weight gain, insomnia, mood swings, short-term memory loss, wrinkly skin and osteoporosis.

- It is not the absolute deficiency of oestrogen or progesterone but rather, the relative dominance of oestrogen and relative deficiency of progesterone that is the main cause of health problems when they are off balance.

- From age 35 to 50, there is a 75% reduction in production of progesterone in the body. Oestrogen, during the same period, only declines about 35%.

- Stress causes adrenal gland exhaustion as well as reduced progesterone output. This tilts the oestrogen to progesterone ratios in favour of oestrogen. Excessive oestrogen in turn causes insomnia and anxiety, which further taxes the adrenal glands. This leads to a further reduction in progesterone output and even more oestrogen dominance. After a few years in this type of vicious cycle, the adrenal glands become exhausted. This dysfunction leads to blood sugar imbalance, hormonal imbalances, and chronic fatigue.

- According to the late Dr. John Lee, the world's authority on natural hormone therapy, the key to hormonal balance is the modulation of progesterone to oestrogen ratio.

For optimum health, the progesterone to oestrogen ratio should be between 200-300 to 1

- Vitamin C comes to the rescue for low progesterone and it has been clinically proven to be effective. At doses of 750 mg/day, vitamin C has been shown to raise progesterone. In a randomized trial, women were randomly assigned to receive either vitamin C or a placebo. Within three menstrual cycles, the group receiving vitamin C saw progesterone levels increase on average from 8–13 ng/ml. The goal with progesterone is to get your levels between 10–25 ng/ml.

- Also, drop the coffee if you want to raise your progesterone levels. Why? Caffeine increases cortisol and high cortisol can block progesterone receptors, a number of studies have linked caffeine with PMS symptoms.

- What is so bad about oestrogen dominance? It is the root cause of a myriad of illnesses. Conditions associated with this include fibrocystic breast disease, PMS, uterine fibroids, breast cancer, endometriosis, infertility problems, endometrial polyps, PCOS, auto-immune disorders, low blood sugar problems, and menstrual pain, among many others.

- High oestrogen relative to normal progesterone is a combination that is common in overweight women, and in women who have been exposed to xenoestrogens. Ovaries are the main source of oestrogen in females, but unfortunately fat cells also make oestrogen, as we have already discussed.

- According to the research, women who gain more than 20lbs from age 18 to mid-life double their risk of post-menopausal breast cancer. That's only a few pounds per year! Oestrogen is 50-100 times greater in overweight menopausal women than in lean women, because as we now know fat cells produce oestrogen, and that probably accounts for the greater risk in breast cancer associated with being overweight.

- Birth control pills lower free thyroid hormones and testosterone. Birth control pills increase thyroglobulin, a protein that binds thyroid hormone. If you are on thyroid medication, you may need to adjust your dose accordingly. Additionally, birth control pills raise sex hormone binding globulin, a protein that binds free testosterone and may make it biologically inert. Let me point out though that if you are considering coming off the contraceptive pill then you should discuss this with a qualified medical professional.

Oral

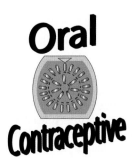

Contraceptive

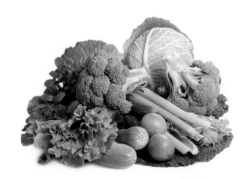

- A report, from the Universities of Southern California and Hawaii, published in the British Journal of Cancer, states that eating grapefruit can increase the risk of breast cancer by nearly a third. The fruit is believed to boost blood levels of oestrogen, the hormone associated with increased risk of the illness. The researchers claim that post-menopausal women who eat as little as one quarter of a grapefruit per day (or juice equivalent) could see their chances increase by 30%.

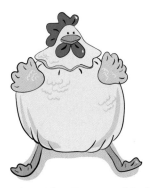

According to a 1976 article in Environmental Quality and Safety, some steroids were so good at increasing levels of body fat that when estrogens were given to broiler chickens, they caused such an increase in body fat that the practice had to be stopped. The levels of fat in the hen's bodies jeopardized their lives.

- Caffeine intake from all sources is linked with higher oestrogen levels regardless of age, body mass index (BMI), caloric intake, smoking, alcohol, and cholesterol intake. Studies have shown that women who consumed at least 500 milligrams of caffeine daily, the equivalent of four or five cups of coffee, had nearly 70% more oestrogen during the early follicular phase (days 1 to 5 of their menstrual cycle) than women who consume no more than 100 mg of caffeine daily, or less than one cup of coffee.

Foods from the brassica family (e.g. broccoli, cauliflower, spinach) help the liver enzymes detoxify excess oestrogen.

- Researchers have found that certain flavnoids such as green tea polyphenols and quercetin, found in onion and garlic, have shown anti-oestrogenic activity.

- Research has concluded that tumeric could be used to inhibit the oestrogenic effects of pesticides and environmental xenoestrogens. Tumeric has also been shown to counter the proliferative effect on oestrogen on cancer cells.

- It is known that the ovaries concentrate a large amount of iodine. After the thyroid, the ovaries have the second largest concentration of iodine in the body. Iodine deficiency produces changes in the ovarian production of oestrogens as well as changes in the oestrogen receptors of the breasts.

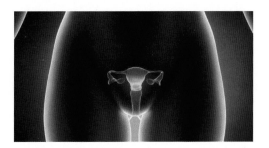

- In an iodine deficient state, research has shown that ovarian oestrogen production increases, while oestrogen receptors in the breast increase their sensitivity to oestrogens. Both of these conditions can increase the risk of developing pathology of the breasts, including breast cancer.

- Iodine affects oestrogen metabolism, reported to transform estrone and estradiol into estriol

- Several varieties of fruits and vegetables have Calcium D-glucarate. This is a botanical extract found in high levels in apples, oranges, broccoli, and brussel sprouts. This extract allows the body to excrete hormones such as oestrogen before they can become reabsorbed.

Conclusion

- Wow! I bet you didn't realise how important cholesterol was in providing the raw materials for all your steroid hormones, which you now understand includes your sex hormones. The key here is to eat high quality proteins, good fats and low glycaemic carbohydrates to optimise your steroid hormone balance. When it comes to stress this must be controlled at all times otherwise your cortisol levels are always going to be high and that is a disaster for your health and body fat levels. When you are stressed always remember Buffalo Bill's story from Habit 3 - that for me always put things into perspective.

- If you want to learn more about these topics then I suggest that you start with the following books;

  - "The Testosterone Revolution" - Malcolm Carruthers
  - "The Secret Life of Your Cells" - Whitford Press
  - "Revitalize Your Hormones" - Theresa Dale
  - "The Anti-Estrogen Diet" - Ori Hofmekler
  - "Oestrogen - the killer in our midst" - Chris Woolliams
  - "The Cortisol Connection" - Shawn Talbott
  - "Overcoming Adrenal Fatigue" - Kathryn Simpson
  - "Super T" - Karlis Ullis
  - "The Testosterone Edge" - Brian O'Neill
  - "The Complete Doctor's Stress Solution" - Penny Kendall-Reed & Dr. Stephen Reed
  - "The Great Cholesterol Myth" - Jonny Bowden & Stephan Sinatra

HABIT 7

THE AWESOME FOURSOME:
Growth Hormone, Insulin, Sunshine & Sleep

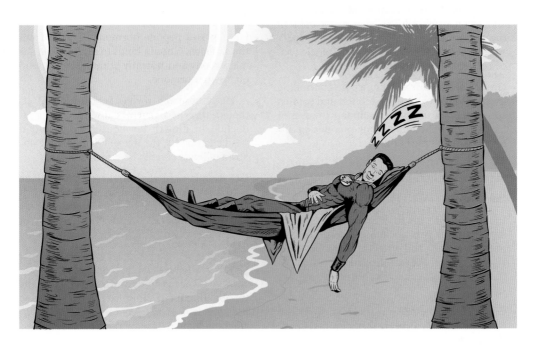

"Phil Richards, in my opinion, pioneered Performance Nutrition in Rugby. His influence on sports nutrition can now be seen across a broad range of sports. If anyone is serious about developing as a nutritionist they need to spend time with Phil Richards."

John Dams
Head of Strength & Conditioning, Harlequins rugby

- Growth hormone, insulin, sunshine & sleep are 4 major players in your ability to lose fat and keep it off for good. That's why I call them the awesome foursome for fat loss. Get it right and the excess fat will literally drop off you, get it wrong and it will pile up on you - the choice is yours. So lets look how to get the awesome foursome on our side, starting with growth hormone.

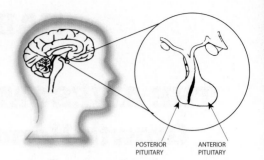

Growth Hormone is synthesised and secreted in the anterior pituitary gland

Growth Hormone

- Growth hormone is a protein hormone made up of about 190 amino acids that is synthesized and secreted by cells called somatotrophs in the anterior pituitary. It is a major participant in control of several complex physiologic processes, including growth and metabolism.

- Growth hormone is well known for controlling longitudinal growth in childhood and is often considered an anabolic hormone. However, it has both anabolic and catabolic actions on different tissues in the body

- For example, GH stimulates protein synthesis in muscle but in fat tissue it promotes lipolysis (breakdown).

- Production of growth hormone is modulated by many factors, including stress, exercise, nutrition, sleep and growth hormone itself. However, its primary controllers are two hypothalamic hormones and one hormone from the stomach.

- Growth hormone-releasing hormone (GHRH) is a hypothalamic peptide that stimulates both the synthesis and secretion of growth hormone.

- Somatostatin (SS) is a peptide produced by several tissues in the body, including the hypothalamus. Somatostatin inhibits growth hormone release in response to GHRH and

to other stimulatory factors such as low blood glucose concentration.

- Ghrelin is a peptide hormone secreted from the stomach. Ghrelin binds to receptors on somatotrophs and potently stimulates secretion of growth hormone.

- A recent research review concluded that although there is a general consensus that a reduction in growth hormone (GH) secretion results in obesity, the role of GH in the metabolism of lipids is yet to be fully understood.

- GH stimulates lipolysis and seems to regulate lipid deposition in adipose tissue. Patients with GH deficiency (GHD) have enlarged fat depots due to higher fat cell volume. The treatment of these patients with GH results in a loss of body fat.

- However, whereas GH replacement in patients with GHD leads to specific depletion of intra-abdominal fat, administering GH to obese individuals does not seem to result in a consistent reduction or redistribution of body fat.

In obese individuals the GH secretory response to a variety of stimuli (e.g. insulin, sleep, exercise...) is impaired compared to normal individuals.

- It has been reported that for every increase in 1 unit of BMI, GH secretion is reduced by 6%. The mechanism behind this is largely unknown. This is reversible though with weight loss

Physiologic Effects of Growth Hormone

- A critical concept in understanding growth hormone activity is that it has two distinct types of effects:

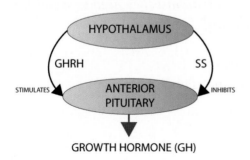

- Direct effects are the result of growth hormone binding its receptor on target cells. Fat cells (adipocytes), for example, have growth hormone receptors, and growth hormone stimulates them to break down triglyceride and supresses their ability to take up and accumulate circulating lipids.
- Indirect effects are mediated primarily by a insulin-like growth factor-I (IGF-I), a hormone that is secreted from the liver and other tissues in response to growth hormone. A majority of the growth promoting effects of growth hormone is actually due to IGF-I acting on its target cells.

- Metabolic Effects: Growth hormone has important effects on protein, lipid and carbohydrate metabolism.

  - Protein metabolism: In general, growth hormone stimulates protein anabolism in many tissues. This effect reflects increased amino acid uptake, increased protein synthesis and decreased oxidation of proteins.
  - Fat metabolism: Growth hormone enhances the utilization of fat by stimulating triglyceride breakdown and oxidation in adipocytes.
  - Carbohydrate metabolism: Growth hormone is one of a battery of hormones that serves to maintain blood glucose within a normal range. Growth hormone is often said to have anti-insulin activity, because it supresses the abilities of insulin to stimulate uptake of glucose in peripheral tissues and enhance glucose synthesis in the liver. Somewhat paradoxically, administration of growth hormone stimulates insulin secretion, leading to hyperinsulinemia.

- The secretion of Growth Hormone decreases by 10 – 15% in each decade of life, but the body can still make large amounts of GH as we age; we have just got to know how to optimise growth hormone naturally so we can stay lean & healthy.
- Growth Hormone Releasing Hormone (GHRH), is produced by the Hypothalamus and induces the Anterior Pituitary to release Growth Hormone.

- Releasing growth hormone: To promote anabolism, first you have to increase output of growth hormone from the anterior lobe of the pituitary gland.
- The four most effective ways to increase growth hormone naturally is high quality sleep, intense physical exercise, control blood sugar and use certain amino acids like arginine and glutamine to help increase growth hormone. This can all be achieved quite easily with a bit of discipline and a real focus to decrease body fat.
- Growth hormone is released into the blood stream in bursts. Some of each burst goes directly to bone and muscle cells where it initiates growth.
- The rest is neutralized by the liver within 60–90 minutes. Before it is neutralized, the growth hormone causes the liver to manufacture somatomedins also called insulin like growth factor (IGF).
- IGF is made by the liver and is triggered by growth hormone. When the liver is damaged or overworked, through our enormously toxic environments, then this potent anabolic hormone decreases.
- Also, if you happen to suffer from fat stores concentrated centrally around abdominal region, growth hormone (GH) secretion will be even more impaired. Fortunately, research indicates that declining GH due to body fat gain is partially reversible with fat loss. So, lose fat to regain your growth hormone benefits.
- As we now know, excess cortisol from stress stimulates the formation of excess fat in the abdominal area. Growth hormone and leptin have a see-saw effect; when leptin levels are high, growth hormone levels are low. Thus, leptin and growth hormone have an ebb and flow relationship, leptin's main effect on growth hormone is to restrict it. Once growth hormone is lacking, there is no metabolic factor to help reduce abdominal fat, and it will keep accumulating as part of leptin and insulin resistance.
- During fasting growth hormone levels rise, but this is not because the brain is stimulating growth hormone production, rather in a fasting state the hunger hormone ghrelin promotes extra growth hormone production. Ghrelin acts to stimulate growth hormone and it loses its effectiveness in overweight individuals. It does this because leptin is too high as soon

as leptin levels come down, ghrelin levels goes back into natural balance. This information means we can restore natural growth hormone function by lowering leptin and getting it back into natural balance.

The Fat Burning Benefits of Ghrelin And the Relationship With Growth Hormone

- Your stomach secretes ghrelin when it's empty, signaling the hypothalamus to turn on your appetite. As a society, we've come to fear hunger and avoid it like the plague. As soon as we feel hungry, we look for ways to satisfy our desire for food.

- But what if you could make friends with hunger and actually learn to enjoy the feeling?

- There are benefits to prolonging eating and staying hungry for a while. You see, ghrelin is a potent stimulator of growth hormone, and growth hormone has profound effect on fat burning and building lean muscle. It is often considered an anti-aging hormone.

- So the next time you get hungry, remember that the longer you hold out (within reason) the more you rev up your fat-burning furnace

Growth Hormone and Protein

- Next to be considered is the relationship of GH to protein intake. GH is released after the consumption of protein. This might signify to the body that it is now an opportune moment to build.

- Moreover, hormonally, protein intake is positively correlated with growth hormone, IGF-1, and glucagons. These hormones collectively,

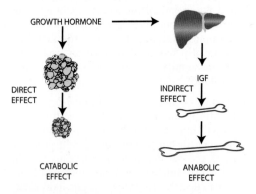

Growth hormone can have both direct and indirect, as well as anabolic and catabolic effects, in the body

exert an anabolic and lipolytic effect (fat burning).

- Increased protein intake will increase GH levels, and increased GH levels will increase the need for protein. Moreover, frequent protein feedings will increase absorption of protein and produce frequent GH spikes.

- So an ideal GH raising diet would include frequent feedings of high quality protein from animal sources (grass fed meat and wild fish). REMEMBER YOU CAN'T ABSORB MORE THAN 30–50 GRAMS OF PROTEIN PER SERVING. Otherwise if you try to eat a cow, at each meal, the excess will be converted in to fat and the excess acid will lower your pH levels.

Growth Hormone and Blood Sugar

- The most important point in regards to growth hormone (GH) and diet is that growth hormone levels increase significantly when insulin levels are low. Glucose inhibits the secretion of growth hormone by acting on specific areas of the hypothalamus.

- Consequently, during the day, when food is consumed periodically, growth hormone secretion by the pituitary is suppressed, and insulin release by the pancreas is increased. What this means is, consuming foods constantly throughout the day will limit growth hormone's fat burning effect and increase insulin's fat storage effect. So, when it comes to growth hormone, you want low insulin.

- However, we need insulin to promote the benefits of growth hormone. Studies show that GH fails to cause growth in Diabetics and it also fails if carbohydrates are restricted from the diet.

- The reason for this could be that a strict low carbohydrate diet would lead to chronically low insulin levels, and insulin is needed to drive amino acids into the muscle cells.

- Moreover, IGF-1 is produced in the body through the combined actions of GH and insulin. And IGF-1 is at least as powerful an anabolic agent as either of its parents. But a low carbohydrate diet would lead to a reduction in IGF-1 levels.

- So a low carb diet is not the answer either. In fact, this relationship of insulin, growth hormone, and IGF-1 is one reason why those following a low carbohydrate diet also often plateau after a period of time. The key word here is TIMING. Time your carbohydrates to enhance insulin's effect on growth hormone by producing IGF-1 to ensure it gets transported from the liver to the tissues to do its magic of burning fat and building muscle. The most beneficial time for this is your pre, during & post workout meal and breakfast. We cover this in great detail in habit 9.

- There is also a relationship with thyroid hormone here as well. Raising GH has a profound effect on normalizing thyroid function.

- Studies show that diets that continuously restrict carbohydrate cause a reduction in T3, and that administering carbohydrate can restore T3 levels after they have declined. This reduction in T3 is another reason people will often plateau on low carb diets.

- So, some carbohydrates must be included in any diet, but not an excessive amount, if the aim is to enhance growth hormone. And the focus would be on the timing of eating the carbohydrates. The best time to consume carbohydrates is after exercise and with breakfast I cover this in habit 9, nutrient timing.

Growth Hormone, Potassium & Sodium's relationship.

- The next dietary nutrient to be looked at is potassium. Medical science has known for some time that even modest potassium deficiency causes growth hormone and IGF-1 suppression.

- The reason for this is related to cellular hydration, which is more complex than simply guzzling water for hydration.

- Fluid is constantly moving in and out of the cell across an electrical gradient bisected by the cell membrane. The key to obtaining the positive benefits of "cell volumization" is to maximize intracellular fluid.

- Water moves in and out of cells with electrolytes. The mineral sodium is the chief extracellular (outside) electrolyte, whereas the mineral potassium is the chief intracellular (inside) electrolyte.

- By increasing your potassium intake and reducing your sodium intake, you can shift water from the extracellular compartments of your body into the intracellular compartments.

- An increased intracellular hydration increases HGH release. And historically, human beings consumed far more potassium than sodium.

- The reason for a change in the potassium to sodium ration is two fold. First, the best source by far for potassium is vegetables, and second fruit. But there has been a trend towards consuming less fruit and veggies than historically were eaten.

- Researchers at the University of Aarhus in Denmark shows that growth inhibition occurs only after a few days of reduced potassium intake - long before there is any significant decline in muscle potassium.

- Potassium deficiency causes profound inhibition of growth because potassium deficiency is required for the development of muscle cells themselves.

- When serum levels of potassium decline, as they almost do immediately on a potassium deficient diet, it is likely that this decline signals your brain to reduce growth hormone output and slow down muscle growth and recovery.

- That way your body avoids forming defective muscle cells because of an inadequate potassium supply.

- Research has also established that activation of the growth hormone releasing hormone, somatocrinin, requires another enzyme called alpha – amidating monooxygenase, which is absolutely limited by the amount of vitamin C available for use as a co-factor. So you better have plenty of vitamin C around if you want to maximize growth hormone output.

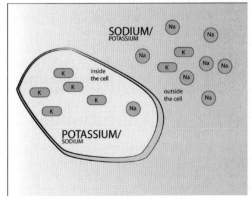

There is naturally more potassium than sodium in the cell. By increasing your potassium intake, and lowering your sodium intake, then you can shift fluid into the cell

Bedtime Growth Hormone Release

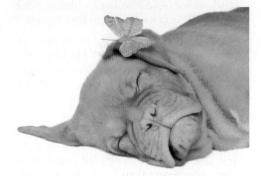

- It is well documented that inadequate sleep, irregular sleeping patterns, and poor quality sleep can substantially inhibit GH secretion. To optimize sleep keep to a regular bedtime and wake up time; do not consume alcohol or caffeine 4-6 hours before bedtime; and keep excess light and noise out of the bedroom.

- There are two times when the release of growth hormone is the greatest. First, the largest burst of GH is released during the early hours of sleep-hence our eating habits are crucial to maximizing this night time secretion

- More specifically, growth hormone is especially dependent on sleep, because a major growth hormone surge occurs during the first episode of slow-wave sleep, approximately 30-70 minutes after falling asleep.

- Sleep is a prime fat burning time especially when one has not eaten after 6 p.m.

- The fastest way to disrupt sleep is to eat after your evening meal, later than 6 P.M., eat too large a dinner, or eat your last meal too late. This forces the body to digest food when it should be performing other functions such as fat burning and body repair. Also, leptin resistance sets in, it causes higher amounts of adrenaline during sleep hours. This causes insomnia, light sleep, restless sleep and a general feeling of unrest. Put alcohol on top of late night eating and from a fat loss perspective it is a disaster. So if you want to drop the fat, drop late night eating and the booze and this in itself will be a massive step in the right direction.

- Ideally, you should be slightly hungry and tired before bed time and resist the urge to attack the fridge and eat it's contents. Avoid emotional stress before bed and this includes watching the doom and gloom of the news. Watch things that make you laugh, don't get into arguments or deep emotional discussions as this will simply put you in fight or flight mode and not into sleep mode.

Here are simple strategies to maximize your melatonin secretion:

1. Go to Sleep Early: Hormone secretion, body temperature, digestion and tissue restoration are governed by 24 hour cycles linked to natural light exposure. Up to 80% of human growth hormone secretion takes place between the hours of 11pm and 1am. Individuals that are in bed by 10pm are maximizing this restorative hormone's ability to heal and regenerate body tissues.

2. Practice intentional quiet time before you go to bed: Utilizing present moment mindfulness or meditation helps boost melatonin. This process speeds up the time from lying down to falling asleep and boosts the quality and satisfaction of the sleep. Take 15-20 minutes before bed and relax your mind and concentrate your breathing.

3. Reduce sugar, artificial flavorings & preservatives, processed foods, alcohol, caffeine and any other sort of stimulant. These reduce melatonin and growth hormone secretion in the body.

4. Hydrate effectively: Dehydration causes chronic stress responses in the body that minimize healthy melatonin and growth hormone secretion.

5. Keep Your Room Dark: Any sort of light stimulation will inhibit the pineal gland from forming melatonin. This will disrupt sleep and minimize melatonin's beneficial effects in the body.

- Melatonin is an important hormone that is released during sleep as well as growth hormone. It must peak at the proper time in order to ensure adequate deep sleep. Melatonin levels decline with age and melatonin released correctly during the night is essential for proper leptin rythym during the day. When melatonin is released incorrectly, leptin is thrown out of balance. It has been shown that supplementing with melatonin can restore normal leptin levels. An animal study showed that melatonin prevents accumulation of stomach fat and lowers leptin, independence of diet. Melatonin improves diabetes in animal studies by eliminating insulin resistance. You cannot buy melatonin supplements in the UK, so we will look at increasing melatonin levels naturally.

First Of All, What Is Melatonin?

- Melatonin is a hormone that is produced from the amino acid tryptophan in minute quantities by the pineal gland when the eyes detect no light (i.e., in darkness or blindness, or during sleep). Melatonin also is produced by the retina and, in vastly greater amounts, by the gastrointestinal system. Light at night, regardless of duration or intensity, inhibits melatonin secretion and phase-shifts the circadian clock, possibly altering the cell growth rate that is regulated by the circadian rhythm. Use black out blinds in your bedroom to increase melatonin production.

- High melatonin concentrations are found in seeds and some fruits such as bananas and tomatoes. Melatonin also is found in food sources such as oats, rice bran, sweet corn, wheatgrass juice, and ginger. The building blocks for natural melatonin production in the body include sufficient amounts of vitamin B6, vitamin B3 (niacinamide), and most important, the amino acid tryptophan, which is found in high quantities in foods such as nuts, seeds, spirulina, beans, and tofu and a product that I have developed called Amino Relax.

Eating before bed

- Plan your last meal of the day carefully. Your last meal of the day is the most important for maintaining a robust GH/IGF-1 axis.

- A medium-protein, low-carbohydrate meal 3-4 hours before bed helps minimize insulin release and allows for maximum endogenous GH secretion.

- Consumption of carbohydrates at bedtime can blunt this crucial release of growth hormone. And the greater the amount of carbs and the higher the glycemic rating of the carbs, the greater will be the increase in blood sugar and the greater the suppression of growth hormone.

- Thus going to bed with a belly-full of carbohydrates is hormonally unwise and may diminish, if not nullify, nocturnal growth hormone release.

- In order to benefit from the night time release of HGH, it is important for you to sleep normally. However, alcohol-induced sleep is not normal. Unlike other hormones, HGH is tied to human circadian rhythms. When alcohol is consumed 1-6 hours before bedtime, it has a disruptive effect on the second-half of sleep. Alcohol can suppress the release of HGH during sleep, and decrease, or eliminate the benefits of the HGH.

How Important is Sleep?

- The longest recorded period that a person has gone without eating is over 40 days. Most people can survive around 3 weeks without food. When it comes to sleep, the longest recorded period a person gone without sleep is just 11 days before death occurred. However, after just 2 days without sleep, concentration levels will be extremely poor and after 4 days, hallucinations occur.

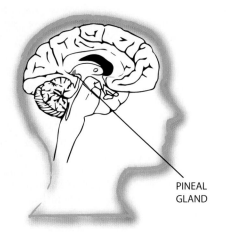

PINEAL
GLAND

Melatonin is produced in the pineal gland when no light is detected by the eyes.

- From this, it seems to make no sense that more attention is often focused on what goes in our mouth than how many hours snooze we get each night

- There are many, many studies showing that sleep deprivation can lead to overeating. In one of them, 26 healthy, normal-weight men and women participated in which they spent either 4 h/night (restricted sleep) or 9 h/night (habitual sleep) in bed. Each phase lasted 6 d, and functional magnetic resonance imaging was performed in the fasted state on day 6.

- Overall neuronal activity in response to food stimuli was greater after restricted sleep than after habitual sleep. In addition, a relative increase in brain activity in areas associated with reward, including the putamen, nucleus accumbens, thalamus, insula, and prefrontal cortex in response to food stimuli, was observed.

- The findings of this study link restricted sleep and susceptibility to food stimuli and are consistent with the notion that reduced sleep may lead to greater propensity to overeat.

St-Onge MP, McReynolds A, Trivedi ZB, Roberts AL, Sy M, Hirsch J. Sleep restriction leads to increased activation of brain regions sensitive to food stimuli. Am J Clin Nutr (2012)

In humans, sleep deprivation has been associated with higher ghrelin levels, increased hunger and higher BMI.

- Even a single night of sleep deprivation appears sufficient to increase ghrelin (an appetite stimulating hormone) and hunger.

- Spiegel et al. found that restricting sleep vincreased ghrelin as well as hunger and appetite, especially for calorie-dense, high- carbohydrate foods.

- Studies have also repeatedly shown that sleep deprivation is strongly correlated with decreased insulin sensitivity and unwanted weight gain.

- One study has shown that one week of sleep deprivation (5 hours sleep a night) can significantly reduce insulin sensitivity

Buxton OM, Pavlova M, Reid EW, Wang W, Simonson DC, Adler GK. Sleep restriction for 1 week reduces insulin sensitivity in healthy men. Diabetes. 2010;59(9):2126-33

- One study even found that insulin sensitivity was reduced after only 1 night of partial sleep

Donga E, van Dijk M, van Dijk JG, Biermasz NR, Lammers GJ, van Kralingen KW, Corssmit EP, Romijn JA. A single night of partial sleep deprivation induces insulin resistance in multiple metabolic pathways in healthy subjects. deprivation. J Clin Endocrinol Metab. 2010 Jun;95(6):2963-8

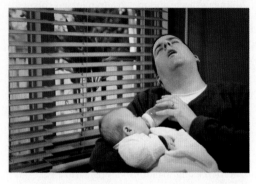

Just one night of sleep deprivation can have detrimental effects on many hormones.

Animal and human studies have shown that just 4 hours sleep for 1 night leads to a reduction in testosterone and growth hormone and increases cortisol levels.

- A research team from Chicago University compared normal sleepers (7.5-8.5 hours per night) to short sleepers (around 6.5 hours per night). They found that those with less sleep secreted 50% more insulin and were 40% less sensitive compared to the group of longer sleepers.

- Before the invention of electric light in 1879, it was estimated that the majority of people got around 10 hours sleep a night. However, since then average nightly sleep time has been reduced by 20% to around 8 hours a night

- One of the reasons for this may be the effect light has on melatonin. When the sun goes down and darkness occurs, the pineal gland is "turned on" begins to actively produce melatonin, which is released into the blood and you begin to feel less alert. Melatonin levels in the blood stay elevated for about 12 hours - all through the night - before the light of a new day when they fall back to low daytime levels by about 9 am. Daytime levels of melatonin are barely detectable.

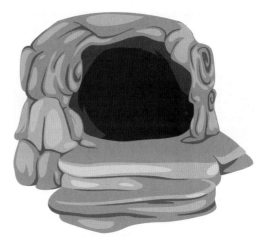

Your bedroom need to be like a cave - dark and quiet - in order to get a good nights sleep.

melatonin suppression. This means that products such as tablets, smartphones, and other devices with self-luminous electronic displays are major sources for suppressing melatonin at night, thereby reducing sleep duration and disrupting sleep.

Sleep deprivation and exercise

- In a 2013 study, 30 healthy football players performed 4 interval sprints on a treadmill at 8am after both a regular night's sleep and a restricted night's sleep. Blood samples showed that plasma concentrations of IL-6 and TNF-α were higher after restricted sleep both during the exercise (i.e., the first and the fourth run) and remained elevated during the recovery period (i.e., 60 min after the exercise). These results showed that sleep restriction increases the pro-inflammatory effect of exercise.

- Bright light directly inhibits the release of melatonin. Even if the pineal gland is switched "on" late in the evening, it will not produce melatonin unless the person is in a dimly lit environment. In addition to sunlight, artificial indoor lighting can be bright enough to prevent the release of melatonin

- It is well established that short-wavelength or "blue" light is the most melatonin-suppressive; this is the type of light typically emitted by devices such as televisions, computer screens, and mobile phones. To produce white light, these electronic devices must emit light at short wavelengths, close to the peak sensitivity of

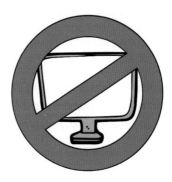

If you are looking for a good nights rest then you need to ensure that you switch off the T.V. or computer at least one hour before you hit the pillow

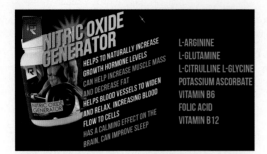

NITRIC OXIDE GENERATOR

HELPS TO NATURALLY INCREASE GROWTH HORMONE LEVELS

CAN HELP INCREASE MUSCLE MASS AND DECREASE FAT

HELPS BLOOD VESSELS TO WIDEN AND RELAX. INCREASING BLOOD FLOW TO CELLS

HAS A CALMING EFFECT ON THE BRAIN. CAN IMPROVE SLEEP

L-ARGININE
L-GLUTAMINE
L-CITRULLINE L-GLYCINE
POTASSIUM ASCORBATE
VITAMIN B6
FOLIC ACID
VITAMIN B12

- A 2005 study looked at how supplementation of arginine can effect Growth Hormone concentrations. The study found that 5g and 9g of supplemental arginine significantly increased GH levels. This rise occurred after 30 minutes and peaked after 60 minutes. 9g supplementation was found to be optimal. Other studies have also noted that supplementing with >9g/day can cause gastrointestinal discomfort and diarrhea

- Although be aware that not everyone is classed as a responder and will not see as much of a benefit as others.   Growth   hormone responses to varying doses of oral arginine, Growth Hormone & IGF Research, Volume 15, Issue 2, Pages 136-139   Scott R. Collier, Darren P. Casey, Jill A. Kanaley

- For the millions of sleepless among us, there may be good news—in the form of an inexpensive, naturally occurring amino acid known as glycine. Within the central nervous system, glycine functions as an inhibitory neurotransmitter, playing a well-documented and critical role in initiating normal patterns of REM sleep. Now, a new study of chronic insomniacs demonstrates that glycine administered orally just prior to bedtime significantly improves sleep quality, shortening the latency between sleep onset and initiation of slow-wave (deep) sleep as measured by polysomnography. Volunteers also reported less daytime sleepiness, a subjective finding that was objectively corroborated by improved performance on cognitive tasks testing memory recognition.

L - Glycine also has a calming effect on the brain and has been found to be an effective in releasing growth hormone.

- L-arginine and Glutamine have been found in many studies to increase levels of growth hormone.

- The effect is accentuated when there is a relatively low blood glucose levels such as after the consumption of a low carb meal.

- This is why a good time to supplement is late in the evening, a few hours after consuming your last meal of the day

- There are a variety of nutrients and supplements that have demonstrated to increase the release of growth hormone. For instance the amino acid

L – Glutamine has been shown to increase growth hormone by 15%.

- The most abundant amino acid in the body is glutamine. Consuming even a relatively small amount of glutamine (2,000 mg) has been shown to increase plasma GH levels. Glutamine has also been shown to help preserve muscle mass in individuals vulnerable to losing lean body mass due to inactivity following surgery. This suggests that glutamine may provide important benefits in maintaining lean body tissue.

- When 9 healthy subjects consumed two grams of oral glutamine 45 minutes after a light breakfast, 8 of the 9 subjects experienced elevated plasma growth hormone within 90 minutes. These findings demonstrate, the study authors wrote, that a surprisingly small oral glutamine load is capable of elevating…plasma growth hormone.

- In the small intestine, glutamine is converted into citruline, which in turn triggers the synthesis of arginine, an amino acid shown to release growth hormone.

- A study on glutamine that produced the most significant elevation of growth hormone administered the amino acid using carbonated water.

- Arginine enhances exercise performance because it is one of the main ingredients, along with glycine, that goes into the biosynthesis of creatine in the liver.

- This means that arginine provides a two-fold boost in exercise performance by stimulating growth hormone levels and creatine synthesis.

- L – Arginine is an amino acid that has the ability to stimulate the secretion of Growth hormone and combined with L – Citrulline helps to produce Nitric Oxide. Nitric Oxide helps blood vessels to relax and widen.

- L - Glycine is an amino acid that has a calming effect on the brain and has been found to be an effective in releasing growth hormone.

- Phil Richards Performance Nitric Oxide Generator is a potent blend of L – Arginine, L – Glutamine, L – Citrulline, L – Glycine, Potassium Ascorbate (Vitamin C), Vitamin B6, Vitamin B12, Folic Acid & Niacin (Vitamin B3).

- Exercise is a significant, natural optimizer of GH secretion. The type of exercise you do, as well the intensity and duration of your workouts, all play an important role in determining to what degree your training regimen contributes to GH secretion.

- Growth hormone is released under intense exercise. You can get some growth hormone release from strength work but it's primarily from lactate driven exercise and that is most potent when the exercises of a novel variety. Once you've acclimated to a particular type of exercise you tend to get less hormone signaling.

- So get plenty of variety in your training and I will cover this in great depth and what are the best exercise to stimulate growth hormone in habit 10.

- One study investigating the effects of three exercise sessions a day with either 1.5 or three-hour recovery periods between them found that the longer recoveries led to the greatest volume of 24-hour HGH) secretion.

- It is also important to drink plenty of water during exercise, as dehydration has been shown to significantly reduce the exercise-induced human growth hormone response.

Insulin: the storage hormone

- What is the purpose of insulin in humans? You may say that it's to lower blood sugar. Insulin's evolutionary purpose, as is known right now, is to store excess nutrients.

- We come from a time of feast and famine when if we couldn't store the excess energy during times of feasting, we would not be here because all of our ancestors encountered famine on a regular basis. We are only here because our ancestors were able to store nutrients, which they were able to do because they were able to elevate their insulin in response to any elevation in energy that the organism encountered.

- When your body notices that sugar is elevated, it is a sign that you've got more than you need; you're not burning it so it is accumulating in your blood. So insulin will be released to take that sugar and store it. How does it store it? Glycogen?

- Your body stores very little glycogen at any one time. All the glycogen stored in your liver and muscle wouldn't last you through one active day. Once you fill up your glycogen stores that excess sugar is stored as saturated fat. So the idea of the medical profession recommending a high complex-carbohydrate, low-saturated-fat diet is insane if fat loss is the goal. A high-complex-carbohydrate diet is nothing but a high-glucose diet, or a high-sugar diet. Your body is just going to store the excess glucose as saturated fat, and the body makes it into saturated fat quite readily.

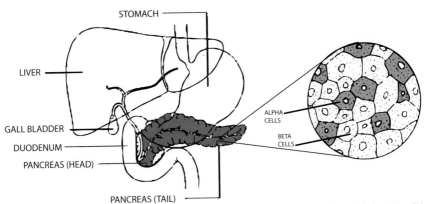

The pancreas is in the upper half of the abdomen. It lies behind the stomach and just in front of the backbone. It's about 15cm (6 inches) long and is shaped like a tadpole. The alpha cells secrete glucagon and beta cells secrete insulin.

Pancreatic Health

- Lets now look at pancreatic health and function, as well as insulin and glucagon's role in fat loss.

- The pancreas has digestive and hormonal functions:

- The enzymes secreted by the exocrine gland in the pancreas help break down carbohydrates, fats, proteins, and acids in the duodenum. These enzymes travel down the pancreatic duct into the bile duct in an inactive form. When they enter the duodenum, they are activated. The exocrine tissue also secretes a bicarbonate to neutralize stomach acid in the duodenum.

- The hormones secreted by the endocrine gland in the pancreas are insulin and glucagon (which regulate the level of glucose in the blood), and somatostatin (which prevents the release of the other two hormones).

- Most people have about one million islets of Langerhand (which secrete insulin) that in total weigh 1 to 2 grams and constitute only 1-2% of the mass of the pancreas.

- Pancreatic enzymes are natural chemicals that help break down fats, proteins and carbohydrates. A normally functioning pancreas secretes about 8 cups of fluid, called pancreatic juice, daily into the duodenum, the portion of the small intestine that connects with the stomach. This fluid contains pancreatic enzymes and helps neutralize stomach acid as it enters the small intestine.

- Dr. Humbart Santillo, M.D., states in his book Intuitive Eating that: "A human being is not maintained by food intake alone, but rather by what is digested. Every food must be broken down by enzymes to simpler building blocks. Enzymes may be divided into 2 groups, exogenous (found in raw food) and endogenous (produced within our bodies.) The more one gets of the exogenous enzymes, the less will have to be borrowed from other metabolic processes and supplied by the pancreas. The enzymes contained in raw food actually aid in the digestion of that same food when it is chewed. One can live many years on a cooked food diet, but eventually this will cause cellular enzyme exhaustion which lays the foundation for a weak immune system and ultimately disease."

- Lita Lee, PhD, in her book The Enzyme Cure, explains that "food enzymes—and only food enzymes— spare the pancreas from having to

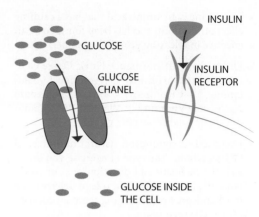

Insulin is the key that unlocks the body cell's glucose channel, allowing glucose to enter the cell. Without the insulin key, glucose is locked out of the cell and must remain in the bloodstream.

compensate for inadequate predigesting." In other words, consuming a predominately "enzymeless" diet of over-cooked foods taxes the pancreas and, eventually, it will become less efficient at enzyme production.

- Insulin is a hormone secreted by the beta cells of the pancreas in response to the ingestion of energy. Insulin helps move macronutrients from the bloodstream into cells for either immediate use or storage. Chronically elevated insulin levels are often associated with elevated leptin and cortisol levels.

- Insulin is the hormone that helps the cells and tissues of the body use glucose. An autoimmune process, whereby the body's immune system attacks the insulin-producing cells of the pancreas, is the defect behind type 1 diabetes. This is a different process from so-called 'adult-onset', or type 2, diabetes.

- Type 2 diabetes in adults represents a metabolic imbalance of both insulin secretion and insulin action at the cellular level, as opposed to the absolute deficiency of insulin observed with type 1 diabetes.

- In patients with type 2 diabetes, a number of factors lead to a poor response to insulin in muscle, fat, and liver. In essence, tissue cells become less responsive to insulin. This triggers the pancreas to overcompensate by producing greater quantities of insulin. Blood levels of insulin double, triple, even quadruple as the pancreas struggles to overpower the body's poor responsiveness to insulin. This is the situation called "insulin resistance.

- For reasons that have yet to be understood, an overworked pancreas cannot meet the increased demand for insulin for long. After just a few years, the insulin-producing beta cells of the pancreas begin to "burn out" and blood sugar rises. Rising blood sugar is therefore a sign of insulin resistance.

- Insulin resistance is present in 90% or more of people with diagnosed diabetes. In all practicality, adult-onset, or type 2, diabetes is synonymous with poor sensitivity to insulin.

- Insulin resistance is an underlying cause of a number of metabolic abnormalities that are grouped together in a condition called the metabolic syndrome.

- This disorder is associated with a host of undesirable consequences such as rising blood sugar, increased triglycerides, which lead to a reduction in beneficial high-density lipoprotein (HDL) and an increase in dangerous, small low-density lipoprotein (LDL) particles, greater risk for blood clotting, and high blood pressure

More About Metabolic Syndrome

- Metabolic syndrome is known by a number of different names—insulin resistance syndrome, syndrome X, borderline diabetes, among others and is typically associated with increased triglycerides, reduced HDL, heightened inflammation, three-fold or greater risk of heart attack, greater risk for stroke, and diabetes.

- Metabolic syndrome can drive the growth of atherosclerotic plaque even when everything else, like LDL, is corrected to perfect levels. Even with excellent LDL levels, for instance, hidden atherosclerotic heart disease can continue to grow at an alarming rate.

- A blood glucose meter can be a useful addition to your home health tools.

- Leptin and insulin resistance almost always occur together most people who are overweight have very high levels of both insulin and leptin. The best treatments for overcoming insulin and leptin resistance is to to focus on improving the receptor that is alleviating the resistance. We will look at some nutrients which help the receptor become more sensitive to the call of leptin and insulin later in this habit.

- Insulin acts on nearly every cell and influences energy storage, cell growth and repair, reproductive function and blood sugar levels.

- When we eat, the carbohydrates in our food get broken down to simple sugars (such as glucose) which end up in the blood stream.

- One of insulin's main functions is to shuttle glucose out of the bloodstream and into the cells so it can be used as fuel. Without insulin, our cells would starve, leaving us feeling tired, hungry and a slower metabolism.

- Consuming too much glucose from a high sugar-diet can make our cells become deaf to insulin's message, making us insulin resistant. When this occurs our appetite increases, we are more likely to be leptin resistant, and our metabolism slows. The more body fat an individual has, and particularly the more abdominal fat they have, the more likely they are to be insulin resistant.

- Insulin resistance makes fat cells produce TNF (tumor neurosis factor), a toxic hormone that causes inflammation. Excess fat, especially in the belly, causes insulin resistance, elevated blood sugar, dyslipidemia, and high blood

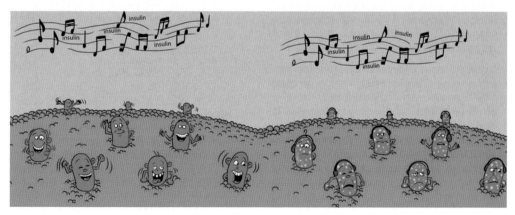

Consuming too much glucose from a high sugar diet can make our cells "deaf" to insulins message. When this happens, no matter how much or how loud insulin shouts its message, the cells can not hear it.

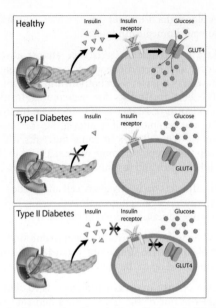

Here's a diagram to show the mechanisms affecting the body in Type I & Type II diabetes. In type I diabetes insulin is not secreted from the pancreas. In Type II diabetes, the cell receptors have gone deaf to insulins message.

pressure and increased inflammation. Therefore obesity causes inflammation and inflammation causes obesity so you must reduce body fat to dampen the flames of inflammatory substances spewing into the body 24 hours a day 7 days a week.

- Although insulin resistance is the most common hormone problem in the world today, most people don't even know they got it. It is the key factor to obesity, type 2 diabetes, metabolic syndrome, polycystic ovary syndrome, high blood pressure, and cardiovascular disease. Since insulin and leptin resistance go hand in hand, as already mentioned, treatments that help one will naturally help the other a win win situation. In fact most fat cell hormones are linked to insulin resistance, so you can see that obesity is a disease that causes many more diseases.

- Insulin resistance makes fat cells dysfunctional in many ways. The normal biological processes that regulate energy balance and metabolism get out of whack. Insulin resistance makes fat cells leak their contents, known as free fatty acids, into the circulation. Its normal to have some free fatty acids in your blood but, if free fatty acids get too high, problems can occur. Free fatty acids have a toxic effect on the insulin receptor. This is called lipotoxicity, which means the toxic effect of fat. The free fatty acids intensify insulin resistance, in a vicious

cycle. Insulin resistance increases levels of free fatty acids, which worsen insulin resistance. The result very high levels of free fatty acids dumb down your insulin to the call let me in.

- All of the following contribute to insulin resistance;

  - Genetics - if you have a family history of diabetes or obesity, you are more likely to have insulin resistance
  - Physical Activity - lack of exercise is a major risk factor of insulin resistance. Just a few weeks of exercise can improve insulin sensitivity
  - Stress - cortisol and epinephrine both promote insulin resistance
  - Diet - eating too much sugar is a huge cause of insulin resistance

- First off, your blood is not a very sweet beverage. Normal fasting blood sugar is slightly less than one teaspoon of sugar in your five or so litres of blood. What happens when you drink a sugar sweetened drink that contains 10 teaspoons of sugar, like many soft drinks consumed today? It causes a tsunami of an insulin wave where the liver converts most of the sugar into triglycerides and slaps it on your ass and your gut!

- Insulin's goal is to take blood sugar, as its passenger, to various locations in your body that want it. It helps if you are active, as some of the sugar is more likely to be wanted by cells in your body, including your many muscle cells.

- In a healthy person, insulin drops 60% of the sugar at your liver, which acts as a warehouse, converting the blood sugar to glycogen for storage

- Insulin is released by your pancreas in two phases. The first phase is from insulin that is already made and stored in your pancreas, which is just waiting for some food to come along. This is your first insulin burst coming to pick up the first set of blood sugar passengers. The release of this insulin triggers your pancreas' beta cells to start making more insulin to deal with the rest of the meal.

- As you are eating, some of the insulin transports blood sugar to your white adipose tissue, or stored fat. The blood sugar is taken up by fat cells, activating their metabolism, in turn producing the hormone leptin. Leptin now enters your blood and begins traveling up to your brain. The more you eat, the more insulin you make, and the more leptin you make.

- When leptin levels get high enough, meaning you have eaten enough, then leptin permeates into your brain and tells your subconscious brain you are full. At the same time, the higher levels of leptin also tell your pancreas that you are full, which turns off the beta cell production of insulin, as no more insulin is required.

- If you ate the right amount of food for your physical activity level, then blood sugar always has some place healthy to go; insulin rises and falls in a controlled manner, as does leptin.

- When insulin is too high, and cells don't need any sugar, then insulin stimulates the production of triglycerides, which can become stored fat. This is how you gain weight through a high carbohydrate diet, along with low activity levels.

- Unfortunately, as triglycerides elevate in your blood they get in the way of leptin getting into your brain. This keeps you eating more than you need to because you don't yet have a full signal, a problem called leptin resistance. This encourages even further insulin driven triglyceride formation, making it more likely you will gain weight.

- If you continually eat too much and gain weight, then cells get tired of seeing insulin and reject entry into the cell. The reason for this rejection of insulin is rather simple. If the cells take in blood sugar when they can't use it, because they already have enough, then the extra sugar will kill the cell. Rejecting insulin is a self defensive measure. This is the mechanism behind basic insulin resistance at the cellular level.

- When insulin levels are elevated, the system shifts to fat storage. As insulin levels fall back to normal, fat can leave fat cells and be used as fuel throughout the body. And, remember as insulin rises, growth hormone lowers, but timing of carbohydrates are essential because as mentioned earlier you need insulin to transport nutrients into cells, including IGF1 which is derived from growth hormone. This is covered in habit 9 on nutrient timing.

- Fat cells don't make any decisions independently. They must be told when their stored fat energy is required. Hormones monitor this situation carefully, and when more energy is needed, insulin is the messenger that communicates with each fat cell about what action is necessary. When insulin levels are high, they tell fat cells to keep fat locked up and not to release it.

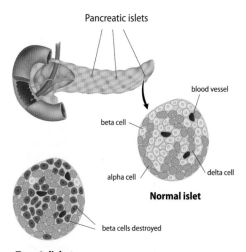

Pancreatic islets

blood vessel

beta cell

alpha cell

delta cell

Normal islet

beta cells destroyed

Type 1 diabetes

The difference between GI and GL

- GI value indicates only how rapidly a particular carbohydrate appears as glucose in the circulation. It does not take into account the amount of the food that is normally consumed

- For instance:

- the GI of a watermelon is high

- but....

- there is not much carbohydrate in it

- Therefore the GL of a watermelon is low

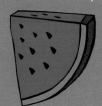

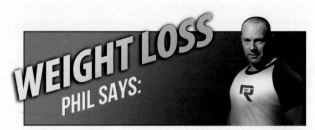

WEIGHT LOSS
PHIL SAYS:

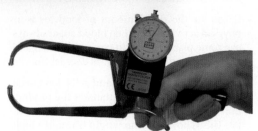

Research clearly shows that 2.0 pounds per week is usually the maximum rate for safe, permanent weight (fat) loss. Don't ever confuse weight loss with fat loss. You can lose weight quickly, but you can't lose fat quickly. If you think you can outwit Mother Nature and you're dead set on losing 4, 5, 10 pounds a week, you're going to lose fat in the beginning, but not all of it. It will be mostly water and muscle dropping off you. Concentrate on dropping body fat % than dropping body weight massive difference. Find a good trainer who can test your body fat every 2–4 weeks. The best trainers for this are those that have been through the Biosignature system that Charles Poliquin has created. I have to commend Charles for doing an incredible job on teaching trainers how to take body fat composition levels not only correctly, but also accurately. I used to have athletes drop no weight on the weighing scales whatsoever but dropped body fat% significantly, which is far more important, in my book, than overall weight.

- What happens if your insulin level stays high most of the day? Your fat cells have no choice but to respond by staying locked in storage mode, and they keep getting larger and larger. Not only that, but because the energy in that stored fat is not available to be properly used, nutrient levels fall, and your brain's appetite centres tell you it's time to eat again.

- The fat storing hormone that farmers also depend on is insulin. Animals are not usually fed a wide variety of foods. However, significant changes occur when they go from grass fed to corn fed. Lets look at how this nutritional alteration makes a big difference to the bottom line in the cattle business. When you crowd animals together so they can't move around, just like they do in feedlots, so they expend less energy, and then most importantly take them from their natural grass fed diet to one which is now derived from corn. As corn is digested, it is converted into sugar, which as we know is a potent signal for our fat storage hormone insulin to come and do its job of keeping the fat storage switch on.

- This is a very effective method for making cattle bigger - after all the farmer gets paid more money the heavier the animal. This type of feeding and environment increases fat storage whilst simultaneously keeping the fat already

in the fat cells from being released. Our bodies work exactly the same way. This is very similar as to why humans are getting fatter less exercise and wrong food choices.

- Insulin and glucagon are oppositional hormones. Insulin is both lipogenic (fat storage) and anabolic (muscle builder), whilst glucagon is both lipolytic (fat burning) and catabolic (muscle breakdown). When insulin goes up glucagon goes down and vice versa, so it is imperative to fat loss that you get these two hormones working for you and not against you if you want to be lean and healthy.

- The human body wants blood glucose (blood sugar) maintained in a very narrow range. Insulin and glucagon are the hormones which make this happen. Both insulin and glucagon are secreted from the pancreas, and thus are referred to as pancreatic endocrine hormones. Insulin and glucagon are hormones secreted by islet cells within the pancreas. They are both secreted in response to blood sugar levels, but in opposite fashion!

- Insulin is normally secreted by the beta cells (a type of islet cell) of the pancreas. The stimulus for insulin secretion is a HIGH blood glucose... it's as simple as that. Insulin has an effect on a number of cells, including muscle, red blood cells, and fat cells. In response to insulin, these

160

cells absorb glucose out of the blood, having the net effect of lowering the high blood glucose levels into the normal range.

- Glucagon is secreted by the alpha cells of the pancreatic islets in much the same manner as insulin...except in the opposite direction. If blood glucose is high, then no glucagon is secreted.

- When blood glucose goes LOW, however, (such as between meals, and during exercise) more and more glucagon is secreted. Like insulin, glucagon has an effect on many cells of the body, but most notably the liver.

- The effect of glucagon is to make the liver release the glucose it has stored in its cells into the bloodstream, with the net effect of increasing blood glucose. Glucagon also induces the liver (and some other cells such as muscle) to make glucose out of building blocks obtained from other nutrients found in the body (eg, protein).

- The effect of insulin and glucagon on body fat is well illustrated by a study published in the journal of comparative and physiological psychology in 1978. In this study researchers injected a group of rats with insulin and another group of rats with glucagon. The rats that received insulin injections gained body fat whilst the rats that received glucagon injections lost body fat.

- The fact is with high insulin levels you can't lose fat, and with insufficient insulin you can't build muscle that will help you burn fat. And with high glucagon levels you will lose body fat but also muscle as well. So you can see managing the yin and yang of insulin & glucagon is very important in maintaining a healthy body fat %. The key word here is timing knowing when you want high levels of either hormone to manipulate building lean muscle tissue and burning fat.

- It is helpful to think of insulin as a storage hormone and glucagon is the key to open the storage room up to release the nutrients to be used as fuel. In addition to insulin being a storage hormone, it is also a anabolic hormone because not only does it shuttles sugar into muscles, but amino acids and other nutrients too. So insulin enhances muscle growth, recovery, and repair by delivering to the muscles every thing it needs for muscle growth.

- Glucagon mobilizes fat for use as energy; in order for this to happen you must ensure the liver isn't full of glycogen as the body will use this source of glucose first before glucagon can convince the fat cells to give up their stash of fat.

- The liver can hold up to 100 grams of glycogen so the body has a constant stream of glucose to feed the brain in between meals.

- As a fat burning hormone glucagon is obviously important in helping you lose excess body fat. However, just like insulin is a double edged sword so is glucagon. For example if you are on a high protein low carbohydrate diet then glucagon will be high and after the liver glycogen stores have been exhausted, the glucagon will simply break down muscle tissue in a process known as gluconeogenesis (the process by which glucose is made, primarily in the liver, from non-carbohydrate sources) and convert to glucose.

- Carbohydrate is the primary trigger for insulin secretion and protein is the primary trigger for glucagon secretion. However, protein also exerts a weak stimulatory effect on insulin approximately 30% of the effect of carbohydrate on insulin.

- If you are wondering about fat, it does not elicit a response either way when consumed alone. When fat is added to a protein or carbohydrate meal it either has no effect on insulin response or slightly increases the insulin response but it does not blunt it. For example if you add butter to a baked potato you will likely experience a greater insulin response than if you ate the potato on its own.

- Carbohydrates will only be converted into body fat when both the muscles and liver are saturated with glycogen (stored carbohydrate), and also if you are insulin resistant. Therefore, to avoid sticking that bread roll on your ass, you must make sure that the cells are sensitive to insulin and there is room for the carbohydrates to be stored. Carbohydrate needs are activity dependent which means lots of activity = lots of carbohydrates needed, little activity = little carbohydrates needed - now it don't get much simpler than that.

- Insulin is the fat storage hormone and that's why if you are trying to lose body fat then snacking between meals, if you are not exercising regularly and with intensity, simply wont cut it as you will constantly have raised insulin even if the snack is pure protein. .

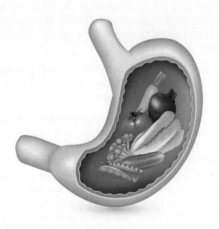

Obesity related diseases:

80% of type II diabetes is related to obesity.

70% of Cardiovascular disease is related to obesity.

42% breast and colon cancer is diagnosed among obese individuals.

30% of gall bladder surgery is related to obesity.

26% of obese people have high blood pressure.

Obese individuals have a 50% to 100% increased risk of death from all causes, compared with normal-weight individuals.

- A Norwegian study in 2005 showed that exercise and diet were more effective for type-2 diabetes than insulin therapy. Those treated with lifestyle changes lost more weight, improved their blood sugar, blood pressure and triglyceride levels. The group receiving insulin therapy actually increased in weight and saw some of their metabolic parameter worsen.

- To begin increasing your glucose sensitivity there are many things that you can do.

- Eat low glycemic load (GL) foods - to do this you need to cut out simple sugars and switch to low GL foods which do not cause large blood sugar spikes. Low GL foods include foods such as oats and berries. You can also combine carbohydrates with proteins which slows down their digestion and therefore further stabilises blood sugar levels

- A 2005 study comparing low GL diets to a conventional low-fat, low-calorie diet found that, after 6 months, those following the low GL diet lost more weight, had lower levels of LDL cholesterol, triglycerides and fasting glucose levels.

- The researchers concluded that "implementation of a low GL diet is associated with substantial and sustained improvements in abdominal obesity, cholesterol and blood sugar control"

- High fibre from nonstarchy fruits and vegetables slow down the passage of carbohydrates through your intestines. This slows blood sugar rises and so will have the effect of improving insulin sensitivy.

- While most of the recent focus has been on increase in abdominal girth, recent research done at the San Francisco VA Medical Center has shown that upper body fat (fat deposits in the upper chest and back), is also associated with insulin resistance, and if fat stores in both the visceral and abdominal area are present, the risk is doubled.

Reduce inflammation

- Inflammation promotes insulin resistance and so must be reversed in order to increase insulin sensitivity. To do this you need to balance your omega-3/omega-6 ratio and reduce you intake of saturated and trans fats. High levels of meat and dairy can cause inflammation as they increase arachadoic acid, so try to reduce your intake of these

- On August 1, 2006 the American Chemical Society published research that showed conclusively that methylmercury induces pancreatic cell apoptosis and dysfunction. Mercury is a well-known toxic agent that produces various types of cell and tissue damage yet governmental health agencies diminish this fact exposing billions of people worldwide to levels of mercury harmful to pancreatic health.

- In the case of diabetes mercury is especially telling for it affects the beta cells, the insulin itself, and the insulin receptor sites setting off a myriad of complex disturbances in glucose metabolism.

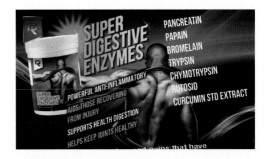

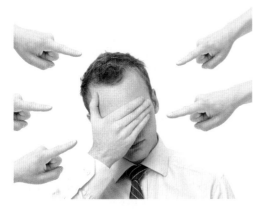

The dental industry who still allow amalgam (50% mercury)and governments who allow mercury in their vaccines need to get their heads out of their arse's and stop poisoning human beings and the sad fact is they know the facts but bury their heads because they hide behind placebo evidence.

Nutritional Supplements for improving insulin sensitivty

- The following supplements can help reduce insulin resistance and inflammation in the body:

- Omega-3 fatty acids contained in fish oil help in numerous ways. Omega-3s effectively reduce the inevitably elevated triglycerides of metabolic syndrome, raise HDL, and reduce inflammation. Of all their benefits, the triglyceride-reducing power of omega-3s represents their most powerful effect, which is likely responsible for the dramatic reduction in heart attack and stroke seen with supplementation.

- USDA scientists have identified unique compounds in cinnamon bark that increase in vitro sugar metabolism "20-fold." According to one government expert, "These polyphenolic polymers found in cinnamon may function as antioxidants, potentiate insulin action, and may be beneficial in the control of glucose intolerance and diabetes."

- Cinnamon is rich in bioactive compounds that help regulate blood sugar levels. This isn't the cinnamon you'd use to flavor your cappuccino, by the way. It's a related species called Cinnamomum cassia (as found in PRP's Super Brain Talk)—and scientists around the world are now discovering its glucose-lowering power.

- Extract of this form of cinnamon triggers cell signaling proteins inside the pancreas, bringing the secretion and regulation of insulin levels into greater balance. This helps to restore your body's natural ability to control blood sugar as you age.

- Cinnamon acts as an insulin sensitizer, triggering proteins that lower insulin resistance at the cellular level. It has also been shown to thwart advanced glycation end products (AGEs) which are implicated in diabetic complications, atherosclerosis, and Alzheimer's disease. A recent in vivo study found cinnamon accomplishes this anti-glycation effect in part through its antioxidant scavenging capabilities.

- Cinnamon also triggers genes in muscle and fatty tissue that transfer glucose out of the bloodstream and into energy producing cells, effectively lowering blood glucose. This quenches the highly reactive oxidant and inflammatory inferno in your body stoked by chronic glucose overexposure.

- An abundance of animal studies published in 2010 confirm that cinnamon polyphenols can significantly reduce fasting glucose levels, improve pancreatic function, and enhance insulin sensitivity—even in diabetic models.

- Curcumin is another nutrient which influences key hormones, supports major body organs, and regulates inflammatory signaling all in ways that help correct or prevent metabolic problems.

- Curcumin helps lower inappropriately high levels of leptin (reducing leptin resistance) while boosting the all-important levels of the adiponectin protein hormone that modulates metabolism including glucose and fatty acid catabolism. High levels are associated with low body fat. (which lowers insulin resistance).

- Curcumin helps activate the fat-burning gene signal PPAR gamma, which also helps to make more new, metabolically-fit fat cells.

- Curcumin directly reduces major inflammatory events from occurring inside white adipose tissue (tumor necrosis factor alpha, interleukin-6, and monocyte chemotactic protein-1). When these inflammatory signals are excessively activated in white adipose tissue they keep sending "EMERGENCY" messages to immune cells around your body to come to the white adipose tissue and join in the inflammatory party. By lowering such inflammation, the source of overweight-induced disease is stopped.

- Curcumin acts directly on liver cells to help prevent them from becoming fatty. And it works directly on pancreatic beta cells to help them produce insulin normally. By helping the liver and the pancreas, curcumin is taking stress off the two most important organs whose function declines before the onset of type 2 diabetes. (This is another reason why I added curcumin to both PRP's Super Digestive Enzymes and Super Brain Talk)

- Chromium has long been known to play a central role in healthy glucose metabolism at the cellular level. It sensitizes cells to insulin and increases the number of insulin receptors in cells. Studies link low chromium levels with increased blood glucose, triglycerides, and cholesterol, increasing the possibility of diabetes and heart disease.

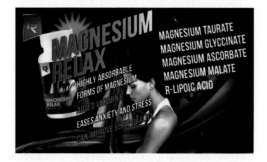

- Chromium works by interacting with cell-signaling receptors that enhance the body's response to insulin. In the presence of chromium

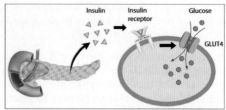

Chromium appears to make insulin function more efficient by enhancing the uptake of glucose from the blood into the cell. Chromium increases the number of insulin receptors on the cell membrane and enhances insulin binding to cells.

cells require less insulin to become activated, resulting in greater overall insulin sensitivity and enhanced glucose control.

- Chromium also aids in the transfer of glucose from the blood into cells by activating insulin-sensitive glucose transport molecules. Its central role in regulating glucose is underscored by the hallmark signs of chromium deficiency which manifest as elevated fasting glucose and insulin blood levels. Some chromium-deficient patients have even developed diabetes that could not be reversed through insulin injections, but subsided when supplemented with chromium. The body absorbs dietary chromium poorly, highlighting the need for supplementation.

- The more efficient your insulin metabolism, the more amino acids get inside the cells and the more muscle you can make. Chromium appears to make insulin function more efficient by enhancing the uptake of glucose from the blood into the cell. Chromium increases the number of insulin receptors on the cell membrane and enhances insulin binding to cells.

- The result from chromium therefore is improved glucose transport into muscle, fat and liver tissue, and therefore better glucose control. Although chromium is present in such foods as whole grains, cheese, liver and meat, the typical Western diet is much lower than the recommended 50–200 mcg per day and if you exercise a lot then you need much more than this. The average intake in the typical Western diet is said to be in the region of 28–35 mcg. One reason for the such low amounts of chromium is processing of foods removes the chromium - another reason to stay away from processed junk foods.

- Chromium picolinate has anabolic effects. Dr Muriel Gilman at Bemidgi State University gave 200mcg of chromium picolinate per day to half of a group of freshmen who had enrolled in weight training classes.

- The study run double blind for six weeks. Freshmen not receiving any chromium made negligible gains, those on the chromium gained an average of 3.5lbs of lean body mass. That's a huge increase in six weeks, even for novices who have not exploited their muscle growth potential. So a larger study was done with trained football players to validate it.

- Over six weeks intensive weight training, the football players receiving chromium picolinate gained 5.7lbs of lean body mass compared with 4lbs for the control group. In addition, the chromium group lost 3.6% of body fat compared with 1% for the control group.

- Of all the trace minerals, chromium may be the most beneficial to diabetes patients. It's an insulin potentiator, so it makes the body's own insulin production go further.

- The results of several studies suggest that chromium may play a role in controlling diabetes and heart disease. For example, in one study, 180 people with type 2 diabetes were randomly assigned to receive 100 mcg elemental chromium, 500 mcg elemental chromium, or a placebo. Four months later, those taking either dose of chromium scored significantly lower on their fasting and two-hour insulin level tests, indicating improvement in their disease. Those taking the higher amount of chromium were also found to have lower total cholesterol levels.

- The average adult body contains between 0.4 and 6 mg of chromium and older people usually have lower levels. There is a wide geographical variation in chromium levels and population studies suggest that the incidence of diabetes and heart disease is lower in areas where chromium intakes are relatively high. In double blind studies, just the addition of chromium supplementation, with no other dietary changes, alters the body fat composition to increase non fat body mass.

- One factor affecting chromium stores in the body is the amount of sugar that an individual consumes. Once chromium has acted as a cofactor in insulin response, it is excreted in the urine. With the high sugar diet of today, the turnover rate of chromium is quite high.

Magnesium Enhances Insulin Function

- Without insulin, magnesium doesn't get transported from our blood into our cells where it is most needed. When Dr. Jerry Nadler of the Gonda Diabetes Center at the City of Hope Medical Center in Duarte, California, and his colleagues placed 16 healthy people on magnesium-deficient diets, their insulin became less effective at getting sugar from their blood into their cells, where it's burned or stored as fuel. In other words, they became less insulin sensitive or what is called insulin resistant. There is a strong relationship between magnesium and insulin action. Magnesium is important for the effectiveness of insulin. A reduction of magnesium in the cells strengthens insulin resistance.

- A less known fact is that insulin also stores magnesium. But if your cells become resistant to insulin, you can't store magnesium so you lose it through urination.

- Intracellular magnesium relaxes muscles. What happens when you can't store magnesium because the cell is resistant? You lose magnesium and your blood vessels constrict. This could lead to cardiovascular problems.

- This causes an increase in blood pressure and a reduction in energy since intracellular magnesium is required for all energy producing reactions that take place in the cell.

- But most importantly, magnesium is also necessary for the action of insulin and the manufacture of insulin. When you raise your insulin, you lose magnesium, and the cells become even more insulin resistant.

- Blood vessels constrict and glucose and insulin can't get to the tissues, which makes them more insulin resistant, so the insulin levels go up and you lose more magnesium.

- Magnesium is also vital for converting glycogen into glucose for use as the body's fuel.

- The interrelationships between magnesium and carbohydrate metabolism have regained considerable interest over the last few years. Insulin secretion requires magnesium: magnesium deficiency results in impaired insulin secretion while magnesium replacement restores insulin secretion. Furthermore, experimental magnesium deficiency reduces the tissues sensitivity to insulin. Subclinical magnesium deficiency is common in diabetes. It results from both inssuficient magnesium intakes and increase magnesium losses, particularly in the urine. In type 2 diabetes, magnesium deficiency seems to be associated with insulin resistance.

- Magnesium is needed for more than 300 biochemical reactions and is recognized as an important mediator of insulin action and in reducing inflammation. In several studies, daily oral magnesium supplementation substantially improved insulin sensitivity by 10% and reduced blood sugar by 37%. The Women's Health Study including nearly 12,000 participants showed that people who fail to take the recommended adequate intake of magnesium of 320-420 mg/day are more prone to have both metabolic syndrome and increased CRP.

- R-Lipoic Acid also significantly increases insulin sensitivity, enhances glucose transport, increases metabolic rate and reduces the gain in body fat from aging. This is why I combined magnesium, chromium and R-lipoic acid in my Magnesium Relax so that I get a product that enhances insulin sensitivity.

The Power Of Sunlight And Vitamin D

- The sun is the ultimate giver of all life and one of the most important anti cancer, anti obesity tools by provding the nutrient Vitamin D. Yes of course respect the sun but ignoring its incredible benefits is not the wisest thing to do.

- Vitamin D is not a vitamin but a hormone. It is unique in that it is made in the skin as a result of exposure to sunlight.

- The skin has a large capacity to make vitamin D. Exposure of a person in a bathing suit to a dose of sunlight, which is typically no more than 15-20 minutes on Cape Cod in June or

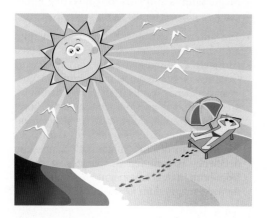

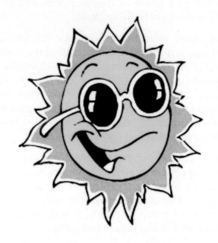

July at noon time, is the equivalent to taking 20,000 IU of vitamin D orally.

- Numerous exciting reports about vitamin D's myriad of beneficial effects include recent observations that vitamin D deficiency contributes to insulin resistance and raises blood pressure (by increasing the blood pressure-raising hormone renin). Vitamin D deficiency is exceedingly common, particularly in northern climates, where up to 90% of people have moderate-to-severe deficiency. In sun-deprived climates, 1,000–4,000 IU/day may be required to raise blood levels to normal, occasionally more. However, adequate sun exposure does not necessarily guarantee optimal vitamin D levels. Vitamin D status can be assessed by having one's blood tested, as discussed in Habit 6.

- High-dose vitamin D supplements may help increase the body's sensitivity to insulin, thus reducing the risk of diabetes, researchers have found. In the current study, conducted by researchers from Massey University, and published in the British Journal of Nutrition, researchers randomly assigned 81 South Asian women between the ages of 23 and 68 to take either a placebo or 4,000 IU of vitamin D once per day. All participants suffered from insulin resistance at the start of the study, but none were taking diabetes drugs or vitamin D supplements larger than 1,000 IU per day. At the start of the study, the average participant had vitamin D blood levels of approximately 50 nanomoles per liter, slightly lower than the average levels in a U.S. adult (60-75 nmol/L). After six months, women in the vitamin D group exhibited significantly more insulin sensitivity and less insulin resistance than women who had received a placebo. The largest effect was seen in women whose vitamin D blood levels had reached 80 to 119 nmol/L.

According to the Vitamin D Council, blood levels should be at least 125 nmol/L for optimal health.

- A 2009 meta-analysis published in the Journal of Clinical Endocrinology & Metabolism found that higher blood levels of vitamin D lowered diabetes risk. Likewise, in a study published in the journal Diabetic Medicine, researchers from the Sitaram Bhartia Institute of Science and Research in New Delhi found that a large dose of vitamin D significantly improved insulin sensitivity after meals in 71 men who were healthy except for central obesity.

- Johns Hopkins University Medical School conducted a ten-year epidemiological study that showed exposure to full-spectrum light (including the ultraviolet frequencies) is positively related to the prevention of breast, colon and rectal cancers. How does this work? There is in fact a scientific answer. The sun stimulates production of a hormone in your skin. Ultraviolet B rays, the kind of rays that give you sunburns, interact with a special cholesterol in unblocked skin. Once stimulated, this cholesterol triggers your liver and kidney to make vitamin D3. Vitamin D3 isn't exactly a vitamin,, but rather a type of steroid hormone that can drastically improve your immune system function.

- Vitamin D 'triggers and arms' the immune system. In particular it triggers and arms the body's T cells, the cells in the body that seek out and destroy any invading bacteria and viruses.

- Scientists at the University of Copenhagen have discovered that Vitamin D is crucial to activating our immune defences and that without sufficient intake of the vitamin, the killer cells of the immune system – T cells – will not be able to react to and fight off serious infections in the body.

- For T cells to detect and kill foreign pathogens such as clumps of bacteria or viruses, the cells must first be 'triggered' into action and "transform" from inactive and harmless immune cells into killer cells that are primed to seek out and destroy all traces of invaders.

- The researchers found that the T cells rely on vitamin D in order to activate and they would remain dormant, 'naïve' to the possibility of threat if vitamin D is lacking in the blood.

- Professor Carsten Geisler from the Department of International Health, Immunology and Microbiology, said: "When a T cell is exposed to a foreign pathogen, it extends a signalling device or 'antenna' known as a vitamin D receptor, with which it searches for vitamin D. This means that the T cell must have vitamin D or activation of the cell will cease. If the T cells cannot find enough vitamin D in the blood, they won't even begin to mobilise. "

- Yes - you can now see how moronic the advice is to stay out of the sun. Sensible advice would be get enough sun exposure that your skin colour takes, then cover up.

- Vitamin D from all sources (sunlight, sun lamps, or supplements) reduces the incidence of respiratory infections. Dutch children with the least sun exposure are twice as likely to develop a cough and three times more likely to develop a runny nose compared with children with the most sun exposure.

- When Russian athletes were given sun lamps to stimulate vitamin D synthesis in the body, there were 50% fewer respiratory infections and far fewer days of absence.

- In Russia, a full-spectrum lighting system was installed in factories where colds and sore throats had become commonplace among workers. This lowered the bacterial contamination of the air by 40%-70%. Workers who did not receive the full-spectrum light were absent twice as many days as those who did.

- Breast cancer is the most common form of cancer in women, causing about 370,000 deaths annually worldwide. Each year some 220,000 women in Europe and 180,000 women in North America are diagnosed with the disease. About 15,000 British women die of breast cancer annually, a death rate that is higher than elsewhere in Western Europe. One in 12 British

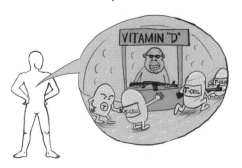

Vitamin D help can help boost your body's defence system by arming your body's T-cells

women will develop breast cancer at some time in their lives and, as we have already seen, the incidence of breast cancer is increasing. The reasons for this are not altogether clear, but lack of sunlight could be a factor. In 1989 the Drs Garland, together with Dr Edward Gorham, published the first ever epidemiological work on the relationship between sun exposure and breast cancer. Their research demonstrated that, as in the case of colon cancer, there was a strong negative correlation between available sunlight and breast cancer death rates. The chances of women from areas of the United States with less available sunlight dying of breast cancer were 40% higher than those of women who lived in Hawaii or Florida.

- Vitamin D is also gaining recognition as a crucial modulator of inflammation. A University of London study demonstrated a dramatic reduction in the inflammatory proteins CRP and matrix metalloproteinase (MMP), after supplementation in 171 healthy adults, with a startling 68% reduction in MMP.

The healing rays of natural sunlight (that generate vitamin D in your skin) cannot penetrate glass. So you don't generate vitamin D when sitting in your car or home.

- It is nearly impossible to get adequate amounts of vitamin D from your diet. Sunlight exposure is the only reliable way to generate vitamin D in your own body.

- A person would have to drink ten tall glasses of vitamin D fortified milk each day just to get minimum levels of vitamin D into their diet. The further you live from the equator, the longer exposure you need to the sun in order to

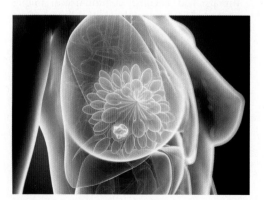

generate vitamin D. Canada, the UK and most U.S. states are far from the equator.

- People with dark skin pigmentation may need 20-30 times as much exposure to sunlight as fair-skinned people to generate the same amount of vitamin D, as we have already discussed. Sufficient levels of vitamin D are crucial for calcium absorption in your intestines. Without sufficient vitamin D, your body cannot absorb calcium, rendering calcium supplements useless. Chronic vitamin D deficiency cannot be reversed overnight: it takes months of vitamin D supplementation and sunlight exposure to rebuild the body's bones and nervous system. Even weak sunscreens (SPF=8) block your body's ability to generate vitamin D by 95%. This is how sunscreen products actually cause disease -- by creating a critical vitamin deficiency in the body.

- The sunscreen industry doesn't want you to know that your body actually needs sunlight exposure because that realization would mean lower sales of sunscreen products.

- It is impossible to generate too much vitamin D in your body from sunlight exposure: your body will self-regulate and only generate what it needs.

- Vitamin D is "activated" in your body by your kidneys and liver before it can be used. Having kidney disease or liver damage can greatly impair your body's ability to activate circulating vitamin D.

Even though vitamin D is one of the most powerful healing chemicals in your body, your body makes it absolutely free. No prescription required.

- On the issue of sunlight exposure, by the way, it turns out that super antioxidants greatly boost your body's ability to handle sunlight without burning. Astaxanthin is one of the most powerful "internal sunscreens" and can allow you to stay under the sun twice as long without burning. Other powerful antioxidants with this ability include the super fruits like Acai, Pomegranates, blueberries, etc.

- According to a new review of research, evidence suggests that adequate treatment of vitamin D deficient athletes could dramatically improve their performance. Activated vitamin

D is a steroid hormone which regulates more than 1,000 human genes.

- Researchers reviewed the world's literature for evidence that vitamin D affects physical and athletic performance. Numerous studies, particularly in the German literature in the 1950s, show vitamin D-producing ultraviolet light improves athletic performance.

- A study in 1945 found that UV radiation for up to 2 minutes, three times a week, improved cardiovascular fitness scores by 19% compared to 2% of students who did nothing.

- Vitamin D also increases the size and number of fast twitch muscle fibers. Most cross-sectional and randomized controlled studies show that vitamin D levels are directly associated with musculoskeletal performance.

- Vitamin D also increases levels of testosterone, which may boost libido. In one study, overweight men who were given vitamin D supplements had a significant increase in testosterone levels after one year.

- A few years back, the recommended level was between 40 to 60 nanograms per milliliter (ng/ml), but more recently the optimal vitamin D level has been raised to 50-70 ng/ml.

How Much Vitamin D Do You Need?

- Dr. John Cannell, MD, is the president of The Vitamin D Council, a non-profit group that advocates higher vitamin D intake. According to Dr. Cannell, adults need to take 5,000 IU a day of vitamin D to put the vast majority of them (97.5%) above the 50 ng/mL level.

- For each receptor for vitamin D there are two receptors for vitamin A on every cell. A relative balance of these two nutrients is essential for health. For example if you take large amounts of vitamin D you will create a vitamin A deficiencies which will be catastrophic for health.

- Recent research from Spain indicates that vitamin A is necessary for both vitamin D binding and vitamin D release to receptor sites. It also turns out that vitamin D is the most potent protector of omega 3 oils, as mentioned previously.

- The best ways to increase your vitamin D levels, in my order of preference, are by:

1. Exposing your skin natural sunlight. Vitamin D from sunlight acts as a pro-hormone, rapidly converting in your skin into 25-hydroxyvitamin D, or vitamin D3.
2. Using a safe home tanning bed to achieve similar results as that from natural sunlight exposure. I use a UVB sunbed three times per week for two minutes each time.
3. Taking an oral vitamin D3 supplement whenever natural sun exposure is not an option.

Vitamain K2

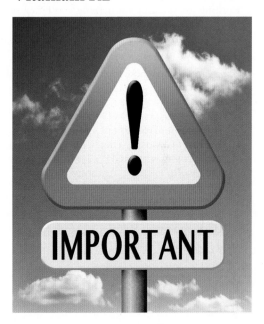

- Dr. Kate Rheaume-Bleue, a naturopathic physician has authored an incredible book which alerted me to the importance of combining K2 with Vitamin D in my Ultimate Fish Oil Blend. Her book is titled Vitamin K2 and the Calcium Paradox: How a Little Known Vitamin Could Save Your Life.

- "K2 is really critical for keeping your bones strong and your arteries clear," Rheaume-Bleue says. This is a really crucial point: If you opt for oral vitamin D, you need to also consume in your food or take supplemental vitamin K2. "There are so many people on the vitamin-D-mega-dose bandwagon, taking more and more of vitamin D. And it could absolutely be causing harm if you are lacking the K2 to complete the job to get the calcium where it's supposed to be," Rheaume-Bleue warns."We don't see symptoms of vitamin D toxicity very often. But when we do, those symptoms are inappropriate calcification. That's the symptom of vitamin D toxicity. And it is actually a lack of vitamin K2 that can cause that..." While the ideal or optimal ratios between vitamin D and vitamin K2 have yet to be elucidated, Rheume-Bleue suggests about 150-200 micrograms of K2 will meet the need for the "average" healthy person.

Conclusion

- There is a very synergistic relationship between the awsome foursome growth hormone, insulin, sleep and sunshine. This habit alone if you follow by enhancing growth hormone, getting insulin working for you and not making you fatter, getting good sleep and adequate sunshine can have a dramatic effect on your health and ability to lose fat. Hopefully though you can see that the 10 habits is like a jigsaw puzzle you need all of the pieces to complete the jigsaw and for maximum fat loss to be initiated.

- In researching for these topics, some of the books that I read included;

-

  - "The Fat Resistance Diet" - Leo Galland
  - "The Vitamin D Solution" - Michael Holick
  - "The Liver Cleansing Diet" - Dr Sandra Cabot
  - "Grow Young with HGH" - Dr Ronald Klatz
  - "The Insulin Factor" - Anthony Haynes
  - "Life Extension Revolution" - Philip Miller
  - "The Primal Blueprint" - Mark Sisson
  - "Enzynes for Health and Healing" - Ellen Culter & Dr Jeremy Kaslow
  - "The Blood-Sugar Solution" - Mark Hyman

HABIT 8

NUTRITIONAL CARDIOLOGY

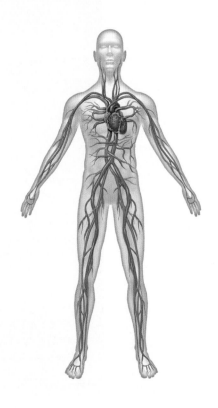

"Thanks to the continued advice from Phil on my strength work, nutrition and supplements, I'm fitter, stronger and leaner than I have ever been! I cannot stress enough the need to be smarter with all aspects of your nutrition and listen to what Phil has to offer......its helped me run personal best times and, at the age of 36, to get into the 2012 GB Olympic's Team".

Stuart Stokes (2012 Team GB Steeplechaser)

- There are not any books that I know on fat loss that would devote so much information about the cardiovascular system. The reason why I wanted to include information about the heart, blood vessels and blood is quite simple - there is no point being lean and dead. With heart disease being the biggest killer in Westernised countries, I wanted to share with you my knowledge on how to have a very healthy and functional cardiovascular system. Also of importance here is that the cardiovascular system is the transportation system of our nutrients, oxygen and hormones. There is no point eating clean if the roads (blood vessels) are clogged.

- The knowledge I'm about to share with you in this habit literally changed my life from the ages of 40 – 45. I had chronic breathing problems where it felt like I had an elephant sitting on my chest, whilst being strangled and drowned at the same time. I was constantly dizzy and felt as if I was going to pass out at any time. I was in a bad way and, through my research, I felt that it was my heart that was the cause and I that needed to increase its energy capacity so it could pump more strongly and efficiently.

- At the time, I felt that my problem was a deficiency in substrates for my heart when I now realise that was just one of the causes. The biggest cause was the accumulation of stress, which had built up over my entire life, which had strangled my heart.

- Nutritional cardiology is essential for the health of our heart, blood vessels & blood. For our 100 trillion plus cells to be kept well nourished, we need a fully functioning cardiovascular system which also must be well nourished for it to function at maximum efficiency.

Your Heart is the Key

- Most of us think of the heart as a pump that propels blood around the body. This is true, of course, but researchers at the leading edge of science are telling us that it is so much more than a mere pump.

- Traditionally, we think of the brain as the central computer of the body. It receives information from the five physical senses and sends information signals to the body to produce the desired actions and to drive physiological functions.

- I suspect that not many of you know that your heart is an organ that can learn, remember,

The Heart can Remember: a heart transplant story

- There are some fascinating stories coming from heart transplant recipients, such as those from Dr Paul Pearsall's book, "The Heart's Code".

- In one example, Pearsall tells of an eight year old girl who received a heart transplant from a ten year old girl who was murdered. After a successful operation, the eight year old began having nightmares about the man who had killed her donor.

- Distressed, the girl's mother took her to see a psychiatrist, who after a couple of sessions, began to think the girl might not just be having a stress response to her life threatening health problems and the major life change of her receiving a new heart. The psychiatrist could not deny what she was being told by the child. The girl's mother too came to suspect that perhaps this information might be useful to the police. It took some time but she finally overcame her resistance and called the appropriate authorities who came and talked to the girl.

- Astonishingly, armed with a description of the man and other information about the murder weapon and circumstances of the crime that the little girl gave them, the police were able to find the murderer, who was eventually convicted.

feel and sense independently of your brain. It's true.

- There are countless studies that have shown a link between mind and body diseases. Here is one just to magnify the huge importance of taking charge of your emotions.

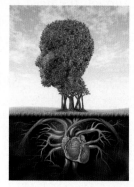

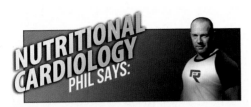

NUTRITIONAL CARDIOLOGY
PHIL SAYS:

When I started my research into nutritional cardiology my health changed. After I started combining high dose CoQ10, L-Carnitine, D-Ribose, Magnesium, Vitamin C, Lysine & Proline - BANG! Within 48 hours I was breathing deep lung-fulls of air which I hadn't been able to do so for years. My dizziness stopped almost immediately - it felt like I had got my life back. This got me more enthusiastic about my research and I developed a number of nutritional products which had a profound effect on my health. I am very excited to share this knowledge with you and the wonderful products which literally give me my life back.

- In a twenty five year follow-up study involving 255 University of North Carolina medical students, Dr. John Barefoot found those who scored highest in hostility on a standard personality test were nearly five times as likely to die of heart disease as their less hostile classmates. They were seven times more likely to die by the age of fifty.

- In 1993, a paper published by the Institute of Heart Math documented the fact that the information coded in our emotions plays a key role in the way the heart tells the brain which chemicals (hormones, endorphins and immune enhancers) to produce in our body at any given time,

- More precisely, our emotions tell our brains what we believe we need in that moment. This heart-brain communication is well document-

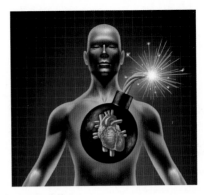

Hostility cripples the heart

ed in the open literature and generally accepted in the progressive medical community.

- Studies by the Institute of Heart Math also show that feelings associated with beliefs (heart-centered beliefs) are transmuted into the heart's electrical and magnetic waves that not only affect our bodies but are also sent out and interact with the physical world.

- Recurring feelings of frustration, worry, stress, and anger cause heart rhythms to become unbalanced and disordered.

- On the other hand, forgiveness, appreciation, and love create coherent, harmonious heart rhythms and affect the physical heart's electrical output, as seen in an ECG.

"Hatred paralyzes life; love releases it. Hatred confuses life; love harmonizes it. Hatred darkens life; love illuminates it." Martin Luther King Jr.

- The most extensive studies on heart disease have shown that a lack of happiness is one of the greatest risk factor for developing heart problems.

- Even remembering an upsetting experience can reduce the heart's pumping efficiency by 5-7% and decrease the immune system's potency for many hours.

The greatest revenge is massive success. Never hold grudges against anyone it will destroy you far more than it will destroy them and especially your heart.

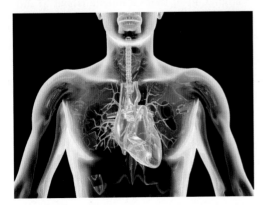

Your heart is a key organ and needs to be nourished, cared for and exercised to function optimumly

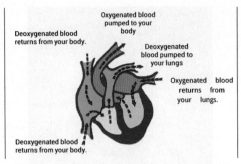

Your heart is a non-stop worker. It pumps deoxygenated blood from the body to the lungs, and then it pumps oygenated blood, it recieves from the lungs, around the body.

- A 9 year study in Finland showed that hostility is a major risk factor and predictor of coronary heart disease. Hostile people were more than three times likely to die from cardiovascular disease than those with a non-hostile approach to life.

- In the book "The Emotional Wellness Way to Cardiac Health", a study on the role of anger is discussed. It found that among 1,600 patients who had previously suffered a heart attack, the risk of another heart attack after an episode of anger was increased by 200%.

- A study at the Johns Hopkins School of Medicine tracked 1,337 male medical students for 36 years after medical school and found that students who became angry quickly under stress were three times more likely to develop premature heart disease and five times more likely to have an early heart attack. Angry young men, it appears, turn into angry old men with heart problems

- A Harvard study concluded that men who showed high hostility at the start of an eight-year investigation exhibited significantly poorer lung function at the end of it. "This research shows that hostility is associated with poorer [lung] function and more rapid rates of decline among older men," notes Rosalind Wright, an assistant professor at the Harvard School of Public Health.

- The biggest surprise that I personally had during my research on finding the most important nutritional factors that cause cardiovascular disease was that the media's and medical professions obsession with cholesterol when, in reality, that is a myth. Stress is undoubtedly the biggest killer when it comes to cardiovascular deaths.

- Of course, you must get good nutritional habits in place, as well as sensible lifestyle factors, but the most important factor is managing your stress factor if you do not want to become another heart disease statistic.

- Remember, you do not catch heart disease; you build it. You build it with the food you eat, your thoughts and the people you live with. Take every opportunity in life to have fun as this is the most therapeutic thing for the heart.

The Heart: a non-stop worker

- The world's most perfect pump is at this very moment right in your chest. The human heart is approximately the size of a fist, and is a pump made of muscle. With its non-stop beating, the heart sends all of your blood around your body some 1,000 times during the course of a single day.

- The heart's most important feature is being able to work without stopping, contracting around 40-70 times a minute (about 37 million times a year). It beats on average around 2.5 billion times during the average human

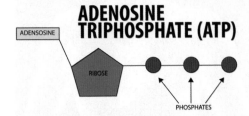

Adenosine triphosphate (ATP) is the energy used by an organism in its daily operations. It consists of an adenosine molecule and three inorganic phosphates. After a simple reaction breaking down ATP to ADP, the energy released from the breaking of a molecular bond is the energy we use to keep ourselves alive

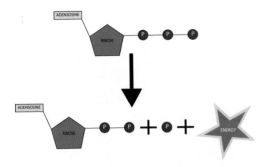

ATP is like a battery containing stored energy within a cell. When the cell requires energy, the bond between the 2nd and 3rd phosphate is broken, releasing some of the stored energy

lifespan and pumps approximately 300 million litres of blood.

- That is the equivalent of the amount of liquid it would take to fill 10,000 oil tankers. Even while you sleep, your heart pumps some 340 litres of blood. To put it another way, your heart could fill a car's petrol tank 9 times over every hour.

- Many of the processes that take place within your body are linked to the circulatory system, thanks to an exceedingly complex structure. A network of arteries and veins nourish the 100 trillion or so cells in your body, visiting every one individually. Many of the needs in all living things—such as carrying nourishment and gasses like oxygen to the cells, and eliminating waste products from the body—are met by substances carried by the circulatory system. In human beings, the liquid that performs all these functions is the blood. Every single cell in your body, from a skin cell on your fingertip to the specialized retinal cells in your eyes, depends on what blood provides.

- The mechanical stress of this non-stop work is a particular challenge to the millions of cells which make up the heart. These cells need an optimum supply of nutrients to ensure their proper functioning and the general health of the heart.

- It's all about ATP - the energy currency of the body (see below). Hearts, skeletal muscles, and every other tissue in our bodies have an absolute requirement for adenosine triphosphate, or ATP, as their primary energy currency.

- ATP molecules are both synthesized and recycled within the body, and supply all of the body's energy.

- Both the total pool of ATP in the cell and the cell's ability to recycle these compounds are fundamental to healthy energy metabolism and cell function.

- If you give your cells the ability to make optimal levels of energy, they can use it to do whatever they want: build and renew cell membranes, create and maintain cell structures, and replicate and protect cell information.

- Our immune function depends on adequate energy production, as does tissue maintenance such as bone building and muscle building. In fact it's impossible to think of any physiological function that is not linked in some way to our energy supply.

- Collectively, heart and circulatory diseases cause more than one in three of all deaths in the UK, accounting for more than 191,000 deaths each year at an estimated cost of £30 billion to the economy.

- Joanne Ingwell, a professor of physiology at Harvard University and an expert on energy metabolism of the heart, informs us that every event in the myocyte (heart cell) requires ATP.

- Diseased hearts are energy-starved, which means they lack enough ATP to fuel healthy cardiac function. Failing hearts lack adequate energy to drive pump function. As the heart is one of the most responsive organs in the body for targeted nutritional supplementation, practicing "nutritional cardiology" is a must.

- By enhancing ATP synthesis and recycling, and promoting more efficient metabolism in mitochondria, the correct nutritional support helps ailing hearts recover

- Nutritional cardiology aims to build up and maintain ATP stores in the heart, and ultimately enhance heart health, by providing the body with the nutrients it needs to make ENERGY.

People with heart disease often exhibit CoQ10, L-carnitine, D-ribose, and/or magnesium deficiencies.

- This information was first brought to my attention following the excellent work of American cardiologist Dr. Steven Sinatra.

CoQ10

- As a nutrient essential to ATP production, co-enzyme Q10 (CoQ10), is a VIP (very important particle) within your body. With the potential to help heal almost all cardiovascular conditions, it is one of the best nutrients you can feed your heart.

- CoQ10 can be synthesized within the body. There are, however, circumstances where the body does not make sufficient amounts. When deficiency occurs the heart may be the most affected leading to serious problems. Why?

Because the heart has such high metabolic (energy) demands.

- Often called the "miracle nutrient" or the "universal antioxidant," CoQ10 exists in the mitochondria of our cells, and scavenges and destroys free radicals that cause cardiovascular problems and heart disease. Hundreds of studies have documented the actions of CoQ10 and how they improve heart health.

- CoQ10 molecules perform a vital role in the production of the body's ATP. This is the key reason CoQ10 is probably the single best nutrient you can take for your heart.

- CoQ10 is an important part of the inner membranes of the mitochondria where the actual production of ATP occurs. Here electrons (negatively charged particles in atoms) are passed around in what is known as the electron

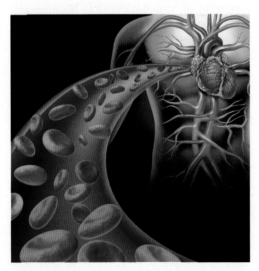

CoQ10, D-ribose, L-carnitine and magnesium all increase the power of the heart to pump blood efficiently

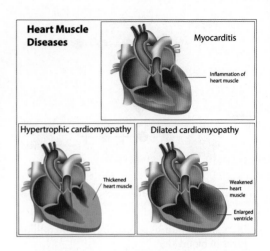

Heart Muscle Diseases

Myocarditis

Inflammation of heart muscle

Hypertrophic cardiomyopathy

Thickened heart muscle

Dilated cardiomyopathy

Weakened heart muscle

Enlarged ventricle

transport chain. CoQ10's job is to collect and transfer these electrons along the chain, which helps power the production of ATP.

- It is believed that CoQ10 is the key nutrient for generating 95% of the total energy required by the human body.

- Your heart muscle consumes huge amounts of oxygen and energy. CoQ10 essentially recharges the energy system in the heart, enabling the heart muscle to pump blood more efficiently.

- One of the most serious heart conditions caused by a CoQ10 deficiency is congestive heart failure.

Congestive Heart Failure

- Congestive heart failure (CHF) is the inability of the heart to pump blood effectively to the body. Congestive heart failure does not mean that the heart has stopped working completely, but does mean that the heart is not pumping as strongly as it should.

- As a result, some of the blood that is normally pumped out of the heart backs up into the lungs and other parts of the body, causing a build-up of fluids in the body (resulting in swelling), shortness of breath and fatigue

- CoQ10 pioneer Karl Folkers claimed that the primary source of CoQ10 in man is biosynthesis. Folkers argues that suboptimal nutrient intake in man is almost universal, causing subsequent secondary impairment in CoQ10 biosynthesis.

- According to CoQ10 expert Peter H. Langsjoen, MD. This means that average or "normal" levels of CoQ10 are really suboptimal and the very low levels observed in advanced disease states represent only the tip of a deficiency ice berg..

- In the early 1980's, Karl Folkers collaborated with Peter Langsjoen, of the Scott and White Clinic in Temple, Texas, in the first well controlled cardiomyopathy (a weakening of the heart muscle or another problem with the heart muscle. It often occurs when the heart cannot pump as well as it should) study of CoQ10.

- The effect of CoQ10 on nineteen patients, all of whom were expected to die of heart failure were astounding. They made an "extraordinary clinical improvement", the researchers said. Heart size decreased and blood pumping improved, regardless of the form of cardiomyopathy.

- If mitochondria are little engines, which use oxygen to burn the organic fuels that come from foodstuffs, then you may think of CoQ10 as the part of the engine that provides the spark for this process. No other substance will substitute for CoQ10. Without CoQ10, there is no spark and therefore no production of energy for the cell. And, without energy, there is no life

- A significant link has been found to exist between low levels of CoQ10 and congestive heart failure. The lower the levels of CoQ10, the more severe the heart failure.

- Depriving the heart of CoQ10 is like removing a spark plug from your engine -- it just won't work. Low levels of CoQ10 are implicated in virtually all cardiovascular diseases, including angina, hypertension, cardiomyopathy and congestive heart failure.

CoQ10 is also known as ubiquinone. That simply means it is found everywhere (in every cell) of our bodies. This fact alone should give us a feel for how important it is to our survival and proper health!

- CoQ10 plays many vitals roles in numerous bodily processes such as: cellular energy production; cell membrane stabilization; prevention of LDL (Low-density lipoprotein: one of the five major groups of lipoproteins) oxidation.

- CoQ10 also plays an important role in reducing platelet size, distribution, stickiness and limiting platelet aggregation and activation.

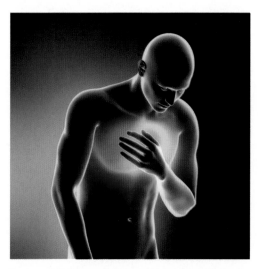

Poorly nourished hearts often become diseased hearts. You need to give the heart a constant supply of oxygen and usable energy.

As well as these it also helps prevent blood clot formations.

- Research indicates that if levels of CoQ10 decline by 25% our organs may become deficient and impaired. If levels decline by 75% serious tissue damage and even death may occur.

Strengthening the Heart Muscle: The Power of CoQ10

- Studies have shown that nutrients and supplements can strengthen the heart muscle, with fewer side effects than the powerful pharmaceuticals often used to treat the condition. CoQ10 is one of the most powerful.

- Present in high quantities throughout the heart muscle, CoQ10 has many beneficial effects, including energy production (Awata N et al 1980; Crane FL et al 1997; Nakamura Y et al 1982; Nayler WG 1980), an antioxidant effect (Frei B et al 1990), and stabilizing the heart membrane (Ondarroa M et al 1986).

Heart muscle requires an incredible amount of CoQ10 to circulate oxygenated and nutrient-rich blood through your body.

- It's well known among integrative cardiologists that heart failure (HF) patients have low blood concentrations of CoQ10. Although CoQ10 is made naturally in the body, production falls off as we age. It is also blocked by certain medications, including statin drugs.

- A group of New Zealand doctors tested the hypothesis that CoQ10 blood levels are a predictor of total mortality in HF. They took blood samples from 236 hospitalized HF patients and then followed them for an average of 2.7 years. The researchers concluded that CoQ10 concentration in the blood is an independent predictor of mortality and that a deficiency is indeed associated with worse outcomes in HF.

- A study conducted at Japan's Toyama University Hospital followed 29 patients with significant coronary artery disease (CAD), none of whom had overt HF. All 29 received either 5 or 10 mg of a well known statin drug once daily for three months.

- At the end of the study, the researchers found that most participants had a lower blood level of CoQ10 than they had at the trial's start. They noted that as cholesterol goes down, so does CoQ10. The greater the reduction in cholesterol levels, the more significant the drop in vital CoQ10 levels.

- This study re-confirms that regular treatment with statins depletes CoQ10.

- *"In fact, I strongly recommend that anyone – and especially those with any known cardiac condition like hypertension, blocked coronary arteries, or arrhythmia – supplement their statin therapy with at least 200 mg of CoQ10 daily, in divided doses."*

  Dr Stephen Sinatra Cardiologist

- More than 35 controlled clinical trials in Japan, Europe and the U.S. have proven that CoQ10 therapy is highly effective in treatment of congestive heart failure, angina and ischemic heart disease, and myocardial infarction.

- One study has shown that CoQ10 reduces oxidative stress (damage from free radicals) in patients with atherosclerosis: Following a placebo-controlled trial, researchers from Taiwan concluded that a daily CoQ10 dose of 150 mg was associated with a 29% drop in a dangerous marker of oxidative stress called malondialdehyde (MDA). MDA has been implicated in cardiovascular disease, specifically in the progression of atherosclerosis.

- In the study, the researchers recruited 51 people with known coronary heart disease and randomized them into two groups: a group receiving either 60 mg or 150 mg/day of CoQ10 and a placebo group. The participants were followed for 12 weeks.

- At eight weeks, MDA levels decreased significantly in CoQ10 group when compared to the placebo group. After 12 weeks, the group receiving the higher dose increased CoQ10 blood levels by 189%

- The authors from Chung Shan Medical University concluded:

- *"We believe a higher dose of CoQ10 supplements (greater than 150 mg/day) might provide rapid and sustainable antioxidant [protection] in patients with coronary heart disease."*

- Heart disease may even be caused by a cholesterol deficiency; According to Dr. Stephanie Seneff:

- *"Heart disease, I think, is a cholesterol deficiency problem, and in particular a cholesterol sulfate deficiency problem..."*

- Through her research, she has developed a theory in which the mechanism we call "cardiovascular disease" (of which arterial plaque is a hallmark) is actually your body's way to compensate for not having enough cholesterol sulfate. She believes that cholesterol combines with sulphur to form cholesterol sulfate, and this cholesterol sulfate helps thin your blood by serving as a reservoir for the electron donations you receive when walking barefoot on the earth (also called grounding). She believes that, via this blood-thinning mechanism, cholesterol sulfate may provide natural protection against heart disease. In fact, she goes so far as to hypothesize that heart disease is likely the result of cholesterol deficiency — which of

---

Getting your daily need of CoQ10

- You can get your CoQ10 through foods you eat such as meat, poultry and fish in that order. 3 ounces of beef for instance will get you about 2.6 mg. of CoQ10. 3 ounces of oily fish such as herring will get you 2.3 mg and 3 ounces of chicken will get you 1.4 mg (nuts, seeds and whole grains also contain CoQ10 to a lesser degree).

- Relatively good food-based sources of CoQ10 include animal products such as beef, pork and chicken with organ meats such as the heart ranking highest.

CoQ10 Typical Daily Dosages

- 90 - 250 mg daily for the prevention of cardiovascular and periodontal diseases;
- 180 - 360 mg daily if you have hypertension and heavy exerciser;
- 300 - 600 mg daily for those with CHF (Start with 180 mg and work up to 300+ mg over three weeks);and
- 600 - 1,200+ mg daily for people with Parkinson's disease and other debilitating illness such as cancer

- Recommended dose: Take at least 100–300 mg of CoQ10 daily if you have any form of heart disease (the most serious cases and those people taking a statin to lower LDL cholesterol levels may require even more). For best results, take CoQ10 in divided doses with your meals. It's more readily absorbed with food (especially some fat). Always consult with your health care provider before taking any supplementation.

course is diametrically opposed to the conventional view.

- High cholesterol is a warning to you to control inflammation. Inflammation in the body generates C-reactive protein, which in turn causes the body to respond with soothing, repairing, life-saving cholesterol. C-reactive protein is a measure of the body's history of inflammation and a far better predictor of heart attacks than cholesterol levels.

- Vitamin C and fish oil have both been proven to reduce your C-reactive proteins better than statin drugs ever will! Tufts University, Berkeley, Seattle's University of Washington School of Medicine, Linus Pauling Institute and others have beaten statin drug statistics with as little as 500 mg a day of vitamin C. When studied, heart attack rates in vitamin C groups have fallen but the statin drug users still had "heart events", fatal heart attacks, and the usual accompanying diabetes risk.

- Peter H. Langsjoen, MD has said, *"We are now in a position to witness the unfolding of the greatest medical tragedy of all time - never before in history has the medical establishment knowingly created a life threatening nutrient deficiency in millions of otherwise healthy people".*

- The deficiency that Peter was talking about was a CoQ10 deficiency.

- You must remember that lowering cholesterol has become a multi-billion pound industry worldwide and there is a lot of misinformation about cholesterol. In my opinion, this is to scare the general public into unknowingly taking statin medication when in reality, they should be questioning the medical profession more on the side effects of statins.

- One in three people over the age of 45 in the UK currently takes statins – that's a staggering 7 million people. It costs the National Health Service £450 million per year to fulfill these prescriptions...which goes straight into the pockets of the drug companies and their consultants in the medical establishment.

- A new born baby that is being breast fed by its mother receives a high dose of cholesterol right from the beginning of its life. Mothers milk contains twice the cholesterol of cows milk. Nature has no intention of destroying a baby's heart by giving it such high amounts of cholesterol. On the contrary a healthy heart consists of 10% pure cholesterol (all water removed).

- Your liver can make cholesterol but it takes a lot of effort. It's a 25-30 step process, very complex and, of course, for this you require various substrates. The liver has a lot of functions. So making cholesterol is just one of the things it does, that's why it is essential to eat foods rich in cholesterol.

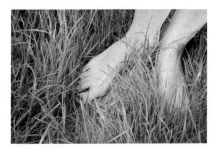

Dr Stephanie Seneff believes that walking barefoot on the earth (or earthing/grounding) can have a great impact on our health

- Every single one of your cells needs cholesterol to thrive, and when your levels get too low, it can wreak havoc on your health, even increasing your risk of cancer. In 2007 a meta-analysis of over 41,000 patient records found that people who take statin drugs to lower their cholesterol as much as possible may have a higher risk of cancer, and research since has confirmed the significant association between low cholesterol and cancer mortality.

- All kinds of other problems can occur as well when your cholesterol levels get too low, including episodes of violent behaviour, depressive symptoms, hormonal imbalances, memory loss, stroke and even Parkinson's disease. This is why keeping your cholesterol levels higher may actually help you to prevent disease.

- Since we cannot possibly eat enough cholesterol to use for our bodies' daily functions, our bodies make their own. When we eat more foods rich in this compound, our bodies make less. If we deprive ourselves of foods high in cholesterol -- such as eggs, butter, and liver — our body revs up its cholesterol synthesis. The end result is that, for most of us, eating foods high in cholesterol has very little impact on our blood cholesterol levels.

- Moreover, cholesterol-rich foods are the main source of arachidonic acid (AA). While AA is often said to be inflammatory, it is actually the most critically essential fatty acid in the body. Healthy adults only need very little, if any, of it, but growing children, women who are looking to conceive or are pregnant or nursing, and people who are body building, suffering from degenerative diseases involving oxidative stress, or recovering from injury need to consume AA in the diet. Strict vegans and those who consume lots of omega-3 fats might also require AA in the diet. Signs of deficiency include scaly skin, hair loss, and infertility.

- The way to bring down your LDL in a healthy way is to get sunlight exposure in the skin. Your skin will produce cholesterol sulfate which will then flow freely to the blood not packaged up inside LDL and therefore the liver doesn't have to make so much LDL. So the LDL goes down.

- In fact, in places that are sunny there is a complete inverse relationship between sunlight and cardiovascular disease – the more sunlight, the less cardiovascular disease.

- It is estimated that most folks don't get more than 10 mg from foods. Since cells will absorb and utilize CoQ10 made available in the blood, consuming foods and supplements with CoQ10 can make up for deficiencies caused by age, malnutrition, or drug interference.

- A healthy, youthful human body can make its own CoQ10. Endogenous production or biosynthesis of CoQ10 has 17 steps, requiring at least seven vitamins (vitamin B2 - riboflavin, vitamin B3 - niacinamide, vitamin B6, folic acid, vitamin B12, vitamin C, and pantothenic acid) and several trace elements.

- Researcher Dr. John Ely, of the University of Washington, holds that CoQ10 supplementation is essential in the aged. Most people make approximately 500 mg of Coq10 daily in the body, at least up until age 21.

- However, between ages 21 and 30, levels of CoQ10 begin to drop, perhaps because of aging. This causes the degeneration of cells, which may contribute to age-related diseases and conditions such as high blood pressure, arthritis, heart disease and the breakdown of skin tissue.

- Statin drugs and deficiencies in several other vitamins also cause blood levels of CoQ10 to drop.

- To reiterate; statin drugs, (as well as tricyclic antidepressants and beta blockers) deplete CoQ10 and if CoQ10 is not given at the same time as these drugs, cardiomyopathy or CHF may result.

- An over-active thyroid or a pulsating heart will also require additional CoQ10.

- Also, if you exercise strenuously you are using your body's supply. High intensity exercise has been shown to lower CoQ10. This is most probably due to the consequence of an excess of free radicals caused by increased metabolic demands of chronically exercising muscles.

- In a double-blind, placebo-controlled study published in 2008 in the Journal of the International Society of Sports Nutrition, Baylor University scientists found that supplements of 100 and 200 milligrams increased CoQ10 levels in muscles and prolonged the length of exercise in healthy adults.

- A double-blind, placebo-controlled study from researchers at the University Graduate School of Medicine, Osaka, Japan, published in 2008 in Nutrition, showed that 300 milligrams of CoQ10 helped exercise bikers achieve higher velocities for longer periods of time and recover from fatigue more rapidly.

L-Carnitine and the Heart

- Combining CoQ10 with another nutrient called L-Carnitine is very effective at improving the heart's function.

- L-carnitine is a compound produced by the liver and kidneys from the biosynthesis of the amino acids lysine and methionine. To form L-carnitine you also need adequate levels of folic acid, vitamin C, B6, niacin, and iron.

- The name carnitine is derived form the Latin 'camus' for flesh as carnitine was first isolated form meat sources.

- Carnitine is the gatekeeper for fat burning, it picks up fat and dumps it into the mitochondria for burning to create ATP. The more carnitine present, the more fat burnt.

- The heart is a fat hog and this is essential for the heart to fire on all cylinders.

- Since the heart is our hardest-working muscle, it is no surprise that carnitine improves myocardial metabolism.

- This is evidenced by increased fatty-acid uptake by the mitochondria, and higher concentrations of ATP and creatine phosphate (a storage form of ATP) in the heart tissue after carnitine supplementation.

- Carnitine's role is to exclusively ferry fatty acids to be oxidized to make ATP. L-carnitine is essential for the transport of fatty acids into the heart muscle and mitochondria for energy production and is sensitive to the level of oxygen in the heart muscle. So the body needs a lot of

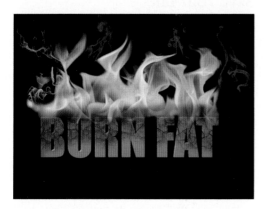

L-carnitine transports fat into the mitochondria to be burnt as fuel.

Chronic Obstructive Pulmonary Disease (COPD)

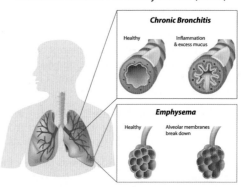

it to be optimally energized. A normal heart muscle derives 60-70 percent of its fuel from fat. That means anyone with heart disease or a weak heart will have a hard time getting better without addressing the problem of fat delivery inside the heart muscle.

- There is also the well-documented finding that L-Carnitine lowers triglycerides, and this alone dramatically lowers the risk of heart disease.

- Lower plasma triglycerides means that blood is less thick with fats, and can move more easily even through the narrow capillaries. And since carnitine also raises HDL cholesterol, blood vessels stay cleaner, again improving blood flow.

- L-carnitine is also a vasodilator meaning it opens blood vessels and increases blood flow to your heart, muscles and other tissues, resulting in better overall oxygen use by your body.

- L-carnitine also addresses two of the most serious problems associated with CHF by improving ejection fraction and preventing enlargement of the left ventricle, .

- Studies have shown that patients with CHF who take L-carnitine have improved ejection fraction (Goa KL et al 1987; Mancini M et al 1992; Pucciarelli G et al 1992).

- In one human trial, carnitine improved exercise tolerance and the strength of respiratory muscles in COPD (Chronic Obstructive Pulmonary Disease) patients; levels of the metabolic by-product lactate, which causes fatigue, were also reduced (Borghi-Silva A et al 2006).

- Equally important, carnitine transports waste material out of the mitochondria, such as toxic metabolites that could otherwise disturb the burning of fats and cause disruption inside of cells.

- The human body is a high energy machine. It creates a lot of toxic waste and accumulates outside toxins as well. In the interest of getting rid of the gunk and maintaining good health over a lifetime, carnitine gives you a huge detoxification weapon.

- In a study published in April, 2003 - L-Carnitine was found to help protect the heart from lack of oxygen and from oxygen free radicals.

- Taking carnitine at 1.5 to 6 grams per day for up to one year resulted in fewer deaths and less heart failure episodes in heart attack patients. Compared to placebo, carnitine use was found to slow heart enlargement over time.

- The typical non-vegetarian, Western diet provides around 100-300 mg of carnitine per day. The amount has decreased by an estimated 20 percent over the last decade, mainly as a result of people eating less red meat. Ovo-lacto-vegetarians (egg and dairy eating vegetarians) have an intake of about 10-40 mg, and strict vegetarians, maybe around 1-4 mg.

Food sources of carnitine include meat, poultry, fish, and dairy products are the richest sources of L-carnitine. Grains, fruits, and vegetables contain little or no carnitine.

- Research indicates that when your muscles are loaded with carnitine, it can help reduce the breakdown of amino acids that make up your muscle proteins for energy production. So preventing the use of amino acids for energy reduces the breakdown of muscles.

- When you exercise, if your body uses amino acids for energy, breakdown of muscle mass invariably occurs. In addition to proper protein intake, higher amounts of carnitine in your muscles can deter the use of amino acids for energy production during exercise, and therefore help protect against muscle breakdown and damage.

According to Robert Crayhon (author of "The Miracle of Carnitine" Due to high consumption of red meat, the Stone Age hunter probably got at least 500 mg of carnitine a day,

Giving your heart the nutrients it needs such as CoQ10, carnitine, D-ribose and magnesium will help keep it stronger for many years to come

and possibly as much as 2 grams.

Today the average carnitine intake is estimated at a mere 30 to 50 mg a day. Strict vegetarians consume practically no carnitine.

- Carnitine is useful in clearing the bloodstream of ammonia and aids in creating glycogen, used to store essential glucose.

- Research has shown that L-Carnitine has the ability to remove lactic acid from the blood and tissues helps promote ATP production, and helps short circuit the exhaustion that comes from strenuous physical activity.

- Studies have shown that, at doses of 1-3 g, carnitine reduces blood triglycerides. Carnitine combines with enzymes found in the mitochondrial membrane to transport fatty acids into the interior of the mitochondria, where they are oxidized to provide fuel for the generation of energy. In the absence of carnitine, fatty acids are not oxidized, but, instead, are transformed into dangerous triglycerides.

D-Ribose: Energize Your Heart, Save Your Life

- While coenzyme CoQ10 and L-carnitine both directly support ATP recycling, the most efficient means of cardiac energy metabolism, D-ribose helps ensure there's enough original ATP synthesized for your mitochondria to recycle.

- Some exciting studies have emerged showing how D-ribose affects active human heart tissue and its function. Investigators have shown how increased ATP levels translate into improved heart muscle function & better blood flow.
Pauly DF, Pepine CJ. Ischemic heart disease: metabolic approaches to management. Clin

Cardiol. 2004 Aug;27(8):439-41. Pauly DF, Johnson C, St Cyr JA. The benefits of ribose in cardiovascular disease. Med Hypotheses. 2003 Feb;60(2):149-51

- There's excellent science to back up the idea that D-ribose is good for working muscles. Exercise physiologists have showed that supplementing the muscles with D-ribose increases the total amount of ATP produced by up to four-fold, providing a substantial "bank" of energy that could be called on for use when needed.

- And when physiologists in Missouri provided D-ribose to working muscles, they demonstrated as much as a six-fold rise in the rate at which ATP components were recycled for use (recycling ATP is much faster and more efficient than building it from scratch).

Humans "burn" an amount of ATP equivalent to their own body weight every day!

What Exactly is D-Ribose

- D-ribose is a 5-carbohydrate monosaccharide (sugar) molecule found in every living organism which facilitates the production of cell energy

- If you can remember from earlier, D-ribose is a part of the ATP molecule which is used as the energy currency of cells.

- The body can manufacture ribose from glucose in something called the Pentose Phosphate Pathway [PPP]- this is a slow process which requires an enzyme called glucose-6-phosphate dehydrogenase (G- 6-PDH), an enzyme that is typically in short supply.

- The Pentose Phosphate Pathway is variable between organs and Glucose-6-phosphate dehydrogenase (G- 6-PDH) is an enzyme that has limited expression in the heart with significant delay in the production of ribose via glucose if there is injury to the heart

- Supplemental ribose by-passes this enzymatic step to rapidly replenish ATP levels in heart and muscle

Increasing ATP using Ribose

- Strenuously exercised muscle may have lowered levels of ATP by 20% and it may then take 3 - 4 days to replenish these ATP levels.

- Supplementing with ribose can increase the replenishment of ATP by up to 4 times

- Human cells can manufacture D-ribose. However, when muscle has been stressed by injury or due to high energy demands, the cells may not be able to produce enough D-ribose for ATP production. In other words, the cells have

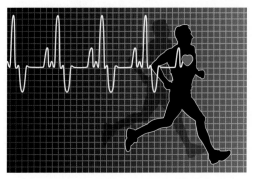

Studies have shown that supplemental D-ribose can increase exercise tolerance, especially in those with cardiovascular problems.

trouble keeping up with the demand for this simple sugar.

- The D-ribose connection to cardiac function was made by the physiologist Heinz-Gerd Zimmer at the University of Munich. In 1973, he reported that energy-starved hearts could recover faster if D-ribose was given prior to, or immediately following, ischemia (oxygen deprivation).

- Five years later, he reported the same effect in skeletal muscle and also showed for the first time that the energy-draining effects of drugs that make the heart beat more strongly (inotropic agents) could be lessened if D-ribose was given along with the drug

- Zimmer and his research colleagues later proved that D-ribose was the limiting element in energy recovery in ischemic tissue and that energy synthesis could not occur without it.

- A clinical study from Zimmer's group in Munich in 1992 showed that D-ribose administration to patients with severe, stable coronary artery disease increased exercise tolerance and delayed the onset of moderate angina.

- Several other notable papers were published in 2003. One study showed that D-ribose improved diastolic functional performance of the heart, increased exercise tolerance, and significantly improved the quality of life of heart patients.

- Every cell in the human body makes some of this simple sugar molecule, but only slowly and to varying degrees, depending on the tissue. The liver, adrenal glands, and fat tissue produce the most—enough to serve their purpose of making compounds involved in the production of hormones and fatty acids.

Red meat, particularly veal, contains the highest dietary concentration of D-ribose, but not significant enough to provide any meaningful nutritional support, especially to unwell individuals.

- Heart, skeletal muscle, brain, and nerve tissue can only make enough D-ribose to manage their day-to-day needs when their cells are not stressed.

- Unfortunately, these cells lack the metabolic machinery to make D-ribose quickly when they come under metabolic stress such as blood and oxygen deprivation (ischemia).

- When oxygen or blood flow deficits are chronic, as in heart disease, tissues can never make enough D-ribose. Cellular energy levels become depleted.

- Ischemia may cause the heart to lose up to 50% of its ATP pool. Even if blood flow and oxygen are restored to normal levels, it may take up to 10 days for an otherwise healthy animal heart to rebuild cellular energy and normalize diastolic cardiac function.

- In studies, when oxygen-starved animals receive D-ribose, energy recovery and diastolic function return to normal in an average of two days. When patients with CAD (coronary ar-

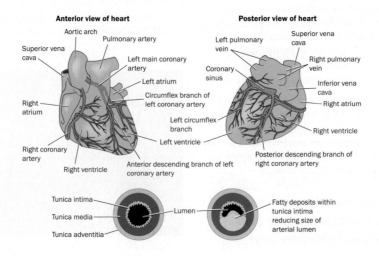

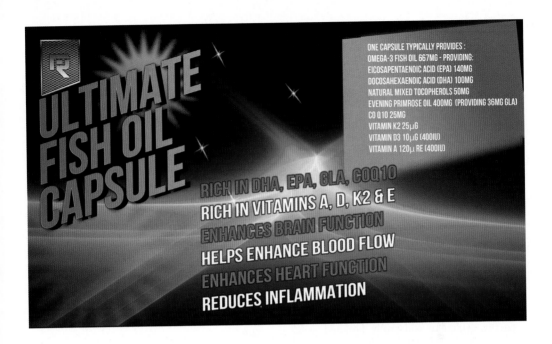

This book is in no way written as an advert for our products. But, I wanted to bring these two in particular to your attention. The whole reason why I developed these products was solely from my research into nutritional cardiology. As you can see from the ingredients, I have included many of the nutrients that I have discussed such as omega-3 fatty acids, CoQ10, hawthorn, taurine and many, many more. The ingredients in these 2 products have made a tremendous difference to my health and many others that I have recommended them to.

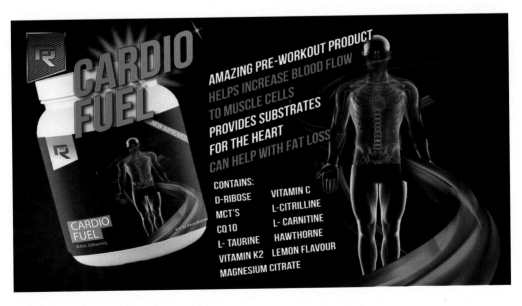

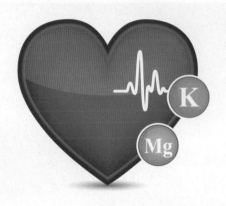

type of muscle tested, and improve the salvage of energy compounds by up to 650%.

- Most amazing is that when muscles are supplemented with D-ribose, they continue to add to their energy stores even while they actively work! Until this study was reported, it was thought that muscle energy stores were only refilled in muscles at rest.

- Patients with arterial and heart disease who chronically choke off oxygen delivery to their tissues need to take a higher dosage simply to allow enough of it to work its way through the clogged vessels into the energy-parched portions of the heart.

- A study published in the International Journal of Cardiology stated: *"Ribose, a pentose monosaccharide, has shown to replenish low myocardial energy levels, improving cardiac dysfunction following ischemia, and improving ventilation efficiency in patients with heart failure."*

- In studies of healthy athletes, supplying fatigued muscle cells with D-ribose quickly restored cell energy to normal levels.
Am J Physiol Regul Integr Comp Physiol. 2004 Jan;286(1):R182-8.

- D-ribose can also actually lower blood glucose levels; therefore, insulin-dependent diabetics should check with their physicians before starting on the supplement.

- As you can see, D-ribose is a very important component of our ATP and so, therefore, an important part of our bodies.

Magnesium

- Since all enzymatic reactions involving ATP have an absolute requirement for MAGNESIUM, it makes perfect sense to include magnesium to any program which wants to enhance heart function.

- Magnesium is vitally important in regulating what goes into and what comes out of all the body's cells. If the level of magnesium within cells fall below normal, calcium and sodium rush inside while potassium and magnesium leak out.

- If this occurs in heart cells' normal function is impaired and there is a tendency towards excess contraction which can cause big problems

tery disease) are treated with D-ribose, symptoms and treadmill time improve significantly within one week.

- Patients with coronary artery disease and persistent symptoms remain in a chronic state of energy depletion, constantly fatigued, weak, and with their heart function progressively worsening. These patients will do well with D-Ribose supplementation.

- These patients will almost certainly advance into congestive heart failure without improvement of the energy state of their heart. Restoration of their energy pool can only be accomplished through the pathway of energy metabolism regulated by the availability of D-ribose.

- *"We cannot overstate the effect of D-ribose supplementation on maintaining energy levels. Any tissue that relies heavily on aerobic energy metabolism, such as the heart and muscles, will be severely affected by any amount of oxygen deprivation. The problem is ATP drain. The solution is to give it back!"* Dr Stephan Sinatra & Dr James Roberts

- Supplemental D-ribose absorbs easily and quickly through the gut and into the bloodstream. About 97% gets through.

- Studies have shown that any amount of D-ribose you give to energy-starved cells gives them an energy boost.

- At the University of Missouri, researcher Ronald Terjung has shown that even very small doses (the equivalent of about 500 mg) of D-ribose increase energy salvage in muscles by more than 100%.

- Larger doses increase the production of energy compounds by 340-430%, depending on the

for the heart. This is what cardiologists refer to as a stone heart

- Magnesium can reduce your risk of sudden cardiac death by nearly 40%, according to a study out of the University of Minnesota. Researchers measured the serum levels of magnesium in more than 14,000 patients. In that group, those who had the highest level of magnesium reduced their risk of sudden cardiac arrest (heart attack) by 38%.

- Magnesium can be amazingly effective at calming down erratic and excitable heartbeats, a leading cause of sudden cardiac arrest.

- A ten-year study of 2,182 men in Wales found that those eating magnesium-low diets had a 50% higher risk of sudden death from heart attacks than those eating one-third more magnesium.

- With insufficient magnesium the muscles stay tense and, through the years, may cause a cramp in the muscle. This could happen when you have too much calcium or too little magnesium. Too much calcium causes the heart to go into a spasm and this can cause a heart attack.

- Magnesium has a stabilizing effect on cell membranes, particularly in heart muscle. A healthy heart generates stable, predictable electrical impulses. Lack of magnesium permits unstable electrical impulses in the heart to emerge, generating abnormal heart rhythms.

Foods rich in magnesium include whole grains, fish and seafood, leafy green vegetables, soy products, brown rice, bananas, apricots, seeds and nuts. The foods highest in magnesium include kelp, tofu, figs and pumpkin seeds

Taurine

- Taurine is the most abundant amino acid in the heart. Taurine has been shown to improve nitric oxide production in the vascular endothelium, which is essential to optimal blood flow, maintaining already normal blood pressure, and overall cardiovascular functioning.

- Taurine is an important amino acid in our body. It is found mostly in our central nervous system, skeletal muscle, and in greater concen-tration in our heart and brain. It is made from two sulphur containing amino acids called methionine and cysteine are found in egg yolk and meat as well.

- Taurine is commonly found in animal protein and not in vegetable protein. Vegetarians with a low intake of protein may have difficulty producing taurine in their bodies

- In the cell, taurine keeps potassium and magnesium inside the cell while keeping excessive sodium out. In this sense it works like a diuretic. But unlike prescription diuretics, it is not a cellular poison.

- There have been studies showing the positive effectiveness of taurine on heart failure. Aside from having diuretic properties, taurine is able to strengthen the heart muscles and maintain proper calcium balance. Together with Coq10 and carnitine, taurine is able to regulate the heart's contractility.

- Working together with magnesium, taurine also is able to regulate heart rhythm and help to stabilize it

- At high taurine concentrations, any access fluid in your blood and tissues surrounding your heart is flushed out, leading to lower blood pressure and reduced cardiac stress.

- Taurine also inhibits the action of angiotensin II, the hormone that increases blood vessel constriction.

- Increased taurine concentration allows blood vessels to expand which further reduces your blood pressure and your risk of strokes and coronary heart disease.

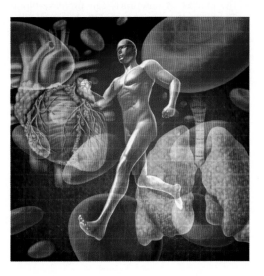

- Taurine must be present to make bile acid, which enables fat and cholesterol metabolism

- Taurine supplementation has been used in combination with coenzyme Q10 to prevent and treat atherosclerosis and hyperlipidemia.

- Taurine is found in abundance in the myocardium of the heart. It helps to modulate the low voltage-dependent calcium channel which allows the transmission of action potential whereby triggering contraction of heart muscles.

- Low taurine levels can reduce the strength of heart muscle contraction and cardiac output. Sustained deficiency can increase your risk of cardiomyopathy

- Taurine also partners with magnesium to maintain proper heart rhythm, and has been used as an effective treatment for cardiac arrhythmia.

- Research on the amino acid taurine suggests that it may be beneficial for those patients with congestive heart failure conditions. In a clinical trial with 14 patients where the patients served as their own control group via a crossover study design, 79% improved with 4 weeks of taurine supplementation compared to 21% on placebo.

Hawthorn

- Another nutrient called hawthorn works with CoQ10 to increase energy in the heart muscle, improves circulation in the coronary arteries and helps to regulate blood pressure.

- The extract of hawthorn can increase blood flow to the heart muscle itself, helping to counteract one of the most common modern causes of death in industrial countries.

- In pharmacological tests on both animals and humans, hawthorn has been shown to improve the contractility of the heart muscle (which can lead to a stronger pumping action of the heart), increase cardiac performance and output, lower the peripheral vascular resistance (reducing the workload of the heart), steady the heartbeat (anti-arrhythmic effect), as well as increasing the heart's tolerance to oxygen deficiency, such as might happen during stress or excitement, or in diseases where the arteries are partially blocked.

- A four year study on the benefits of hawthorn, commissioned by the German Ministry of Health, found that it improves contractions in the veins and heart while dilating the heart. This increases blood flow in the heart as well as flow speed throughout the body for increased circulation to organs and musculature. The researchers concluded that hawthorn is best used for low heart function, congestion, arrhythmia and tightness in the chest and no side effects were noted (Hoffmann 1995).

- A German clinical trial with 18 healthy patients found that hawthorn lowered heart rate and blood pressure during exercise and maintained resting heart rate while elevations were noted in the control group (Hellenbrecht, et. al. 1990).

- Chinese laboratory and clinical trials have reported that hawthorn lowers cholesterol and triglycerides by improving excretion (Chang & But 1986). Hawthorn is also reported to increase urination (DJumlija 1994) (Hoffmann 1995), often an important modality in heart conditions.

Omega-3

- We have talked extensively about the benefits of omega-3 but here is just another sampling, this time in regards to the health of the cardiovascular system:

  - Anti-arrhythmic: counteracting or preventing cardiac arrhythmia
  - Anti-thrombotic: tending to prevent thrombosis (a blood clot within a blood vessel)
  - Anti-atherosclerotic: preventing fatty deposits and fibrosis of the inner layer of your arteries from forming
  - Anti-inflammatory: counteracting inflammation (heat, pain, swelling, etc.)

- Omega-3s also improve endothelial function: a major factor in promoting the growth of new blood vessels.

- Researchers have found that omega-3 oils stop the build up of fatty deposits in the arteries, which is why oily fish and fish oils protect against heart disease and stroke.

- Researchers at the University of Edinburgh suggest that fish oils prevent the platelet activa-

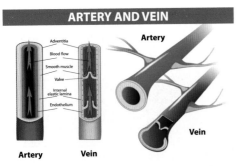

ARTERY AND VEIN

Artery

Adventitia
Blood flow
Smooth muscle
Valve
Internal elastic lamina
Endothelium

Vein

Artery   Vein

Our arteries carry oxygenated blood and our veins carry deoxygenated blood.

tion involved in the formation of atherosclerotic lesions and blood clots (thrombosis).

- A recent study in The European Journal of Clinical Nutrition found that increasing the omega-3's from fish and fish oil reduce the risk of heart failure by 25%.

- Borage oil helps in regulating blood circulation in the arteries and veins. It also prevents the internal clotting of blood. Regular use of borage oil helps in reducing the danger of diseases like high blood pressure and hypertension. The GLA present in this oil reduces body serums and thus protects the body from high cholesterol and heart diseases.

Our Arteries

If you took all of the blood vessels out of an average adult, and laid them out in one line, the line would be around 60 000 - 100 000 miles long!

- Blood vessels are structures that carry the blood from the heart to all the tissues of the body and then back to the heart.

- As such, they must be constructed for carrying fluids over long distances, allowing for exchange of materials to and from the blood, and for vasoconstriction/vasodilation to alter blood flow.

- There are three varieties of blood vessels: arteries, veins, and capillaries.

- Arteries carry blood full of oxygen, picked up in the lungs after you inhale, away from the heart to every tissue of the body.

- As the blood travels further from the heart, the arteries get smaller and smaller. Soon they are

so tiny, they are just one cell thick. Now they are called capillaries.

- There are capillaries lying right next to all of the tissues in the body. They will give off their oxygen and nutrients then take on carbon dioxide and wastes for excretion.

- Now the blood is "oxygen poor" and will start its trip back to the heart. The blood travels back to the heart in veins.

- Probably the major underlying condition leading to cardiovascular disease is atherosclerosis, also known as hardening of the arteries. In time, this degenerative disease can narrow or block arteries in the heart, brain, and other parts of the body. It may begin early in life. The linings of the arteries become thickened and roughened by deposits of fat, cholesterol, fibrin (a clotting material), cellular debris, and calcium. As this build up on the inner walls becomes hard and thick, arteries lose their ability to expand and contract. The blood moves with difficultly through the narrowed channels. This makes it easier for a clot to form that will block the channel (lumen) and deprive the heart, brain, and other organs of the necessary blood supply.

- Cells of the blood vessel walls: The endothelial cells form the barrier or protective layer between the blood and the blood vessel wall; moreover, these cells contribute to a variety of metabolic functions, such as optimum blood viscosity. The smooth muscle cells produce collagen and other reinforcement molecules, providing optimum stability and tone to the blood vessel walls.

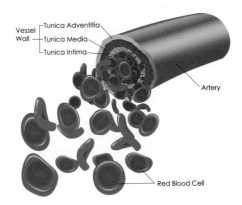

Vessel Wall
- Tunica Adventitia
- Tunica Media
- Tunica Intima

Artery

Red Blood Cell

The different components of artery walls. Our arteries are the blood vessels which carry oxygenated blood around the body.

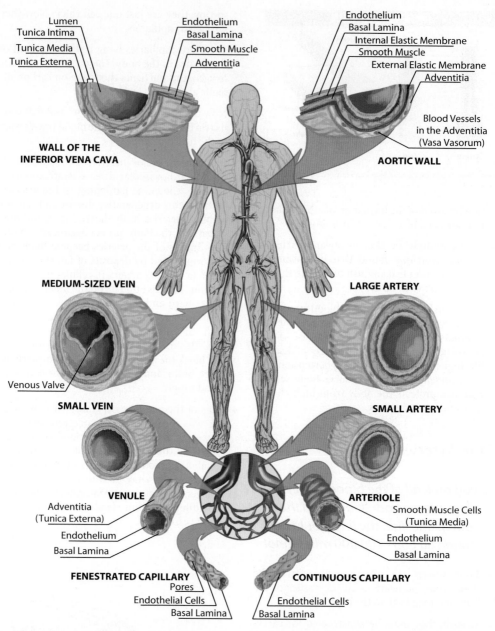

WALL OF THE
INFERIOR VENA CAVA

Lumen
Tunica Intima
Tunica Media
Tunica Externa

Endothelium
Basal Lamina
Smooth Muscle
Adventitia

Endothelium
Basal Lamina
Internal Elastic Membrane
Smooth Muscle
External Elastic Membrane
Adventitia

Blood Vessels
in the Adventitia
(Vasa Vasorum)

AORTIC WALL

MEDIUM-SIZED VEIN

LARGE ARTERY

Venous Valve

SMALL VEIN

SMALL ARTERY

VENULE

Adventitia
(Tunica Externa)

Endothelium

Basal Lamina

ARTERIOLE

Smooth Muscle Cells
(Tunica Media)

Endothelium

Basal Lamina

FENESTRATED CAPILLARY

Pores
Endothelial Cells
Basal Lamina

CONTINUOUS CAPILLARY

Endothelial Cells
Basal Lamina

Our blood vessels are the "pipes" which carry all of our blood through out the body. Rather than just having one layer, like a plastic pipe, these blood vessels have different layers as you can see. Damage to the inner layers can cause plaque build up which can then lead to various cardiovascular related health issues.

- Every second man and woman in the industrialized world dies from the consequences of atherosclerotic deposits in the coronary arteries (leading to heart attack) or in the arteries supplying blood to the brain (leading to stroke).

- Conventional medicine is largely confined to treating the symptoms of this disease. Calci-

um antagonists, betablockers, nitrates, and other drugs are prescribed to alleviate angina pain. Surgical procedures (angioplasty, bypass surgery) are applied to improve blood flow mechanically.

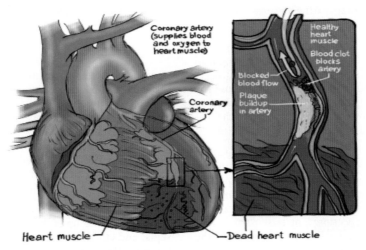

Coronary artery (supplies blood and oxygen to heart muscle)

Coronary artery

Healthy heart muscle

Blood clot blocks artery

Blocked blood flow

Plaque buildup in artery

Heart muscle

Dead heart muscle

Damage to the inner most lining of an arterial wall can lead to a build up of plaqua which can then restrict blood flow. The chances of this occuring are increased when there is insufficient lysine, proline and vitamin C in the body

How to build healthy blood vessels

- When the intercellular glue in your arteries becomes watery due to the lack of vitamin C, the first step of atherosclerosis has taken place.

- In contrast, a continuous and generous supply of vitamin C to the arterial linings keeps the ground substance in it's healthy, gel – like state.

- That means…"The solitary root cause of all coronary arterial blockages is a vitamin C deficiency in the coronary arteries". Dr. Thomas Levy Cardiologist

- Homo Sapiens, like the guinea pig, fruit bat and the high-order primates, cannot synthesize vitamin C because of a missing enzyme. These species must obtain the vitamin in the diet or die of scurvy.

- Here is the main reason why animals don't get heart attacks: With few exceptions, animals produce vitamin C in their bodies. The daily amounts of vitamin C produced vary between1000 mg and 20,000 mg, when compared to the human body weight.

- In contrast, we human beings cannot produce a single molecule of vitamin C ourselves. Our ancestors lost this ability generations ago when an enzyme that was needed to convert sugar molecules (glucose) into vitamin C became defunct.

- This change in the molecules of inheritance (genes) of our ancestors had no immediate disadvantage since, for thousands of generations, they relied primarily on plant nutrition such as vegetables and fruit, which provided the daily minimum intake of vitamins for them.

- Nutritional habits and dietary intake of vitamins have changed considerably in this century. Today, most people do not receive sufficient amounts of vitamins in their diet. To make matters worse, food processing, long-term

How hormones work

Hormone   Target cell

Remember, it is our blood vessels that are used to transport our hormones, oxygen, nutrients and much more. Without having health blood vessels, it is difficult to gain overall health.

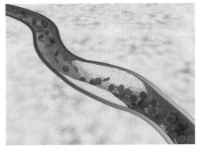

Plaque build-up in a blood vessel. As you can see, as plaque builds up, blood flow is restricted

storage and overcooking destroy most vitamins in the food.

- A mere 10 mg of vitamin C prevents acute scurvy in humans resulting in the long-held hypothesis that ascorbic acid is a vitamin, required only in minuscule amounts. Those few species that fail to synthesize ascorbic acid all suffer similar heart disease, a form of the disease that is not prevalent in other species.

- The arterial intima is especially prone to this localised deficiency. Whenever any toxins are released into the blood, the inner lining of the arteries is logically one of the first destinations for the toxins to gather and start neutralizing local vitamin C stores, at least partially explaining why arterial scurvy is probably the most common form of focal scurvy.

- The anatomy of the artery is fairly straightforward. The thickness of the arterial wall is composed of three basic layers: the intima, the media and the adventita.

- Another important point about the anatomy of the arterial wall is that all three layers in the wall require the normal formation and maintenance of collagen in order to be an anatomically normal structure.

- Vitamin C is absolutely essential for the normal formation of collagen throughout your body. Collagens are the most abundant proteins in the human body, constituting about 30% of the body's total protein content.

- Linus Carl Pauling (Feb 28, 1901 – Aug 19, 1994) was an American chemist, biochemist, peace activist, author, and educator. He was one of the most influential chemists in history and ranks among the most important scientists of the 20th century.Pauling was one of the founders of the fields of quantum chemistry and molecular biology. For his scientific work, Pauling was awarded the Nobel Prize in Chemistry in 1954. In 1962, for his peace activism, he was awarded the Nobel Peace Prize. This makes him the only person to be awarded two unshared Nobel Prizes. He is one of only four individuals to have won more than one Nobel Prize. He is also one of only two people to be awarded Nobel Prizes in different fields, the other being Marie Curie (Chemistry and Physics).

- So you can hardly say Linus Paulin was a rogue scientist, though you will find him getting a battering by the medical profession on many fronts for his theory on Vitamin C and heart disease. You can understand why, as Vitamin C costs pennies. Heart disease drugs and treatments are some of the biggest businesses in the world.

- Pauling's revolutionary concept is that lipoprotein-(a) cholesterol in the blood is an evolutionary adaption for, and a symptom of, low vitamin C. After crucial experiments, Dr. Pauling believed that the vitamin C/lysine protocol would save lives by: a) Preventing chronic scurvy, b) Strengthening and healing blood vessels, c) Keeping Lp(a) blood levels low and d) Inhibiting the binding of Lp(a) molecules to blood vessel walls.

- Due to the build up of damaged collagen, the Lp(a) and other blood clot forming factors increase at the site of damage as well. When this collagen damage continues to grow, so too does the size of the internal scab or plaque that is there to protect the vessel.

- Pauling's crucial insight is that our diets lead to heart disease, but not in the way most people think. Our diets have sufficient vitamin C to prevent scurvy, but less than what we need to function optimally and keep our blood vessels flexible and strong. The result is a sub-clinical form of scurvy, i.e., chronic scurvy.

- Those few species that fail to synthesize ascorbic acid (vitamin C) are prone to a form of heart disease that is not prevalent in other species. The theory that Cardiovascular Disease (CVD) is related to a deficiency of vitamin C was first proposed by the Canadian physician G. C. Willis in 1953.

- If the arteries become abnormal because of inflammation, the whole body becomes abnormal as well. If the arteries become healthy, so will the body.

- He found that atherosclerotic plaques form over vitamin-C-starved vascular tissues in both guinea pigs and human beings. In 1989, after the discoveries of the Lp(a) cholesterol molecule (circa 1964) and its lysine binding sites (circa 1987), Linus Pauling and his associate Matthias Rath formulated a unified theory of heart disease and invented a cure.

- The Lp(a) binding inhibitors become the Pauling Therapy for heart disease only at high dosages, between vitamin 3 to 18 g ascorbic acid and 3 to 6 g lysine. In his video, Pauling recounts the first cases where his high vitamin C and lysine therapy quickly resolved advanced cardiovascular disease in humans. The effect is so pronounced, and the inhibitors are so non-toxic, that Pauling doubted a clinical study was even necessary.

- An optimum supply of lysine, proline, and vitamin C is a decisive factor for the optimum regeneration of the connective tissue in the artery walls and, therefore, for a natural healing of cardiovascular disease.

- Recently, the amino acid proline was found to be an effective Lipoprotein A (a major risk factor of heart disease and similar in structure to LDL) binding inhibitor. Adding between 0.5-2 g proline may be of significant additional benefit.

- In 1970, Dr. Pauling published his first book "Vitamin C and the Common Cold". Following this, vitamin C consumption in the U.S. rose by 300%. Mortality from heart disease then decreased by 30% making the U.S. the only country with a significant drop in heart disease fatalities.

- *"Now I've got to the point where I think we can get almost complete control of cardiovascular disease, heart attacks and strokes by the proper use of vitamin C and lysine. It can prevent cardiovascular disease and even cure it."*
  Linus Pauling, British Journal of Optimum Nutrition (JON), Aug. 1994

- *"You need lysine to be alive, it is essential, but you can take lysine, pure lysine, a perfectly non toxic substance in food [as supplements], and that puts extra lysine molecules in the blood. They enter into competition with the lysyl residues on the walls of arteries and accordingly count to prevent lipoprotein-(a) from being deposited or even will work to pull it loose and destroy atherosclerotic plaques."* [Linus Pauling, JON, Aug. 1994]

- 1997 British Medical Journal: "Vitamin C deficiency, as assessed by low plasma ascorbate concentration, is a risk factor for coronary heart disease." Men who were deficient in vitamin C had 3.5 times more heart attacks than men who were not deficient in vitamin C.

- Vitamin C is the cement of the artery wall, and optimum amounts of vitamin C stabilize the arteries. And, surprisingly, we human beings cannot produce a single molecule of vitamin C ourselves.

Stability of the artery wall through optimum collagen production

- The collagen molecules in our bodies are proteins composed of amino acids. Collagen molecules differ from all other proteins in the body in that they make particular use of the amino acids lysine and proline.

- Collagen molecules differ from all other proteins in the body because they make particular use of the amino acids lysine and proline.

- We already know that vitamin C stimulates the production of collagen in the cells of the artery wall. An optimum supply of lysine, proline and vitamin C is a decisive factor in the optimum regeneration of the connective tissue in the artery walls and therefore the natural healing of cardiovascular disease.

- A deficiency of Vitamin C in the innermost lining of the arteries can initiate what is called atherosclerosis (build up of plaque in the arteries).

- This innermost lining of the arteries is called the intima. Once damaged by a lack of vitamin C, plaque-building processes are initiated and stimulates a host of different as a healing mechanism.

- Atherosclerosis can be readily characterized as arterial scurvy because of the lack of vitamin C in the arterial linings appears to always be the first identifiable starting point for the development of coronary heart disease.

- In almost every case the cause of low vitamin C levels in the arterial linings is a significant daily toxin exposure.

- These toxins keep neutralizing (oxidizing) the body's stores of vitamin C, making the maintenance of active Vitamin C levels in the various tissues of the body a tough task.

- Vitamin C has a short half-life in the blood. A "half-life" is the amount of time it takes for half of the vitamin C to be depleted from the blood stream. The half-life of vitamin C in the blood is 30 minutes. This means that, every 30 minutes there is only one-half of the vitamin C left!

- For example, let's say you have an amount of vitamin C in your blood, we'll say this number is 100 (don't worry about any units). After 30 minutes, if you do not consume any more, you will only have 50 left. After another 30 minutes you would only have 25 left and so on and so on until you take on board more vitamin C.

- *"Vitamin C is essential for the building of collagen, the most abundant protein built in our bodies and the major component of connective tissue. This connective tissue has structural and supportive functions which are indispensable to heart tissues, to blood vessels, —in fact, to all tissues. Collagen is not only the most abundant protein in our bodies, it also occurs in larger amounts than all other proteins put together. It cannot be built without vitamin C. No heart or blood vessel or other organ could possibly perform its functions without collagen. No heart or blood vessel can be maintained in healthy condition without vitamin C."* Roger Williams (Pioneer in Biochemistry, Nutrition, Biochemical Individuality, and Public Education)

- Thomas E. Levy, M.D., J.D. - a practicing physician for 25 years, a board-certified internist, a fellow of the American College of Cardiology, and author of Curing the Incurable: Vitamin C, Infectious Diseases, and Toxins - states as follows:

- *"I never cease to be amazed at the number of persons who remain unaware that vitamin C is the best broad-spectrum antibiotic, antihistamine, anti-toxic and antiviral substance there is."*

- A study conducted at the University of Maryland School of Medicine examined the effects of a high dose of vitamin C on the functioning of the endothelium.

- Healthy volunteers were given either (a) a single high fat meal consisting of 50 grams of fat, (b) a low – fat meal with 0 grams of fat, or (c) a

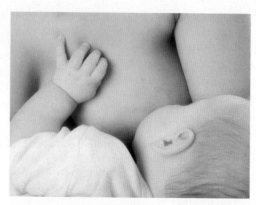

Early exposure to the high cholesterol content of breast milk may improve fat metabolism in later life. In which case, there may be a strong argument for the content of formula feeds to match that of human milk. The highest concentrations of cholesterol are found in breast milk, where it is essential for infant nourishment and brain development.

high fat (50 grams) meal after taking 1000 mg vitamin C and 800 IU of vitamin E.

- In the high fat meal group without the anti oxidants, measurements with ultrasound scans showed that the enormous fat intake interfered with the normal dilation of their arteries and their blood flow, known as the endothelium dependent artery vasodilation ,for up to four hours.

- The group eating the same fat laden meal but taking the vitamins did not experience any such negative effects. These individuals had normal dilation and normal blood flow to the heart.

- As the researchers concluded, a single high fat meal reduced endothelial function for up to four hours in healthy people with normal cholesterol levels. This decrease can be blocked by taking high dose vitamin C & E.

- Weight-loss: A study led by nutrition researchers from Arizona State University found that too little vitamin C in the blood stream correlates with increased body fat and waist measurements. The scientists report that the amount of vitamin C in the blood stream is directly related to fat oxidation – the body's ability to use fat as a fuel source – during both exercise and at rest. The controlled four-week study involved 20 obese men and woman. Half of the participants were given a 500 mg vitamin C capsule daily and the control group took placebos

- Heavy Metal Poisoning: Vitamin C is a surprisingly good chelator of heavy metals. Researchers from the University of California,

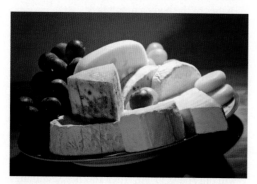

A diet that is low in fat is not the one that is optimal for heart health. You need to include foods such as full-fat, unprocessed dairy products. This will ensure you achieve your nutritional needs for things such as vitamin K2.

San Francisco looked at blood levels of lead and ascorbic acid (vitamin C) and found that those with the highest levels of ascorbic acid were 89% and 65% less likely to have elevated blood lead and ascorbic acid levels, respectively. Some physicians with experience of heavy metal toxicity will administer intravenous Vitamin C to get mercury out as quickly as possible, as this antioxidant helps to minimize the impact of mercury entering the bloodstream after diagnosed mercury toxicity or after the removal of amalgam dental fillings.

- NOTE: Individuals who are suffering from Hemochromatosis should realize that Vitamin C increases the amount of iron absorbed from foods which puts them at risk of excess iron in their blood. Any supplementation with Vitamin C should, therefore, first be discussed with health care providers. On the other hand - since Vitamin C stimulates the absorption of non-heme iron it reduces iron deficiency in those suffering from it.

Cholesterol

- Cholesterol is only a secondary risk factor for heart disease, hundreds of millions of people have elevated blood levels of cholesterol, triglycerides, LDL (low density lipoproteins), lipoprotein (a) and other risk factors.

- The liver manufactures something like 1,000 mg of cholesterol per day, even if you consume no cholesterol at all. Of that amount, about 800 mg becomes bile salts, which is necessary for the digestion of fats. That leaves about 200 available for other functions.

- The formation of cholesterol involves a series of complicated biochemical reactions that begin with the widespread 2-carbon molecule Acetyl CoA: Acetyl CoA (C2) --> mevalonate (C6) -->

isopentenyl pyrophosphate (C5) --> squalene (C30) --> cholesterol (C27). Cholesterol is made primarily in your liver (about 1,000 milligrams a day), but it is also created by cells lining the small intestine and by individual cells in the body

- Vitamin C is a "natural" HMG-CoA (or 3-hydroxy-3-methylglutaryl-coenzyme A to give it its full name. It is a liver enzyme responsible for cholesterol production) reductase inhibitor. It was observed experimentally that when vitamin C levels are low, cholesterol becomes elevated, and when more vitamin C is consumed, cholesterol levels decline. The mechanism by which vitamin C lowers cholesterol was discovered 1985.

- High Vitamin C levels inhibit the same the HMG-CoA Reductase enzyme as the statin drugs. The inescapable conclusion is that vitamin C does what statins do - lowers cholesterol -- without side-effects.

- If statin drugs were patterned after Vitamin C, they lack many other benefits of the vitamin. For example, vitamin C promotes the production of coenzyme Q10 and lowers Lp(a).

- The majority of people who use statin cholesterol-lowering drugs are doing so because they believe lowering their cholesterol will prevent heart attacks and strokes. How many of these people do you think would continue to take them if they knew these very same drugs have been linked to decreased heart muscle function and increased risk of stroke?

- Not very many, right? Well, you may need to reconsider your use of statins, as this study in Clinical Cardiology found that heart muscle function was "significantly better" in the control group than in those taking statin drugs! The researchers concluded:"Statin therapy is associated with decreased myocardial [heart muscle] function."

- Contrary to what the pharmaceutical companies selling cholesterol- lowering drugs want to make you believe – there is nothing wrong with cholesterol levels of 220 or 240. Remember, cholesterol is a "secondary" risk factor because the primary risk factor determining your cardiovascular status is the weakness and instability of your blood vessel walls.

- Elevated blood levels of cholesterol and other blood risk factors are not the cause of cardiovascular diseases, but are the consequence of developing disease.

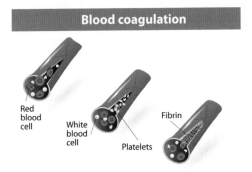

Blood coagulation

Red blood cell

White blood cell

Platelets

Fibrin

The different components of the blood.

- Cholesterol, triglycerides, low density lipoproteins (LDL), lipoprotein (a) and other metabolic products are ideal repair factors, and their blood levels increase in response to a weakening of the artery walls due to a nutrient deficiency of Vitamin C, Lysine & Proline.

- Cholesterol is essential for the formation and maintenance of cell membranes (helps the cell to resist changes in temperature and protects and insulates nerve fibers). It also plays a role in the formation of sex hormones (progesterone, testosterone, estradiol, cortisol) Production of bile salts, which help to digest food

- Conversion into vitamin D in the skin when exposed to sunlight.

- Cholesterol is a health-promoting substance. It is a critical component of cell membranes, the precursor to all steroid hormones, a precursor to vitamin D, and a limiting factor that brain cells need to make connections with one another called synapses, making it essential to learning and memory.

- Some of the most nutritious foods like egg yolks and liver are also the foods richest in cholesterol. The anti-fat, anti-cholesterol campaign has demonized these foods for decades without any evidence they cause disease. To the contrary, they promote health.

- When your diet contains cholesterol, the liver makes a little less. The typical Western diet contains 250-350 grams per day, depending on your sex, but only a third to half of that is absorbed, so out of the 1,000 mg, only 10-15% comes from diet. Even if you eliminate the dietary intake, a healthy liver simply makes more to make up the deficit.

- Eliminating saturated fat from your diet doesn't help either, because the liver will make cholesterol out of sugar and starch. It's that necessary for life.

- When the liver isn't functioning well, dietary intake of cholesterol is essential. A study at the University of California, Berkeley found that dietary cholesterol improved mental ability in the face of advancing age and declining memory.

- The effect of vitamin C on the blood levels of cholesterol and other blood fats has been documented in numerous clinical studies. More than 40 of these studies were evaluated by Dr. Hemilä from the University of Helsinki, Finland. In patients with high initial cholesterol

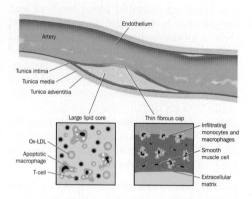

values (above 270 mg per decilitre) vitamin C supplementation decreased cholesterol levels up to 20%.

- Dr. Jacques and his colleagues showed that people taking 300 mg of Vitamin C per day and more also had much higher HDL blood levels than people taking less than 120 mg per day. This is important since HDL (high-density lipoproteins) are fat-transporting molecules that pick up cholesterol and other fats from the artery walls and carry them back to the liver for removal.

Testosterone

- In one study published in the Journal Metabolism in March of 2004, researchers found that low testosterone levels posed the greatest risk for men and was the greatest predictor of heart attacks and clogging of the arteries.

- NOT high cholesterol, not diabetes, not smoking, not high blood pressure, not even being fat

- In the study, researchers analysed 3,484 Italian men who were already being treated for erectile dysfunction (ED). They found that those who were taking statins for their cholesterol had significantly lower testosterone levels than men who weren't on statins.

- The researchers also found an increased incidence of hypogonadism in those taking statins. Hypogonadism is a condition in which the body doesn't produce enough testosterone, which may lead to erectile dysfunction, as well as a decrease in muscle mass and body-hair growth.

- Another study, published in November 30, 2007, has also concluded that - "High endogenous levels of testosterone in men are associated with low mortality from all causes, cardiovascular causes, and cancer".

- The authors suggest that low testosterone may be a predictive marker for those at high risk of cardiovascular disease.

- Lead author Dr Kay-Tee Khaw (University of Cambridge School of Clinical Medicine, UK) commented to heartwire :

- "This is the largest study of testosterone levels ever conducted. We don't know whether the association shown between higher levels of testosterone and lower mortality is causal or just a marker of something else, but regardless of this, it appears that low testosterone levels do identify a group at increased risk of cardiovascular death."

- Low levels of testosterone appear to be correlated with several cardiovascular risk factors, including atherogenic lipid profiles, insulin resistance, obesity, and a propensity to clot (Jones et al 2005).

- In addition, recent research is showing a clear relationship between low testosterone levels and increased incidence of cardiovascular disease and mortality in men (Malkin et al 2010).

- Studies show that those who exercise while on a higher-cholesterol diet gain more muscle mass and strength than those who eat less cholesterol. Foods like egg yolks, liver and red meat are good sources.

Inflammation

- The fixation on cholesterol is not only completely wrong, it supports the sale of statin drugs that has led to enormous profits for pharmaceutical companies for decades, profits that have come at the expense of your health.

- When inflammation, the real cause of elevated cholesterol is treated, cholesterol becomes what it should be—a non-issue in heart disease. It is not the reason millions are dying from heart disease.

- In 2000, doctors at Harvard University published the first of a series of landmark studies revealing the central role of inflammation in cardiovascular disease (CVD).

- People with the highest level of CRP had five times the risk of developing CVD and four times the risk of a heart attack or a stroke compared to individuals with the lowest level.

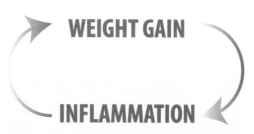

Inflammation increases with weight gain, and weight gain promotes inflammation. The result is a vicious cycle of metabolic lethargy and increased insulin resistance. Medical evidence suggests that obesity-related insulin resistance may be due, in part, to chronic inflammation.

- In obese people, CRP can be chronically elevated. This is because fat cells produce pro-inflammatory signalling molecules called cytokines that in turn stimulate production of CRP.

- A high CRP means that inflammatory processes are active in your body. You might have an obvious source, like a recent bout of viral bronchitis, painful arthritis in your left knee, or gout in the right big toe. However, an increased CRP also tells you and your doctor that inflammation may be active in your blood vessels.

- Increased CRP (>3.0 mg/L) doubles or triples heart attack risk, regardless of LDL levels. When CRP is high, coronary atherosclerotic plaque is more prone to rupture, the feared event that triggers a heart attack. When high CRP occurs in the company of small LDL particle size, one of the phenomena associated with insulin resistance (a lipoprotein measure, the risk of a heart attack risk is nearly seven-fold greater.

- The high-sensitivity C-reactive protein (hs-CRP) blood test is the best method for measuring the body's general level of inflammation. It does not, however, identify the cause of inflammation. The levels can be elevated in patients with metabolic syndrome, insulin resistance, food allergies, toxicity and a host of other diseases. People with high CRP levels typically have problems losing weight.

- C-reactive protein is released into the blood by the liver shortly after the start of an infection or inflammation. CRP is an early indicator of these problems because its levels usually start to rise in the blood before symptoms, such as fever and pain, appear.

  - If CRP level is lower than 1.0 mg/L, a person has a low risk of developing cardiovascular disease.

- If CRP is between 1.0 and 3.0 mg/L, a person has an average risk.
- If CRP is higher than 3.0 mg/L, a person is at high risk.
- C-reactive protein must be viewed in the context of other measures of health and disease. If elevated, the risk of multiple conditions escalates.
- C-reactive protein (CRP) is a protein produced by the liver when there is inflammation somewhere in the body.
- Mounting evidence underscores the critical role that inflammation plays in the development and continuation of diabesity. In fact, those who have a high C-reactive protein blood level have a 1,700% increased probability of developing diabetes.
- Vitamin E and CoQ10 were found to lower CRP by an average of 30% in research with baboons fed a high fat and high cholesterol diet.
- A recent study showed that women with high levels of EPA and DHA fatty acids in their blood had 56% lower CRP.
- Curcumin keeps the heart healthy by preventing a plaque build-up in the arteries, which can lead to atherosclerosis. In one study, participants taking just 500 milligrams of curcumin each day significantly reduced their cholesterol levels in as little as 10 days
- Researchers have found that populations with the highest amount of vitamin E in their blood plasma had the lowest death rate from heart disease. The most dramatic study to date attesting to the benefits of Vitamin E was performed on patients who had already been diagnosed with one heart attack.
- The Cambridge Heart Antioxidant Study was a double blind, placebo controlled study of 2,002 people with diagnosed heart disease. Patients were either given Vitamin E 400 – 800

IU supplements or a placebo. Within 510 days, researchers found that patients who had been taking the vitamin E had an amazing 77% fewer heart attacks than those who did not take the vitamin E.

Homocysteine & heart disease

- Elevation of the homocysteine level in the blood is an independent risk factor for coronary heart disease and arteriosclerosis.
- What this means is that regardless of the cholesterol level, if the homocysteine level is elevated, it is associated with increased risk of arteriosclerosis and coronary heart disease.
- There are many different factors that are related to elevation of the homocysteine level. As we understand it now, perhaps the single most important factor is a dietary imbalance between too much methionine from dietary protein and too little of the three B vitamins which are needed to break down or get rid of excess levels of homocysteine; namely vitamin B-6, vitamin B-12 and folic acid.
- Homocysteine is an amino acid that inflicts damage to the inner arterial lining (endothelium) and other cells of the body.
- A study published in the British Medical Journal (Wouter de Ruijter et al, British Medical Journal, 9th January, 2008) shows that your homocysteine level, a simple blood test, predicts risk of death from cardiovascular disease in older people better than any conventional measure of risk including cholesterol, blood pressure or smoking
- When the body's stores of B6 (pyridoxine), folic acid, and B12 fail to bring this homocysteine down to normal values, there is a three times

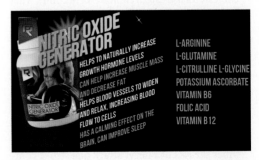

This product is amazing at lowering homocysteine levels and for recovery from exercise

greater risk of heart attack than in males with normal homocysteine values.

- Homocysteine levels can be checked with a simple blood test performed at doctor's offices, hospitals or you can purchase home testing kits.

- A Norwegian study discovered that in 587 patients with coronary heart disease, the risk of death within four years was proportional to total plasma homocysteine level.

- The risk rose from 3.8% with homocysteine below nine micromols per liter to 24.7% in patients with homocysteine levels above 15 micromols per liter.

- A study analysed blood levels of homocysteine and C-reactive protein in heart attack patients compared with a control group who had no symptoms of heart attack. The groups were matched for serum cholesterol, HDL, triglycerides, age, sex, body mass index, and blood pressure. The results showed that compared with the control patients:

  - 32% more heart attack patients had homocysteine levels above 10 μmol/L
  - 500% more heart attack patients had homocysteine levels above 15 μmol/L
  - 572% more heart attack patients had C-reactive protein levels above 3.00 mg/L

- This study demonstrates the importance of keeping homocysteine below 10 μmol/L (optimal levels are below 7-8 μmol/L) and C-reactive protein as low as possible (optimal levels are below 0.55 mg/L for men and 1.5 mg/L for women).

Jarosz A, Nowicka G. C-reactive protein and homocysteine as risk factors of atherosclerosis. Przegl Lek. 2008;65(6):268-7223

Taurine and Homocysteine Reduction

- Supplementing with the amino acid taurine can protect against coronary artery disease by favourably modulating blood levels of homocysteine. Research suggests that taurine can block methionine absorption from the diet, thereby reducing available substrate for homocysteine synthesis (Zulli A 2009).

- A study of 22 healthy middle-aged women (33 to 54 years) found that after taurine supplementation (3g per day for 4 weeks), plasma homocysteine levels exhibited a significant decline, from 8.5 μmol/L to 7.6 μmol/L. The investigators concluded that sufficient taurine supplementation might effectively prevent cardiovascular disease (Ahn 2009).

- A growing body of research on marine lipids, rich in omega-3 polyunsaturated fatty acids (PUFAs), reveals that omega-3 rich fish oil supplementation can reduce elevated homocysteine levels:

- In 1998, the Nobel Prize was awarded to three Americans (Robert Furchgott, Ferid Murad and Louis Ignarro) for their work in the discovery of nitric oxide as a key messenger in the cardiovascular system.

- They had discovered that several important functions relating to the health of the lining of the arteries were initiated by nitric oxide signals. They had also found that nitric oxide was produced in the cells that line the arteries (endothelium).

- Nitric oxide released by the endothelium works to prevent red blood cells from sticking together, or aggregating, and attaching to the vessel wall. It can also work to control vascular tone, allowing the arteries to relax and stay clear.

- The main strategy from reading the research on how to increase nitric oxide seems to focus on L – Arginine, an amino acid the triggers e – NOS (the enzyme endothelial nitric oxide synthase) to make more nitric oxide.

- L-Citrulline is an amino acid that turns into L-Arginine in the body and evidence from Dr. Nathan Bryan and other scientists shows that L-Arginine made from L-Citrulline is much more effective in raising nitric oxide levels than taking L-Arginine directly.

- That's because the L-Arginine made from L-Citrulline is directed toward the nitric oxide making pathway-whereas when you take an L-Arginine supplement, there are eight different metabolic pathways the amino acid can wander down, with only about 3% of the L-Arginine used for Nitric Oxide production. To summarize by providing L-Citrulline the supplement allows the body to more effectively use L-Arginine to produce Nitric Oxide.

- Clinical trials in universities in California have established the effective amount of L-citrulline at 1,000 mg per serving. These studies showed that L-citrulline is critical in the production of nitric oxide because it acts like a catalyst when combined with L-arginine and extends the

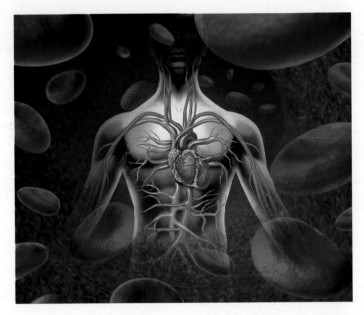

body's production of nitric oxide to over twenty hours. Compared to just 30 min – 2 hours with just using L-Arginine.

- Phil Richards Nitric Oxide Generator is a potent blend of L – Arginine, L – Glutamine, L – Citrulline, L – Glycine, Potassium Ascorbate (Vitamin C), Vitamin B6, Vitamin B12, Folic Acid & Niacinamide (Vitamin B3).

- Its best to take this product before retiring to bed. Our Vascular endothelial cells produce less Nitric Oxide during sleep than when we are awake and moving around. Body Movement stimulates Nitric Oxide production. Most heart attacks occur at night, during the early hours of the morning when we produce the least amount of Nitric Oxide.

- We now know there are pathways in the body that are not dependent on L-Arginine to generate Ntric Oxide. These pathways can convert foods rich in nitrate & nitrites such as kale, spinach, broccoli & beetroot into nitric oxide.

- Dark green leafy vegetables are among the foods richest in nitrate and nitrite, two dietary compounds that create NITRIC OXIDE in the body. Research has shown that Leafy greens have been shown to lower heart disease by 18 % and the risk of stroke by 21%. KALE!!!

- Fish oil boosts Nitric Oxide: In a study conducted by researchers at the University of Kansas 29 people took fish oil and had an increase in their excretion of nitrate, a sign of increasing NO production. Fish oil stimulates nitric oxide production which suggests another mechanism where fish oil prevents heart disease.

Vitamin K2 & heart disease

- Arteries with no plaques have a 20 to 50 fold increase in Vitamin K2 concentration when compared to arteries with arterial plaques. The

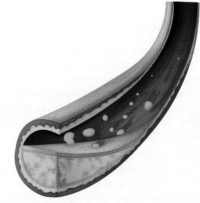

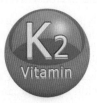

Vitamin K2 helps to de-calcify blood vessels

high K2 content arteries were noted to be more flexible and elastic than arteries lacking K2.

- Lack of Vitamin K2 causes calcium to fail to be deposited in bones where it belongs and to be deposited instead in arteries, aorta, soft tissues including muscle, breast, kidneys and in heel spurs.

- A protein called osteocalcin transports calcium to bone. Vitamin K2(menaquinone-7) is used to solidify this calcium into the bone matrix.

- When Vitamin K2 is lacking the calcium remains in the blood and ends up getting deposited in the walls of arteries and other sites which is very undesirable.

- Vitamin K2 is a critical nutrient for patients with arteriosclerosis as it has the potential to prevent and remove calcium from arteriosclerotic plaques thus making plaques easier to dissolve and less dangerous..

- A large epidemiological study from the Netherlands illustrates this point well. The researchers collected data on the vitamin K intakes of the subjects between 1990 and 1993 and measured the extent of heart disease in each subject, who had died from it and how this related to vitamin K2 intake and arterial calcification.

- They found that calcification of the arteries was the best predictor of heart disease. Those in the highest third of vitamin K2 intakes were 52 percent less likely to develop severe calcification of the arteries, 41 percent less likely to develop heart disease, and 57 percent less likely to die from it. (Geleijnse et al., 2004, pp. 3100-3105) However, intake of vitamin K1 had no effect on cardiovascular disease outcomes.

- It was once erroneously believed that intestinal bacteria are a major contributor to vitamin K status. However, the majority of evidence contradicts this view. Most of the vitamin K2 produced in the intestine are embedded within bacterial membranes and not available for absorption. Thus, intestinal production of K2

likely makes only a small contribution to vitamin K status. (Unden & Bongaerts, 1997, pp. 217-234)

- On the other hand, fermented foods, however, such as sauerkraut, cheese and natto (a soy dish popular in Japan), contain substantial amounts of vitamin K2. Natto contains the highest concentration of K2 of any food measured; nearly all of it is present as MK-7, which research has shown to be a highly effective form. A recent study demonstrated that MK-7 increased the percentage of osteocalcin in humans three times more powerfully than did vitamin K1. (Schurgers & Vermeer, 2000, pp. 298-307).

Blood is the fluid of life

- Blood is the fluid of life, transporting oxygen from the lungs to body tissue and carbon dioxide from body tissue to the lungs

- Blood flows through the arteries and veins that interpenetrates the body like a transport network or river delta, visiting every single corner of the body. During its travels through the arteries, that river carries numerous substances that the cells require.

- We can think of these as cargo packages carried by the river, containing food, water and various chemical substances. The most urgent package to be delivered is oxygen, because if deprived of oxygen, cells will soon die. Thanks to the specially constructed system in your body, however, the packages are delivered to every cell in time and to the correct "addresses."

- Substances of all kinds that the body requires are carried to the relevant organs by the blood. Nutrients such as glucose, amino acids and minerals—and most importantly, oxygen—are just a few of these. In addition, the blood works like a waste disposal system, collecting unwanted substances from every cell. And each of the 100 trillion or so cells in the body produces waste products as a result of its daily functions. These waste products, including such potentially toxic compounds as carbon dioxide and urea, are removed from the cells by means of the bloodstream.

- The blood carries the non-gaseous wastes to the kidneys, where they are distilled. The carbon dioxide produced in the cells is carried to the lungs, from where it is expelled from the body. It is unconscious blood cells that do all this. However, these cells can, in a very con-

Foods high in vitamin K2	
- Natto	- Chicken liver
- Hard cheese	- Salami
- Soft cheese	- Chicken
- Egg yolk	breast
- Butter	- Ground beef

THE ELEMENTS OF BLOOD

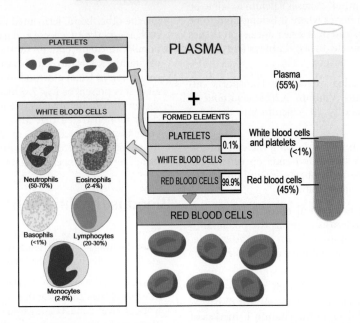

scious manner, distinguish between waste and useful substances carried in the blood, and know which are to be deposited where. For example, they never carry toxic gasses to the kidneys, nor metabolic by-products to the lungs.

- Another of the blood's duties is to carry the cells of the immune system that fight disease.

- Any foreign bodies like viruses and bacteria that enter the body are neutralized by the antibodies and leukocytes in the blood. In addition, immune system cells patrol the bloodstream and so monitor the entire body.

- The blood also constitutes one of the body's main avenues of communication. There is a magnificent communications system among the cells in the human body. They exchange information with one another, just as if each one were truly conscious. The cells send to one another chemical messages in the form of hormones, carried by the blood.

- One of the blood's most miraculous features is its clotting mechanism. Thanks to this clotting, or coagulation, blood loss from a damaged vessel is reduced to the minimum possible. During the clotting process, dozens of proteins, enzymes and vitamins serve in regimented order.

- One of the vital cargo packages carried by the blood is heat. Arteries filled with blood spread heat through the body, just like the piping that carries hot water throughout a building. But unlike the pipes in a building, the body's heat source is not a single boiler, but all the many cells in the body. Thanks to the blood, heat produced by each cell is distributed equally to all the others. Were there no heat distribution system in your body, you would experience grave problems. As the result of any muscular activity you perform running for instance, or carrying a heavy load your legs or arms would overheat, and other regions of your body would remain close to room temperature—an imbalance that would inflict serious damage on your metabolism. For that reason, the equal distribution of heat is of the greatest importance.

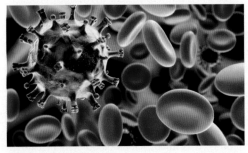

Your blood plays a huge role in making sure that any foreign bodies that enter the blood are neutralised.

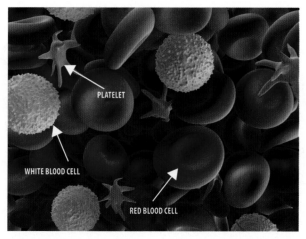

A closer look at some of the components of our blood

- Structurally, the blood is very different to the other fluids in the body. In one sense, blood is actually a tissue, just like bone or muscle. However, while the cells that comprise these other tissues are bound tightly together, cells composing the blood are not attached to one another. Individual blood cells—known as erythrocytes, leukocytes and thrombocytes—move freely distributed within the blood plasma. Blood consists of 55% plasma and 45% blood cells. Water comprises from 90 to 92% of the plasma, the rest consisting of plasma proteins, amino acids, carbohydrates, fats, hormones, urea, uric acid, lactic acid, enzymes, alcohol, antibodies, and elements such as sodium, potassium, iodine, iron and bicarbonate. The blood cells float in this complex fluid.

- Under normal circumstances, some 2.5 million erythrocytes are produced in the body every second. It is not enough for the body's transportation system for red blood cells to be flat. Erythrocytes that carry oxygen would be pointless if they could not offer it to the cells in a usable manner. The cells of the body require molecules to bind oxygen to them—molecules that must combine with the oxygen in the ideal manner, in a three-dimensional form, and carry the oxygen safely. However, they must not bind too tightly to the oxygen, and when they arrive at the cell to which they will release the oxygen, they must separate from it with no difficulty. In short, in order for the oxygen to be transported and used where necessary, a very special molecule with a most particular creation is needed. That molecule is haemoglobin, which gives the erythrocyte and thus, the blood itself its red colour.

- Since haemoglobin performs two entirely separate functions, it has been described as an extraordinary molecule. As haemoglobin deposits carbon dioxide in the lungs, it takes up oxygen and moves from there to the muscles, which oxidize nutrients and produce carbon dioxide. When the haemoglobin reaches the muscles, it carries out a reverse procedure, depositing oxygen and taking up carbon dioxide—all in a seemingly conscious and disciplined manner. In 1996, scientists discovered that in addition to carrying oxygen, the haemoglobin molecules in the erythrocyte structure also carried another molecule of vital importance: nitrogen monoxide.

- There is a very important reason why haemoglobin carries this gas. With the assistance of NO, haemoglobin monitors how much oxygen is to be provided to the tissues. Therefore, haemoglobin's transportation of nitrogen monoxide is of the very greatest importance to human health.

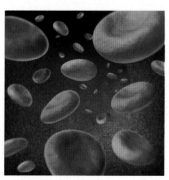

The shape of red blood cells allows them to carry upto 300 million molecules of heamoglobin

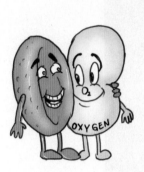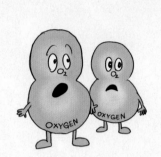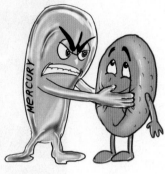

Red blood cells carry oxygen around the body. The oxygen molecules are attracted to red blood cells and are attached to them to be transported around the body. However, mercury can suffocate red blood cells and reduce their ability to carry oxygen molecules

- Haemoglobin does not only carry oxygen; when it passes by a muscle in urgent need of oxygen, it also immediately realizes that it must deliver that oxygen, and acts in the knowledge that it needs to collect the carbon dioxide being released, and heads directly for the lungs to deposit its new load. The haemoglobin never confuses oxygen and carbon dioxide, and always moves to the correct destination. An average of 900 million erythrocytes are produced in the human body every hour, and each erythrocyte cell contains some 300 million haemoglobin molecules.

- Mercury in the bone marrow becomes incorporated into the haemoglobin of the red blood cells and also inhibits the synthesis of the constituent molecule, heme.

- Mercury vapour is attracted to, and can enter, the red blood cells. So it accumulates within the red blood cells and can destroy their membranes causing rupture and the formation of blood clots (thrombi).

- Mercury binds with haemoglobin, which is located inside the red blood cell and carries oxygen for transport to tissues.

- Mercury bound to haemoglobin results in less oxygen carrying capacity of the red blood cell and therefore less oxygen will reach the tissues.

- The body senses the need for more oxygen and compensates for this by increasing more red blood cell production which can increase the viscosity of blood leading to circulation problems.

- Toxins such as mercury interfere with B12's ability to cross the blood brain barrier and reach the neurons where it is needed.

- An average filling contains an estimated 800 milligrams of amalgam, with the average middle-aged adult having 8 fillings. The average adult has 3.2 grams or mercury (8 fillings x 800 mg per filling x 50% of total amalgam is mercury) of potential mercury vapour to go into the lungs, blood, and brain from dental fillings alone! That's going to bite somewhere!

- A single dental amalgam filling can as much as release 15 micrograms of mercury per day. The average individual has eight amalgam fillings and could absorb up to 120 micrograms of mercury per day.

- A mild alkali can absorb 100 times more oxygen than a mild acid. When your body becomes too acidic it develops a lack of oxygen, which is the perfect breeding ground for disease. Blood must retain a pH of approximately 7.4 or it can't hold oxygen.

- The average level of oxygen in the blood is approximately 96% and if this lowers over time, your health can be affected.

- Plasma is the liquid portion of the blood. Blood cells like red blood cells float in the plasma.

- Plasma distributes the substances it contains as it circulates throughout the body.

Plasma Proteins

- Plasma proteins constitute 7-9% of plasma

- There are three types of plasma proteins: albumins, globulins, & fibrinogen

  - Albumin - accounts for 60-80%; creates colloid osmotic pressure that draws H20 from interstitial fluid into capillaries to

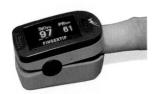

You can purchase an oxymeter online which you can use as a quick measure of the oxygen levels in your blood

maintain blood volume & pressure
- Globulins - carry lipids; gamma globulins are antibodies
- Fibrinogen - serves as clotting factor; converted to fibrin.
- Also dissolved in plasma are electrolytes, nutrients and vitamins (absorbed from the intestines or produced by the body), hormones, clotting factors, and proteins such as albumin and immunoglobulins (antibodies to fight infection).
- Fibrinogen is a protein found in blood plasma which plays a vital role in blood clotting. This protein is produced by the liver.
- Fibrinogen is thought to play a direct role in coronary artery thrombosis. Ideally, therefore, when fibrinogen levels are high, reducing those levels should be the goal of therapy.
- Elevated fibrinogen levels have also been associated with a number of other diseases, including cancer, diabetes and hypertension   (N Engl J Med, 1987, 317: 521; The Framingham Study. JAMA, 1987, 258: 1183).
- Fish oil taken in daily doses of 3000 mg or greater has been shown to lower fibrinogen levels. It may be no coincidence that fish oil has also been shown to reduce heart attack risk
- Excessive homocysteine blocks the natural breakdown of fibrinogen by inhibiting the production of tissue plasminogen activator (tPA). Folic acid, trimethylglycine (TMG), vitamin B12, and vitamin B6 reduce elevated homocysteine levels.
- Vitamin C may help reduce fibrinogen. In one study, heart disease patients were given either 1000 or 2000 mg a day of vitamin C to measure the fibrinogen breakdown effect. At 1000 mg a day, there was no detectable change in fibrinolytic activity or cholesterol. At 2000 mg a day of vitamin C, there was a 27% decrease in the platelet aggregation index, a 12% reduction in total cholesterol, and a 45% increase in fibrinolysis (fibrinogen breakdown) activity.

- What are platelets? Platelets are tiny cells that circulate in the blood and whose function is to take part in the clotting process.
- What happens when we are stressed to affect the heart? Adrenaline & Cortisol is known to increase stickiness of platelets which tend to be blood clotting fragments.
- Stress causes the blood to clot more, this serves you well if it's a life or death situation like being in battle, you want more clotting as this can slow down any potential wounds inflicted in battle.
- However constantly being in a stressed scenario be it through financial, relationship or excess toxicity the blood becomes more of a consistency of red ketchup rather than a vintage red wine an analogy created by cardiologist Kenneth R Kensey, a pioneer in the study of blood viscosity as a risk factor for CVD. The thicker and stickier the blood becomes, the greater the risk for cardiovascular disease.
- Researchers at the University of Edinburgh suggest that fish oils prevent the platelet activation involved in the formation of atherosclerotic lesions and blood clots (thrombosis).
- Vitamin C increases the production of prostacycline, a small molecule that not only relaxes the blood vessel walls, but also keeps blood viscosity at optimum levels.
- Studies have shown that moderate to high intensities of aerobic exercise increases the hematocrit, or blood cell volume in athletes.

What are the effects of low oxygen?

- Low oxygen levels are associated with poor health:
- Poor concentration and forgetfulness
- Easily stressed and anxious
- Shortness of breath when walking short distances

- Cramping of leg muscles
- Swollen ankles
- General fatigue, particularly after eating
- Re-occurring chest infections
- Blueness of fingertips and lips

- Hyperbaric oxygen therapy saturates the blood plasma and haemoglobin with oxygen. The red blood cells become more malleable as well, increasing their ability to penetrate restricted blood vessels. Healing time is reduced significantly, and athletes get back into play faster.

- Breathing high levels of oxygen under hyperbaric conditions causes greater uptake of oxygen by the bodily fluids and so more can reach areas where the circulation is diminished or blocked and therefore improve recovery.

- Sunlight also increases both the oxygen content of human blood and its capacity to deliver oxygen to the tissues; in much the same way that exercise does.

- Essential fatty acids (EFA's) have tremendous oxygenating capabilities. The presence of EFA's in the cell membrane is especially important because they are there to help absorb oxygen.

- For the bone marrow to manufacture new blood cells it needs to be at the right body temperature. The generally low level of red cell production that is, anaemia, which won't respond to vitamins or iron, but only to thyroid production.

- Anaemia occurs when your blood doesn't have enough haemoglobin. Normal levels are 120 - 160 g/L for women and 140-180 g/L for men.

- Red blood cells, or erythrocytes, are the most numerous cells in the blood. Their job is to transport oxygen, the most essential material for the survival of all the body's cells

- They go further than this, however, and in order to purify the body, also carry away the carbon dioxide that accumulates in the cells as a by product of metabolism.

- There are around 25 trillion of these erythrocytes in our bodies. Stretched end to end, these cells would form a tower 50,000 kilometres (or 31,070 miles) high .

- During its four-month lifespan, a single red blood cell travels between the lungs and the other tissues of the body 75,000 times

- Pernicious anaemia is a condition in which the body does not make enough red blood cells (erythrocytes) due to a lack of vitamin B12 in the body. It usually occurs in people whose bodies have lost the ability to absorb vitamin B12 from food.

- In pernicious anaemia, the blood cells do not divide normally and are too large. They have trouble getting out of the bone marrow. The problem is due to a lack of vitamin B12 in the body.

- People who have pernicious anaemia often feel tired and weak because the body is not getting enough oxygen.

- B12 deficiency attacks the nerves, stripping them of their protective myelin coating and disrupting the communication between cells in the brain or other parts of the nervous system.

- B12 deficiency can affect your nervous system in other ways as well. Because the nerve cells in your brain control how you feel, think, and behave, B12 deficiency can cause severe mental illness, including depression, paranoia, and even symptoms resembling schizophrenia.

- B12 plays a crucial role in melatonin production, which is another reason it is important to make sure you're receiving an adequate amount of this vitamin into your blood

- If you have a short supply of vitamin B12, your body won't make as many red blood cells, they will be abnormally large and won't last for as long as they should.

- Pernicious anaemia is a disease in which the red blood cells are abnormally formed, due to an inability to absorb vitamin B12.

- True pernicious anaemia refers specifically to a disorder of atrophied parietal cells leading to absent intrinsic factor, resulting in an inability to absorb B12.

- Besides a lack of intrinsic factor, pernicious anaemia can be caused by Crohn's disease, stomach surgery, or a strict vegetarian diet. Breast-fed infants of vegan mothers are particularly at risk of vitamin B12 deficiency.

- Vitamin B12 deficiency is certainly the etiology of the macrocytic anaemia, macrocytic red blood cells are a common finding in people who drink alcohol to excess..

- Testosterone deficiency also cause anaemia because the hormone helps stimulate kidneys and bone marrow to produce erythropoietin and stem cells.

- If you don't have enough red blood cells, the tissues and organs of your body may not be getting enough oxygen. This leads to the symptoms of anaemia.

- *"During the early stages of pregnancy it soon became apparent that yet again my HB levels were dropping below normal levels. Determined not to undergo the same interventions I had first time around, I began taking Phil's Nature's Multivitamin product. In the space of just 3 weeks of taking the supplement, my HB levels increased from 8.3 – 10 which amazed my midwife. So much so that she questioned me at length as to how I had managed such an improvement. Apparently such an improvement had been unheard of!"* Amy Nicols (Mother)

- Heme iron is from meat sources and non-heme iron is from plant sources, such as cereal grains, legumes, and leafy greens.

- If you are vegetarian/vegan and/or are diagnosed anaemic, then you may want to place some restrictions on your tea drinking. Here's why: Tannins chelate non-heme iron.

- Iron is essential for making haemoglobin, a mere 10% drop in haemoglobin levels can decimate endurance by 20 – 25

- That doesn't sound like much until you understand that only 10% of the iron in a good diet is bioavaliable. So to get sufficient iron, a male athlete in heavy training needs to eat a minimum of 35 mg of iron, and a female 40 mg – every day.

- Research would indicate that vitamin C increases iron absorption when iron is needed. It seems to increase excretion of iron when there is an excessive amount of iron. Therefore, vitamin C might be a good treatment of Hemochromatosis.

- There is only one problem iron by itself hardly works at all to raise your haemoglobin.

- The body cannot make Haemoglobin without Vitamin B6 Pyridoxine.

- Not only does the body need Vitamin B6 Pyridoxine to make Haemoglobin, but Vitamin B6 Pyridoxine will help Haemoglobin to carry more oxygen.

- Studies also show that pyridoxine deficiency impairs vitamin B12 absorption and reduce the function of this essential nutrient for blood formation. Exercise and a high protein diet increases demand for vitamin B6 (pyridoxine).

- Folate is essential for the formation of both red blood cells (erythrocytes) and white blood cells in the bone marrow, and for their development. Folate deficiency greatly affects red blood cell formation

Conclusion

- I hope you know understand just how important it is to have a healthy cardiovascular system and more importantly how to build a healthy heart, blood vessels and blood. This is a habit which I believe is the key for all the other habits to function efficiently. On the back of the research that I did for this habit I developed a number of products which I believe are fundamental for heart, blood vessel and blood health. Remember also the key to a healthy cardiovascular system is happiness and we all deserve to be happy.

- I highly recommend the books written by Dr. Thomas E. Levy, a book written by Owen Fonorow called "Practising without a licence" and one by Matthias Rath entitled "Eradicating Heart Disease".

HABIT 9

NUTRIENT TIMING

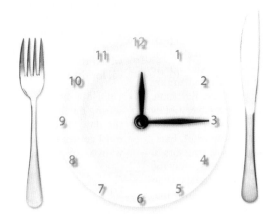

Since I first met Phil in 2010 my life has changed immensely. I had been a Strength & Conditioning coach in professional sport for 10 years and thought my knowledge was at a decent level but within the first half hour of his seminar I knew my knowledge of health and nutrition was a long way off what it should be.

The way in which he researches and presents his findings makes it easy to listen and learn, and he is so free with what he knows that you know he just wants to help rather than wanting to make money. He is the first person I call whenever I have any health or fitness related issue, and he has helped with any issue, from health to Strength & Conditioning to motivation.

His products are outstanding and have literally changed my whole health status. My body fat has dropped, concentration is high and testosterone through the roof. I could not recommend his products highly enough whether you are a sportsman or someone who just wants to improve their health.

Ross Dewar Head Of Strength & Conditioning Worcester County Cricket

- In this habit, I want to cover the importance of breakfast as wells as pre-, during and post-workout nutrition. If you get these factors right everything else falls into place and you can train with much more intensity, which will increase your metabolism and enhance fat loss. You will also increase your ability to recovery, so you can train more frequently and effectively. At the end of this habit there are plenty of nutrition & supplement plans that I have used with my athletes/clients and myself with great success.

- It never ceases to amaze me the amount of people I see beast the shit out of themselves in the gym or other training activities who ignore eating a quality breakfast and not consuming any pre-, during or post- workout nutrition. This will eventually make progress very slow or can make you fatter. Yes, exercise can make you fat if you don't get everything right. Exercise is stress and if you have lots of stressors in your life then adding another stress into the mix will add more problems with exercise than benefits. That's why I am a huge believer that to get any benefits out of exercise, you have got to be healthy first.

- I also want to get this point across on nutrition and biochemical individuality which Dr. Roger, J Williams, PhD Pioneer in Biochemistry, discovered. We are all unique in our nutrient requirements. I can use a great example here: a female bodybuilder that I worked and consulted with got incredibly lean with high amounts of carbohydrates. Whereas, if I ate the amount that she consumed when I was just strength training, I would have made a sumo wrestler look lean. We will also have different times when we need more fats, proteins and carbohydrates and times when we need less, this can take place even in a 24 hour cycle. For example, after 25 years of lifting weights, I have decided to run a mountain marathon and I have given myself 6 months to prepare. My carbohydrate intake has increased significantly to not only fuel my runs but allow me to recover faster from the extreme training. The point I want to make is that if I had consumed this amount of carbohydrates whilst I was only strength training, which was 4–5 times per week, I would have probably gained 40 pounds. So you must tune into your body's needs on what are the most appropriate foods to consume depending for your circumstances. Nothing is set in stone, everything is constantly changing so listen to your body's needs.

- When I first work with an athlete I explain to them that I want them to concentrate on chasing one rabbit at a time. They usually reply, "why?", I then reply, "what happens if you try to catch two rabbits at a time?" The athletes who have a functional brain usually reply, "you catch none". If you zone in on one thing and ignore the other and put all your effort into one rabbit, the chances of you catching it will improve enormously. I look at nutrition, lifestyle and exercise like this; you must decide what rabbit is going to give you the biggest bang for your buck for the effort you put in. With nutrition it is getting the first meal of the day right, which usually sets you up to for how you will eat for the rest of the day.

- Let's look at breakfast and its importance in setting our brain chemistry and hormones for the day. I can't emphasize enough that you must get your first meal right for the day if you want to drop fat and be healthy.

- If you eat a very high carbohydrate breakfast, typical of most breakfast cereals and milk, then you are most likely to become fat and sleepy. Why? Breakfast cereals and milk are full of sugar which increases insulin (remember insulin is a fat storage hormone and when high inhibits the body from burning fat, it will also increase tryptophan levels in the brain which increases serotonin which can leave you feeling sleepy). Also,having breakfast cereal with milk is probably the most allergenic breakfast you can eat as it combines gluten (wheat protein) with casein (milk protein). This are two of the most allergenic proteins in the human

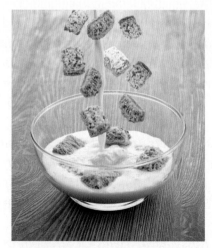

This may look like a nutritious breakfast but we have been brought up in societies that insist that we stick to cereals and milk almost everyday. This breakfast combo contains two of the most allergenic proteins (gluten and casesine).

Eat Like a Sumo Wrestler if you want to look like one

- Sumo wrestling is an ancient Japanese sport; where the heavier you are the better! Here are some Sumo Wrestlers' tricks for getting big:

1. Don't eat breakfast: Sumo wrestlers never eat breakfast. This is a great way to slow your metabolism way down and will definitely ensure over eating later in the day.

2. Exercise on an empty stomach: When you exercise without proper fueling, your metabolism will conserve every ounce of energy you have left to get you through the activity. So you end up burning far less calories than you would have had you eaten prior to exercising. That's why I pre load with amino work capacity this forces the body to use fat as fuel and saves your muscles being used.

3. Eat only 1-2 meals each day: Sumo wrestlers get up early, work out and then don't eat until late in the day. This way they will be starving and will eat anything they can grab and in enormous amounts. This ensures a great calorie surplus and maximum weight gain. When you eat a large amount of calories in one sitting, the body will use up what it can and then fill your extra energy reserves for later. When your storage gets full, everything left over is stored directly as fat.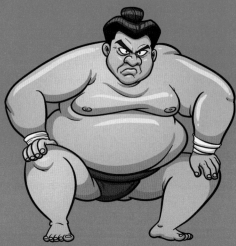

4. Drink beer: Sumo wrestlers drink large amounts of beer with their meals. For a sumo wrestler, the bigger the belly the better! In my next life I'm coming back as a Sumo Wrestler it seems so much fun:)

5. Eat out: Many studies have found that people eating in a restaurant will eat 40% more food and 30% more fat then they would if they were at home.

6. Sleep after eating: When they finish their large meals, the wrestlers will take a long nap. Going to sleep on a full stomach forces the body to store most of the calories as fat because it doesn't have the ability to metabolize large amounts of food while sleeping. This is another reason why eating late at night makes you gain weight.

diet. And food allergies can cause inflammation which can lead to obesity.

- On the flip side, you have got the meat and nuts brigade, munching on their steak whilst flipping almonds in their mouth's frowning on the cereal brigade as if they are lepers. If I had a choice between cereal and milk or meat and nuts I would have to go for the latter no doubt about that. However, I think we can be smart here and have a breakfast that contains a high quality protein source, vegetables or salad, a carbohydrate source from either fruit or gluten free grains and some good fats from a combination of coconut oil and omega 3 fats. Some people frown when you explain that this is an ideal breakfast not only for fat loss but also brain chemistry and multiple reasons which I will explain very shortly.

- When I'm told, "I haven't got time for that sort of breakfast" I reply "make time of find another coach," because I will not work with athletes who won't get breakfast right. You must make time for breakfast. Get this meal right and all the other meals throughout the day usually fall into place quite nicely.

- A study, published in the AMA Journal, compared three diets: a low-fat diet, a low-glycemic/Mediterranean diet, and a low-carb/Atkins-like diet. Although participants burned the most energy on the low-carb diet, researchers found that it came at a cost of increases in cortisol, a stress hormone we discussed earlier, and C-reactive protein which, in excess, binds to leptin - not a good scenario if weight loss is your long term goal.

- Another essential point to make about breakfasts is to rotate them regularly - I never eat the same breakfast for at least 5 days. Remember, we evolved on a massive variety of food choices and we are still genetically a huntergatherer. Eating the same breakfast every morning is probably the quickest way to build allergies to those food sources you are constantly eating.

- This is why the 4 most allergenic foods are:
  - Cow's Milk
  - Gluten (in wheat, oats, rye and barely) - that's 99.9% of breakfast cereals and bread covered
  - Yeast
  - Eggs

- Well I think it's no coincidence these are amongst the most allergic foods for us today. Why? Because we eat them every day, in quantities which we are not genetically adapted to.

- I will always remember taking over as Head of Strength & Nutrition at a very famous rugby team. One of the promising young players there was about to get his contract terminated because of his constant injury problems. Whilst working with this player I got him to fill in a seven day nutrition and lifestyle diary (which is found at the end of this habit). As I analysed the content of the players food diary, my jaw nearly hit the floor. He ate the same breakfast every day, and had done so for the last five years on the recommendations he had been given by a nutritionist. To make things more interesting, the breakfast might look quite nutritious to the layperson as it consisted of scrambled eggs followed by a big bowl of porridge. Now the twist to this is still to come - the breakfast was also cooked in the microwave. On explaining to the player that if I wanted to make someone fat, sick and injury prone I would prescribe that exact breakfast. After putting him in a head lock and making him repeat 100 times "I will never eat that breakfast again", we started our nutritional plan, which was no different to the nutrition plans in this book. He was banned from eating eggs, milk and anything with gluten in. The results were absolutely incredible; from

nearly being told to leave the club, the player returned literally within weeks to full fitness, with no injuries (apart from the obvious ones you would pick up from contact in professional rugby). He was leaner than he had ever been in his life and played for another 10 years. And the biggest change was, no doubt, getting his breakfast right and respecting the healing benefits that the right nutrients can have on health and performance.

- On the next page are some breakfast choices I used when I was working with a world champion boxer and needed to get him as lean as possible. On weigh-in before fight day I had him at around 4–5% body fat. You will see the full plan at the end of this habit, but pay attention to the variety of breakfasts and the combination of protein, carbohydrates and fats. Remember, rotate your breakfasts; that is extremely important.

- Britons are consuming 600 fewer calories a day than they were around 30 years ago but are actually getting fatter because of sedentary jobs and a lack of exercise, a respected think-tank has found. On average adults weigh up to 30 pounds (14kg) more than they did 30 years ago, despite a 20% drop in daily calorie intake.

- Although they are consuming the equivalent of a burger and chips or three pints of Guinness less, they are also less active than those of the same age were in the 1980s, the Institute of Fiscal studies claims.

The average adult is putting on weight at an average of just over half a pound (0.25kg) a year.

A man in his twenties weighs around 15 lbs (7kg) more than a man in his twenties three decades earlier, while someone in their 50s weighs 30 lbs more.

- Report author Professor Rachel Griffiths told industry journal The Grocer: "The drop in calories consumed would have been expected to have caused a weight loss of 1kg per year over the period."

- Well remember from Habit 1, the further you move away from nature the fatter we become. Go back to eating organic foods, grass fed meat, wild fish, limit grains, drop the booze, drink clean water, exercise regularly and have love and happiness in your life in abundance and bingo you will drop the fat.

Thermogenesis the science of using foods to increase metabolism.

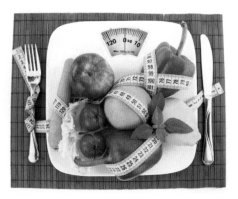

- Thermogenesis (or thermic effect) refers to the calorie burn associated with digestion and assimilation of food. When you sweat after eating a big meal that's thermogenesis kicking in right there and you will notice it more the higher the protein content of the food.

- The thermogenic effect of food peaks within one hour after a meal is consumed, and can be quite substantial in terms of the amount of energy dissipated. The magnitude of the thermogenic effect of food ranges between 10–35% of ingested nutrients, and varies depending on the type of food eaten.

- Of the three macronutrients, protein is the front runner when it comes to thermogenesis, then carbohydrates and a slowly fat meanders across the finishing line. Protein outdistances itself from carbohydrate and fat due to the caloric cost incurred in processing amino acids.

- A meal of pure protein elicits a thermogenic effect amounting to approximately 30% of the meal's total calories, about twice as much as carbohydrate and more than three times as much as fat. So you can now see the value from a fat loss perspective to including high quality protein to each meal. Now, before you try to consume a whole cow with your baked potato and vegetables, your body will not be able to use more than 30–50 grams of protein per meal, anymore than this can be used to create more body fat.

- Fruits and vegetables are also thermogenic because non-processed carbohydrates are moderately thermogenic, but fiber is highly thermogenic. Cruciferous vegetables like broccoli and cauliflower are very thermogenic and therefore need to be consumed often.

- In one study, medium-chain fatty acids (such as those in coconut oil) were found to increase metabolism by between 48-65% in obese patients. This thermogenic effect also lasted 24 hours after ingesting medium-chain fatty acids. Experts agree that, on average, medium-chain fatty acids triple the rate of metabolism compared to long-chain fatty acids. This means that medium-chain fatty acids aren't just a healthy energy source, they also help burn off stored fat.

These are excellent thermogenic carbohydrate fruits:

• Apples	• Blueberries	• Grapes	• Rasberries
• Apricots	• Cherries	• Peaches	• Strawberries
•			

Vegetables with the highest thermogenic properties:

• Asparagus	• Cauliflower	• Mushroom	• Spinach
• Broccoli	• Celery	• Raddish	
• Cabbage	• Lettuce	• Peppers	

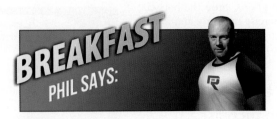

BREAKFAST
PHIL SAYS:

The following would be a typical breakfast for myself or one of my athletes on a non training day. Below is a breakfast schedule that I would suggest for a training week, where high performance and reducing body fat % are the aims.

Non-training day

• Fried Wild Salmon in cast iron pan with 2 tablespoon's of Coconut Oil
• Steamed Vegetables
• Cup of cooked brown rice
• Bowl of Blueberries

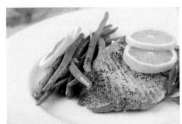

Now isn't that simple - takes about 12 minutes to prepare and will have huge effect on enhancing brain chemistry and stabilizing blood sugar for hours. So, come mid morning you will not be attacking the snack box looking for a sugar fix.

The reason I include a small-to-medium amount of carbohydrates at breakfast is that it can help to reduce cortisol levels and help fuel your brain. When the brain senses low glucose levels it becomes agitated and this can cause stress hormones to be released, leading to a sense of anxiety - not a good start to the day.

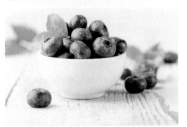

I would also take a number of supplements with my breakfast, as would my athletes. During this habit, there are lots of example nutrition and supplement plans you can look at.

DAY 1	DAY 2	DAY 3	DAY 4
BREAKFAST Stir Fry Vegetables Fish Choice 1-2 TBSP Coconut Oil Nuts & Seeds	BREAKFAST Greens/Veggie Choice Dairy Choice 1 TBSP Extra Virgin Olive Oil	BREAKFAST Greens/Veggie Choice Meat Choice 1 TBSP Extra Virgin Olive Oil	BREAKFAST Greens/Veggie Choice Poultry Choice 1 TBSP Extra Virgin Olive Oil
Fruit Choice	Fruit Choice	Fruit Choice	Fruit Choice
SUPPLEMENTS	SUPPLEMENTS	SUPPLEMENTS	SUPPLEMENTS

DAY 5	DAY 6	DAY 7
BREAKFAST Stir Fry Vegetables Fish Choice 1 TBSP Coconut Oil	BREAKFAST Greens/Veggie Choice Meat Choice 1 TBSP Extra Virgin Olive Oil	BREAKFAST Porridge Coconut Milk 1 Desert spoon of Coconut Oil
Fruit Choice	Fruit Choice	Fruit Choice
SUPPLEMENTS	SUPPLEMENTS	SUPPLEMENTS

Nutrient timing

- You need to deliver the right nutrient mixture, at the right time to enhance recovery from exercise and improve muscle growth, strength and power. There are three phases that you need to maximise during a 24-hour growth cycle -

  a. Energy phase: release sufficient energy to drive muscle contraction during training.
  b. Anabolic phase: 0–45 minute window following a workout; with right combination of nutrients initiates repair of damaged muscle protein and replenishment of muscle glycogen.
  c. Growth & Recovery phase: from the end of the anabolic phase to the beginning of the next workout.

- Combining protein, carbohydrates and fat at each meal will ensure blood sugar levels don't become spiked and that there are building materials to keep muscles in an anabolic state. The ratio of protein, carbohydrates and fat can change from meal to meal. For example, if you have had an extremely intense exercise session then you can add some extra carbohydrates to your post-workout meal. In regards to protein, remember you can't absorb more than 30–50 grams of protein per meal.

- So, in regards to protein consumption, spread it out for maximum absorption and get the thermogenic effect that high quality protein offers.Of the three macronutrients, protein is the one that is least easily converted into fat, but it can happen if you over consume at each meal thinking more is better.

- Also more frequent smaller meals not only maximises more efficient protein absorption, but also the absorption of other nutrients. And, very importantly, it also neutralizes cravings for junk foods; this promotes fat loss and muscle gain. In both animal and human studies more frequent eating is associated with less fat storage at a given caloric intake. Small meals eaten more frequently, instead of the same calories being consumed in bigger meals, increases thermogenesis and leads to more hormonal control, so less is likely to go into fat storage. In one study with boxers, subjects were divided into two groups and were placed on a calorie restricted diet. While both groups consumed 1,200 calories a day, the group that had their 1,200 calories divided in two meals lost signif-

icantly more lean body mass (muscle) than the group who had their 1,200 calories divided into six meals a day. More frequent meal timings also lowers cortisol levels, which explains why the 6 meal group lost less muscle than the two meal group did.

- However, if you are someone who only exercises three times per week, then I believe, from my research, you would be better off sticking to the philosophy, "Eat breakfast like a king, lunch like a prince, and dinner like a pauper". And, before you train, take your pre-workout drink and, immediately after, take your post-workout drink. This way you will keep your fat burning switch on, which in my opinion would be switched off if you were constantly snacking between meals. This is different if you are a professional athlete who is training up to 10–14 times per week; then you have to snack between meals otherwise you crash.

- So make sure you don't get confused in this habit. You need to know what is relevant in terms of nutrient timing for your activity levels. If you train a little, eat a little. If you train a lot, eat a lot. You can't justify eating 6 times per day when you only train 3 times per week. I have spent 30 years training people, from soldiers who wanted to join special forces, professional athletes in multiple sports and members of the public, and trust me, if you are a member of the public and you exercise 3–5 days a week, just make sure you get your pre-, during and post-workout nutrition right. Then get your breakfast right, don't eat within 3 hours before bed time and stay well hydrated and happy. If you apply all this; results will happen, unless you have a major health/hormonal issue or are living with someone you don't like!

Carb-to-Protein Ratio

- Let's now look at the importance of getting the right ratios of carbohydrates and proteins in regards to nutrient timing from both a training and recovery perspective. I have covered the importance of getting the right fats quite extensively throughout this book so you should understand the importance of getting high quality omega 3 and 6 oils and monounsaturated fats from sources like extra virgin oil and avocado oil into your nutrition plan. Get your saturated fats from grass fed meats, organic dairy and coconut oil. Remember, your body makes its own saturated fats but I do advise good sources of saturated fats in your diet, especially during heavy periods of stress, which include hard training. This is to help the body have increase cholesterol which, as you know, is the substrate for our steroid hormones. Yes, the body makes its own cholesterol (actually up to 1000 mg per day - that's how important cholesterol is) but, as explained earlier, you can help the liver, which makes cholesterol, by providing cholesterol through food sources.

- There is an incredible amount of nonsense written about how low carbohydrate diets are the best way for fat loss. In reality, low carbohydrates lead to low glycogen levels.When you consider that glycogen is the optimum fuel for muscles, then does this low-carb crave make sense? Yes, eating high amounts of carbohydrates with every meal and doing very little activity will make you have higher levels of body fat.

- But, eating carbohydrates (and when I mention carbohydrates I want the sources coming from gluten free grains, fruits and vegetables and not shitty breakfast cereals and jammy dodgers) in the right amounts and at the right times can be one of the most important nutritional considerations for fat loss and achieving maximum productivity from your exercise regime. Why? Without high levels of glycogen you will not be able to maintain intensity during weight train-

ing; so the stress and stimulus you put on your muscles, to spark growth, will be limited.

- Studies with athletes have confirmed thatt the level of glycogen in the muscles before they start exercise, is one of the most important factors of performance! Optimal health & sports performance depends on optimal energy. The type of fuel your body uses depends on the energy demands of a given sport (see the table).

- During anaerobic exercise which uses only carbohydrates as fuel, energy requirment jumps 5 times the amount that fat can generate in such a short period of time. Carbohydrates are the highest energy fuel, get it right and you will perform at the highest level. Get it wrong you will become inflamed and have a physique which resembles a swiss ball.

- You need to make a clear distinction between nutrients that are building materials, and nutrients that are fuel.

- Proteins, vitamins, minerals and essential fats are predominately building materials. They are used long term for building a better body whilst all carbohydrates are primarily used as fuel.

- Carbohydrates are used short-term like fuel in your petrol tank. So the amount you have available for your journey is paramount in providing an optimum amount for any particular

Duration	Classification	Energy Supplied By
1 to 4 seconds	Anaerobic	ATP (in muscles)
4 to 10 seconds	Anaerobic	ATP + CP
10 to 45 seconds	Anaerobic	ATP + CP + Muscle glycogen
45 to 120 seconds	Anaerobic, Lactic	Muscle glycogen
120 to 240 seconds	Aerobic + Anaerobic	Muscle glycogen +Lactic acid
240 to 600 seconds	Aerobic	Muscle glycogen + fatty acids

This table shows the primary fuel sources during exercise of different durations. As you can see, during shorter durations, the main source comes from anaerobic sources (meaning without oxygen).

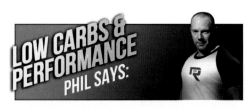

I want to share with you an excellent example of how putting athletes on a low carbohydrate diet to lose body fat can be a disaster. I was working with elite professional rugby players and can you guess what happened to their physical performances? Well, in one word - disaster! It was the biggest lesson I have ever had as a nutritionist, that's for sure.

I had been brought in by this very famous rugby union team to get their players leaner during the 2006–2007 season. At that time everything was about cutting carbohydrates to get lean. Yes, the first 8 weeks worked like a dream - the players were lean and mean. However, a rugby season is almost 11 months long, when you include pre season, and the longer we kept the carbohydrates low, the worse the players felt and performances were starting to falter.

I had to drive over 2 hours to the club, 2/3 times per week; so I had a lot of time to think on these journeys. I was trying to get my head around why the players were starting to lose strength, power and confidence. What the hell was I doing that I hadn't done at my previous clubs where I had been massively successful? Then it was as if I had been hit in the head by a cannon ball moving very quickly - it was carbohydrate timing. I had removed carbohydrates from their breakfasts and recovery drinks. Yes, the players had nice little six packs but were weak as piss. So eureka moment - I got the carbohydrates back into breakfasts; which included things like brown rice, boiled potatoes, gluten free pasta and organic fruits, along with organic meats and wild fish. All the players had breakfast together and I supervised this to make sure everything was in place. Then with the post-workout drinks, we had a trainer who's full time role was getting the post-workout drink ready for the players. I worked out the amount of carbohydrates I wanted in the post-workout drink for each player depending on bodyweight, and we combined this with protein, glutamine and creatine. Bingo - the results were literally astonishing - bigger, leaner and faster - the best season they've had.

So remember, if you do little exercise then you need a little amount of carbohydrates, if you do a lot then you need a lot. Simple really isn't it.

performance to succeed. Carbohydrates are always the limiting fuel, because no matter how lean athletes are, they always have fat calories to spare. With carbohydrates however, you can run out very quickly.

- The primary fuel for exercise is ATP; it's a lot easier for the body to break down muscle glycogen and blood glucose into ATP than it is to break down fat. Consequently, ATP is formed a lot faster from carbs than from fat.

- For low intensity exercise (distance running etc.) glycogen stores can last for as long as 90 minutes. For prolonged high intensity exercise, glycogen stores can provide energy for approximately 20 minutes.

- Your body burns carbohydrates and stores fats; the metabolic cost of converting carbohydrates into body fat is 23%. Excess dietary fats are easily stored as body fat; the metabolic cost of converting excess dietary fat into body fat is 3% (Sims & Danforth, 1987)

- Fat burns in a carbohydrate flame, thus when muscle glycogen is depleted, the ability of the muscles to use fat as an energy source is severely compromised. Fat actually burns in the flame of oxaloacetate, which can be derived from either glucose or amino acids.

- If you have low glycogen stores and aren't eating enough carbs, your body will use protein as an alternative source of energy, and when you're burning protein as a fuel, it means you've got no chance of growing or recovering!

- When you use fat as a fuel, it yields at least 9 calories per gram. But it doesn't work that way in the human body. Despite its high caloric content, in muscles, fat burns very slowly for energy. This is why you use other energy sources during anaerobic exercise.

- Some researchers have made big news on the discovery that the higher the level of an athletes conditioning, the more fat he can use for fuel. Although this is true, I know that if you

217

feed him properly on carbohydrates, he will beat his fat burning performance every time.

- A non-trained person will store around 400 grams of glycogen, whilst a well-trained athlete can store as much as 900 grams!

- If your brain senses that the glycogen levels are too low, it will actually reduce the number of muscle fibres that fire. So, you will not only feel weaker, you will literally be weaker, and eventually you won't be able to move at all. The brain will shut down your muscles before all the glucose supplies (including its own) get completely used up.

- Your brain runs almost exclusively on glucose and uses more than 20% of your body's total energy, even though it only weighs a few pounds. Yet your brain has no place where it can actually store glucose. We use around 120 grams per day for brain function alone.

- Muscle damage, either through body contact and bruising or through eccentric exercise, causes a delay in the recovery of muscle glycogen. This damage causes a disruption of the muscle fibres and physically interferes with their glycogen storing capabilities. Furthermore, the white blood cells which rush to the area as part of the immune system mopping up brigade uses up glucose for their fuel needs.

- Studies show that problems with glycogen storage following muscle damage can at least be partly overcome by increasing carbohydrate intake in the first 24 hours after the event has finished. Therefore, make sure that your nutrition is spot on after intense training or performance.

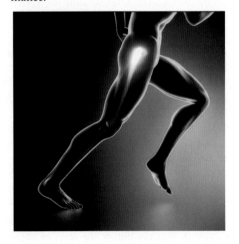

- The glucose that is stored in your muscles, as glycogen, attracts water to the muscle like a magnet. For every gram of glycogen stored in muscles you also store 2.7 grams of water this helps keep you hydrated and in a very anabolic state. This is a very important consideration to take in when preparing athletes who have to make weight for a competition, like a boxer. If, for example, a few days before the fight a boxer is 7 pounds over his fighting weight, I would advise reducing carbohydrates significantly and just have a small amount with breakfast. Also, do not include any creatine in the supplement program as this substrate will also hold water as well as sodium. However, remember that this is only a short term weight loss effect.

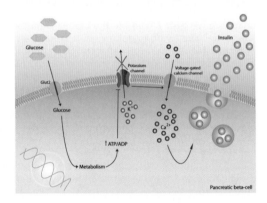

Insulin

- Insulin is probably the most misunderstood hormone among athletes and the general public due to its association with carbohydrate. As we now know, high levels of insulin with high levels of carbohydrates over a prolonged period of time, with little physical activity, will usually increase fat storage and decrease fat breakdown. However, the degree to which insulin promotes fat storage depends on the person's individual body state.

- The most important factor is usually the relative degree of insulin sensitivity in fat cells versus muscle cells: the more insulin sensitive the fat cells are, the more insulin will promote fat storage. The more insulin sensitive the muscle cells are, the more insulin will act to promote muscle glycogen storage and increase protein synthesis.

- Muscle cells are very sensitive to insulin after exercise; if glucose and amino acids are avail-

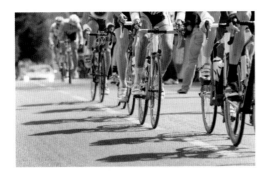

How Much Protein Should You Consume Each Day?

- Evidence for protein needs of athletes has been accumulating since 1974. Dr. I. Gontzea and colleagues at the Institute of Medicine in Bucharest were the first to show that exercise causes the body to use protein at a much faster rate. In one study they instructed their athletes to stop exercising and remain sedentary for two weeks. They were given a daily ration of 1.0 grams per kilogram bodyweight (33% over the RDA). As long as they remained sedentary, this level of of protein intake maintained a positive nitrogen balance. Then, when they were given workouts of 2 hours per day, nitrogen balance dropped to negative within 2 days - meaning they were in a catabolic state.

- Gontzea fed another group of athletes a higher level of protein at 1.5 grams per kilogram of bodyweight (twice the RDA) as long as they remained sedentary, nitrogen balance was positive. But, when they were given the same 2 hour workouts as the first group, nitrogen balance dropped to negative within 4 days.

- Excellent studies that simulated the Tour De France show that, if you increase the intensity and duration of endurance exercise, protein needs increase even further. The Tour De France cyclists doing five hours of intense riding per day, required up to 1.8 grams per kg of bodyweight to remain in nitrogen balance.

- During a study analyzing Romanian Weightlifters over three months of training, the weightlifters increased their protein intake from 2.2 g/kg/bw/ per day to 3.5 g/kg/bw per day. Even though these athletes were already near the top of their potential, they made huge gains of 6% in muscle mass and 5% in strength.

- Before you start guzzling protein, you must remember that they were training 5 times per day. If you want gains, exercise is the key that creates the demand for new structure. Protein does nothing to stimulate growth, it simply provides the building materials.

- Also of importance is the macronutrient (carbohydrate, protein & fat) ratio you eat before you train or compete. A typical meal I would have my rugby players eat pre-match would be the following, and would be consumed at the latest 3 hours before kick off!

able, insulin will help increase the synthesis of muscle proteins and muscle glycogen at a very rapid rate (slowing the synthesis and storage of fat); also slowing the degradation of muscle after exercise.

- Activation of protein synthesis by amino acids is most responsive immediately following exercise; amino acid uptake is 2x greater; muscle protein synthesis will be 3x greater when a carbohydrate/protein supplement is taken immediately versus two hours later.

- So exercise and moderate carbs that are rich in fiber, preferably from vegetable sources and low glycaemic fruits, can increase insulin sensitivity. Alternatively, a low carbohydrate, high fat diet can have a negative effect on muscle mass and performance as I witnessed with the professional rugby team I mentioned earlier in this habit.

- Although we usually think of insulin as just transporting glucose into cells, most are not aware that insulin also increases amino acid uptake into muscle. For example researchers from the University of Texas found, that following insulin infusion, protein synthesis in the muscle cell increased by 67%. Another study at the University of Texas showed that the infusion of insulin into healthy volunteers increased the rate of transport of key amino acids into the muscle from 20% to 50% and this increase was associated with enhanced protein synthesis. Insulin has also been shown to suppress protein degradation following exercise, thereby increasing net protein gain. So you can now see how a low carbohydrate diet can become very counter-productive, if your goal is to increase lean muscle. So once again, carbohydrates are not the enemy - it is the timing and the quality of the carbohydrate that is exceptionally important.

- Fish, Steak or Chicken
- Steamed Vegetables
- Salad
- Rice or Potatoes
- Extra Virgin Oil & Coconut Oil
- Large Selection of Fruit

- And that's as good as it gets folks! Remember, this is eating for performance and nothing else. In terms of quantity the players know better than me how much they need. Then 45 minutes before kick off the pre-workout supplements are consumed. I will explain at the end of this habit what I recommended.

Pre-exercise Nutrition

- In a study published in the British Journal Of Nutrition the effects of exercise before and after meal ingestion on fat metabolism in overweight men was investigated. They found that men performing 60 minutes of walking prior to a meal (fasted state) burned 20% more fat than those who did 60 minutes walking after the meal. And this was just walking! Imagine how much more fat you would burn with higher intensity work.

- What I recommend for maximum fat loss is to load up on amino acids (like Phil Richards Performance Amino Work Capacity). Taken on empty stomach, you will not only burn more fat but, from my research and experience, you will not lose muscle, as would be the case if you exercised regularly in a fasted state. In a purely fasted state, muscles can get broken down to provide fuel during intense exercise. Yes, a form of self-canabolism and a great way to decrease metabolism and become a smaller fatter version of yourself.

- Pre-workout drinks are absolutely essential if you are looking for an edge. If training early in the morning, before 8 a.m., then I advise my athletes to drink Phil Richards Amino Work Capacity as it provides the substrates to tell the body you are in a very anabolic state. Why? The consumption of amino acids on empty stomach triggers the release of anabolic hormones - it senses this is an opportunity to grow. The body senses that there are lots of building materials available and that this is a good time to build. The amino acids will also stimulate glucagon (as mentioned earlier in the book). This will force the body to use stored

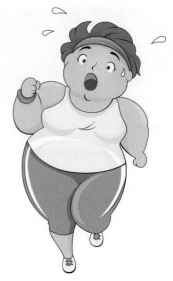

Try to limit dehydration during exercise. Post-exercise, it is important to rehydrate and replace the fluids lost through sweat. Try to drink 150% of the water lost in order to maintain adequate hydration levels

body fat as fuel, especially if taken on empty stomach.

- I know this to be true not only from the science but also from the feedback from all the elite athletes that have taken this product. One that comes to mind is an elite weightlifter who is also an Olympian. He put 10 kgs on his clean & jerk after consuming 2 scoops of Amino Work Capacity - now that's what you call a RESULT!

- It appears that pre-workout amino acid drinks enhance the availability of amino acids to the muscles via enhanced blood flow (from the exercise) during a workout, which prevents, or reduces, the body from breaking down muscle tissue, as it normally does during an intense workout.

- I personally combine my Cardio Fuel and Amino Work Capacity 45 – 60 minutes before training and recommend my athletes do the same but remember; the emptier the stomach, the better the absorption. Cardio Fuel, if you remember from habit 8, contains substrates which help with energy production and vasodilatation to improve blood flow.

- Many athletes dehydrate during training and competitive events, especially long ones, even when it's not particularly hot. You can't rely on feeling thirsty as a reminder to replace fluid lost through sweating - one of nature's dirty tricks is that exercise suppresses thirst. Dehydration impairs both physical and mental performance in most types and levels of sport, yet it can be avoided (or at least minimised) by appropriate drinking strategies before, during and after training. When I worked with teams/athletes I monitored their urine with a specialist hydration testing machine. The biggest lesson I learnt was that the athletes thought that they were hydrated but were often not. In one professional rugby team I worked with, the first time I carried out hydration tests, over 90% of the players were dehydrated and this was before the training session. And the players were informed that they were going to be hydration tested that morning and were told drink plenty!!!

- Not everyone can afford to get one of these pieces of kit. However, urine colour can also be used as a guide to measure hydration levels.

- Although sweat rates are highest under conditions of high-intensity exercise in heat and high humidity, total fluid losses can be appreciable in very prolonged events, whatever the conditions. Unless fluid losses are replaced by drinks, sweating causes progressive depletion of circulating blood volume, leading to hypohydration (commonly called dehydration) and a thickening of blood. This places a strain on the cardiovascular system, with a rise in heart rate in order to maintain adequate blood flow to exercising muscles and vital organs. As blood volume depletes, blood flow to the skin is reduced. As a result, sweating decreases and heat dissipation from the skin is impaired, causing body core temperature to rise, potentially leading to heat stress, collapse and even death.

- Even low levels of dehydration have physiological consequences. A loss of 2% bodyweight (just 1kg for a 50kg person) causes an increase in perceived effort and is claimed to reduce performance by 10-20%. A fluid loss exceeding 3-5% bodyweight reduces aerobic exercise performance noticeably and impairs reaction time, judgement, concentration and decision making - vital elements in all sports, from pole-vaulting to football. A particular issue for boxers is that dehydration increases risk of brain injury.

- The two main factors influencing early fatigue and impaired performance (both physical and mental) in all types of sports and exercise are depletion of body levels of carbohydrate and/or fluid. Maintaining adequate carbohydrates and fluid intake optimises training benefits by enabling athletes to train harder and for longer. This can make a difference between winning and losing. The opportunity and ability to eat and drink during training and competition depends on the sport; sports drinks may not be the only feasible option but most of them do provide a convenient supply of carbohydrates and fluid simultaneously, are well tolerated if used appropriately, and can be adapted to suit individual needs in varying circumstances.

- Whatever the environmental conditions, sweat losses are probably greater than many athletes appreciate. The highest reported sweat rate wass 3.7 litres/hour for Alberto Salazar during the 1984 Olympic marathon. Sweat rates of 2 to 3 litres/hour can be expected during short periods of hard exercise in the heat, and in excess of 1.5-2 litres/hour during endurance events. Even in cooler conditions, losses are appreciable. During a football game on a cool day (10 deg. C), players can lose up to two litres of sweat, and runners are estimated to lose around 1.2 litres/hour at 6 minute/mile pace on

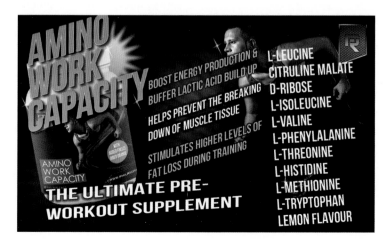

a cool, dry day (double this amount on a hot, humid day). Additionally, fluid is lost via moisture in exhaled air.

- Before any exercise it is important to drink sufficient fluids so as not to be dehydrated. Around 500-750ml of fluid 2 hours before exercise and 300–500ml an hour before then 125-250ml immediatley before exercise is one recommended method for endurance training/competition.

- However, it is of no advantage to drink excess amounts in order to "store" water. This will typically lead to abdominal pains and will probably result in the urge to urinate.

- During exercise it is important to limit fluid loss to less than 2% body mass. The best way to do this is through practice. Nude weight before and after training can help you calculate water loss rate (1litre water loss = 1kg body mass loss). Try to consume 1 litre per hour if the training/competition is intense.

- Replacing just the water that you have lost is not enough. Studies have shown that around you need to drink around 150% of the fluids lost in order to reach hydration following exercise. Any more than this offers no additional benefits. e.g. lose 1kg replace with 1.5 litres of fluids.

- With my athletes, their pre-workout supplements would depend on the situation e.g. the time of day, any meals already eaten. One of my olympic athletes, who was a 3000m steeplechaser, would train exceptionally early, around 5:30a.m., and he swore by the alkalising salts I developed. He would consume 1 teaspoon of the salts in a pint of reverse osmosis water. Boom - he's on the road and has had tremendous results.

- When I was training a world class boxer who had to make weight for fight night I would usually train him twice per day most days. In the first session in the morning I would pre-load him on free form and branch chain amino acids (like my Amino Work Capacity). After training, if we were a few weeks out from the fight I would give him a combination of protein, carbohydrates, creatine and glutamine (like my Anabolic Drive) to ensure maximum recovery. If we were 2 weeks out from fight and he was 5–7 pounds over weight, then I would drop the amount carbohydrates, creatine and glutamine, as this would also hold water, and replace it with the free form branch chain

drink. This always did the trick for getting bang on the weight come weigh-in, which was the day before the fight.

- Many of the rugby teams I worked with usually trained at 10 a.m. and 3 p.m. so the players would have usually had eaten a solid breakfast. There is no point amino loading when there is food in the gut so the emphasis here was their post-workout drink. The players would have lunch and by the time that was digested we were back on the field training - so, again, no point amino loading. When training was complete, they got their recovery drinks and that's it - tommorow we do it all again. But least I knew their tanks were full so they could be pushed to the max in training.

Alkalising Buffer

- Researchers from Loughborough University gave sodium bicarbonate to nine elite swimmers, finding that eight of them reduced their time in a 200 meter race by an average of 1.5 seconds. At the 2008 Olympics, the top four swimmers in the men's 200 meter freestyle were separated by just 1.4 seconds. So, in theory, it could be the difference between winning a medal and not.

- So strong is the effect that athletes can notice the difference in their breathing as more oxygen is carried throughout the system and as more acids are neutralized.

- As hydrogen ion concentrations increase the blood and muscle become acidic. This acidic environment will slow down enzyme activity and ultimately the breakdown of glucose itself.

- By buffering acidity in the blood, bicarbonate draws more of the acid produced within the muscle cells out into the blood and thus reduces the level of acidity within the muscle cells themselves.

- Bicarbonate can be taken frequently throughout the day with half teaspoons amounts, though for long term use lower doses are safer.

- A mild alkali can absorb 100 times more oxygen than a mild acid. When your body becomes too acidic it develops a lack of oxygen, which is the perfect breeding ground for disease. Blood must retain a pH of approximately 7.4 or it can't hold oxygen. The average level of oxygen in the blood is approximately 96% and if this lowers over time, your health can be affected.

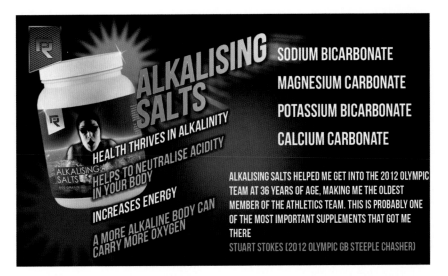

- What are the effects of low oxygen?

  - Poor concentration and forgetfulness
  - Easily stressed and anxious
  - Shortness of breath when walking short distances
  - Cramping of leg muscles
  - Swollen ankles
  - General fatigue, particularly after eating
  - Re-occurring chest infections
  - Blueness of fingertips and lips

- When your body does not have enough alkaline minerals to neutralise the acids you consume, it is catastrophic to your body. This over-acidity leads to a whole host of symptoms including fat gain, muscle loss, fatigue and premature aging.

During Exercise

- It has been shown that when athletes were given a 6% carbohydrate solution during exercise, cortisol levels dropped by almost 80% compared to subjects receiving water. In one study conducted, cyclists drank a fluid containing carbohydrate and protein in a 4:1 ratio, they saw improved endurance of 57% compared with water and 24% compared with a carbohydrate drink. Bishop & colleagues from Lough-borough University England showed that carbohydrate alone during exercise could reduce the biochemical markers of inflammation by almost 50%. So you can start to see how carbohydrates during exercise can increase the quality of the exercise. However, again, each situation warrants its own specific strategy. If you were doing 60 minutes of yoga, then do you think you would need a carbohydrate drink? NO!

Post Exercise

- Research has shown that a carbohydrate intake of 0.8-1.2 grams per 1 kilogram of body weight maximizes glycogen synthesis and accelerates protein repair. However, unless you've had a very long, intense workout, 1.2g/kg may be a bit excessive as excess carbohydrate can be converted to body fat.

- Researchers have used anywhere from 0.2g - 0.4g of protein per 1 kilogram of body weight

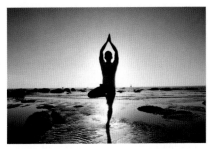

Fuel your exercise appropriately. If you are doing, light-intensity exercise then you do not need to worry about taking on carbohydrates during it.

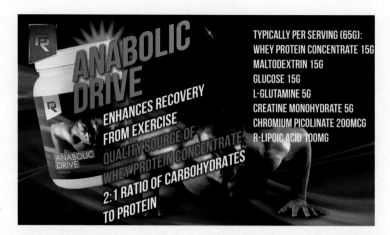

ENHANCES RECOVERY FROM EXERCISE

QUALITY SOURCE OF WHEY PROTEIN CONCENTRATE

2:1 RATIO OF CARBOHYDRATES TO PROTEIN

TYPICALLY PER SERVING (65G):
WHEY PROTEIN CONCENTRATE 15G
MALTODEXTRIN 15G
GLUCOSE 15G
L-GLUTAMINE 5G
CREATINE MONOHYDRATE 5G
CHROMIUM PICOLINATE 200MCG
R-LIPOIC ACID 100MG

to demonstrate the effectiveness of adding protein to a post-workout carbohydrate drink (van Loon et al 2000b, Roy et al 1998).

- Just as you don't need to take in excess protein throughout the day. You also do not need to following exercise. In one study, protein was fed in doses from 0 to 40 g and after resistance exercise and muscle protein synthesis (MPS) was measured. Muscle protein synthesis showed a dose-response increase from 0 to 20 g but, despite doubling the protein intake, at 40 g there was no difference in MPS. Instead, the excess amino acids were oxidised. The conclusion from these data was that an intake of protein of 20 g in larger men (85 kg) was sufficient to maximally stimulate MPS, but that higher intakes would not offer any further benefit and the excess amino acids were oxidized (Moore et al., 2009). This is something you need to consider if you are looking to add a post-workout protein drink into your program. Begin to read labels and check to see how much protein is in the product you take.

- Following a glycogen depleting exercise bout, subjects were given either a carbohydrate or a carbohydrate/protein/antioxidant glutamine beverage.Following a 4 hour recovery period, the subjects completed an exercise bout to exhaustion. The subjects who received the carb/protein/antioxidant/glutamine drink, their performance was 55% better than when they received the carbohydrate only supplement.

- A high glutamine level in a muscle cell stimulates the entry of other amino acids into the cell. Thus glutamine is anti-catabolic and can be considered an anabolic amino acid.

- Glutamine functions as a source of energy for the white blood cells. Eric Newsholm, Phd from Oxford University, suggests that glutamine supplementation can lessen the effects of overtraining. This evidence is supported by a study, in which athletes took 5 grams of glutamine in the first two hours after a marathon. These athletes showed a 32% reduction in infection rate during the seven days following competition.

- Glutamine is classified as a "non-essential amino acid." This label may mislead some people into believing that we don't need it. But, in essence, "non-essential" means that the body can synthesize this amino acid. It does not mean "unimportant". However, there are times when our body may not make sufficient amounts and we may need to supplement.

- In fact, glutamine is of crucial importance; we are lucky that we do not have to depend totally on dietary sources. It seems that every cell in the body uses glutamine. Some tissue types, however, depend on glutamine much more than others. Specifically, glutamine is utilized as a source of energy and for nucleotide synthesis by all rapidly dividing cells, such as the cells of the intestinal lining and certain immune cells (lymphocytes and macrophages). Without sufficient glutamine, the intestines atrophy and the immune function breaks down.

- Thus, to say that glutamine is important for our health is an understatement. In view of its multiple functions, it is no surprise that glutamine is the most abundant free amino acid in the serum, muscle and cerebrospinal fluid. It constitutes 50% of all amino acids in the serum, and more than 60% of free amino acids within the body.

- Glutamine is plentiful in both animal and plant protein. The typical Western diet provides between 3.5 g and 7 g of glutamine; more is synthesized according to need. Even so, heavy stress, such as strenuous exercise, infectious disease, surgery, burn injury or other acute trauma leads to glutamine depletion with consequent immune dysfunction, intestinal problems and muscle wasting. Consequently, it has been proposed that glutamine should be classified as a "conditionally essential amino acid.

- People who use glutamine virtually ensure superior health of their intestinal lining. They need not worry about the "leaky gut syndrome" and all of its troublesome consequences, including allergies, the "leaking out" of pathogens and possible arthritis. In fact, when it was first discovered, glutamine used to be called "intestinal permeability factor." It is by far the most important nutrient for intestinal health.

- The importance of glutamine for the intestines is enormous - glutamine is the chief source of energy for the cells of the intestinal lining. Most glutamine in the diet (and also most dietary glutamate and aspartate) is metabolized by the intestines, both to serve as intestinal fuel and also to produce glutathione, nitric oxide, polyamines, nucleotides and the amino acids alanine, citrulline and proline, making these available to the rest of the body. Glutamine also maintains the structural integrity of the intestinal lining, supporting its quick turnover.

- Glutamine is the primary source of energy for the various cells of the immune system, including T cells and macrophages. Strenuous exercise, viral and bacterial infections, and stress and trauma in general cause glutamine depletion that starves the immune cells. They decline in number and/or show diminished activity. Athletes may want to increase their dosage on an as-needed basis if they tend to succumb to infections after heavy exercise, such as marathon running.

- In addition, glutamine is a substrate for glutathione, a tripeptide amino acid that acts as one of our master antioxidants, and also helps enhance the immune function. Though large doses of glutamine stimulate the immune response even under heavy stress, it is important to reduce stress as much as possible. Stress hormones may interfere with glutamine metabolism in the immune cells

- Glutamine is very important for those who exercise a lot. In its role as a carbon donor, glutamine helps to replenish glycogen. But actually the function of glutamine as a nitrogen-donor

might be even more important. Strenuous exercise such as weight lifting, sprinting & contact sports causes micro-injuries to the muscle tissue. By donating nitrogen, glutamine helps build proteins and repair the muscle. I recommend 5–10 grams of glutamine after high intensity training or competition.

- The more efficient your insulin metabolism, the more amino acids get inside the cells and the more muscle you can make. Chromium appears to make insulin function more efficient by enhancing the uptake of glucose from the blood into the cell. Chromium increases the number of insulin receptors on the cell membrane and enhances insulin binding to cells.

- Chromium picolinate has anabolic effects; Dr Muriel Gilman, at Bemidgi State University, gave 200mcg of chromium picolinate per day to half of a group of freshmen who had enrolled in weight training classes.

- The study ran double-blind for six weeks, freshmen not receiving any chromium made negligible gains, those on the chromium gained an average of 3.5lbs of lean body mass.

- That's a huge increase in six weeks, even for novices who have not exploited their muscle growth potential. So a larger study was done with trained football players to validate it.

- Over six weeks intensive weight training, the football players receiving chromium picolinate gained 5.7lbs of lean body mass compared with 4lbs for the control group. In addition, the chromium group lost 3.6% of body fat compared with 1% for the control group.

- One of the forgotten supplements of recent years seems to be creatine. An interesting effect of creatine supplementation appears to be that it enhances the ability of the muscle to store glycogen. This will help increase recovery.

- Creatine has been shown to pull water into your muscle cells, which increases the recovery of our muscles. New research has also shown that creatine can help buffer lactic acid that builds-up in the muscles during exercise.

- After 28 days of supplementation, creatine supplementation improved body composition, bench press, squat, power clean and 6s sprint time compared to placebo in professional American Footballers

- Most dosing strategies start with a "loading phase" using 20-30g/day for 5-7 days. This will cause a rapid rise in intramuscular creatine that can then be maintained by reducing the creatine intake to just 2-5g/day.

- However, supplementing with lower doses has found to increase intramuscular stores to the same degree. This increase occurs more gradually, taking around 28 days.

- Alpha Lipoic Acid significantly increase insulin sensitivity, enhances glucose transport, increases metabolic rate and reduces the gain in body fat.

- A smart post workout drink from my research would combine carbohydrates, protein, creatine, glutamine, chromium picolinate and alpha lipoic acid and as if by magic I have created this drink Anabolic & Vegabolic Drive.

Conclusion

- You can now see how important it is to get breakfast, as well as pre-, during and post-workout nutrition, right. This is true not only for fat loss, but, also, our overall health. When you get these meals correct, you will get much better results from your exercise program. If you ignore the science on what you have just read, there is a strong likelihood that the exercise that you do will increase body fat and decrease your performance.

- Now that we have looked at the science of having a good breakfast, staying hydrated and what to eat before, during and after training I know want to share with you some of the nutrition and supplement plans I used with my athletes. Remember before embarking on any nutrition and supplement plan always consult with your health care provider.

- Over the years I have read many books that have helped me further my knowledge of nutrition and nutrient timing. In particular, I must give credit to Michael Colgan and his book "Optimum Sports Nutrition" and "Nutrient Timing" by Robert Portman and John Ivy. Remember; never stop reading and never stop learning.

PHIL RICHARDS PERFORMANCE

NUTRITION FOOD CHOICES TABLE

Food group choices:

- ■ Foods which improve our health
- ■ Every opportunity - buy certified organic foods
- ■ Consume food from this group only if you digest Legumes well

MEATS
Beef, Buffalo, Elk, Heart, Kidney, Lamb, Liver (Beef), Rabbit, Venison

POULTRY
Chicken, Hen, Duck, Goose, Pheasant, Quail, Turkey, Ostrich

DAIRY & EGGS
Eggs (Chicken - whites), Eggs (Chicken - yolks), Eggs (Duck - whole), Feta, Goats Cheese, Whey Protein Concentrate, Cottage Cheese

GRAINS
Amaranth, Buckwheat, Kamut, Millet, Quinoa, Rice (basmati), Rice (brown), Rice (white), Spelt, Triticale, Wild Rice, Rice Cakes

FISH
Mackerel, Salmon, Sardine, Anchovy, Bass (Freshwater), Sea Bass, Perch, Catfish, Rockfish, Caviar, Cod, Crayfish, Grouper, Halibut, Herring, Mahi-Mahi, Octopus, Oysters, Mussels, Shark, Squid, Swordfish, Tuna, Shrimps / Prawns, Scallops, Snapper, Trout, Whitefish, Clams, Crab, Lobster, Roughy, Pompano, Cockles

GREENS
Arugula, Beet Greens, Dandelion Greens, Endive, Kale, Lettuce (Bibb), Lettuce (Iceberg), Lettuce (Romaine), Mustard Greens, Radicchio, Rocket, Spinach, Sprouts (Alfalfa), Sprouts (Bean), Swiss Chard, Turnip Greens, Watercress, Pea Shoots

VEGETABLES
Artichoke, Asparagus, Bamboo Shoots, Beet, Bok Choy, Broccoli, Brussel Sprouts, Cabbage, Carrot, Cauliflower, Celery, Cucumber, Corn, Fennel, Garlic, Ginger Root, Jerusalem Artichoke, Leek, Olive (all varieties), Onion, Radish, Eggplant (Aubergine), Jicama, Kohlrabi, Okra, Parsnip, Peppers, Peppers (Hot), Rutabanga, Shallot, Water Chesnuts, Zucchini (Corgette), Potato (all varieties), Pumpkin, Squash (Summer), Squash (Winter), Sweet Potato (Yam), Turnip, Mushrooms

LEGUMES
Adzuki Beans, Black Beans, Black-eyed Peas, Fava Beans, Garbanzo Beans, Green Beans, Green Peas, Lentils, Lima Beans, Mung Beans, Navy Beans, Pink Beans, Pinto Beans, Red Beans, Soy Beans, Tofu, White Beans, Chick Peas

SEA VEGETABLES
Agar, Dulse, Irish Moss, Kelp, Laverbread

NUTS & SEEDS
Almonds, Brazil Nuts, Cashews, Chesnuts, Macadamia, Pecans, Pine Nuts, Pistachios, Poppy Seeds, Pumpkin Seeds, Sesame Seeds, Sunflower Seeds, Walnuts

OILS & FATS
Almond Oil, Blackcurrant Oil, Borage Oil, Coconut Oil, Evening Primrose Oil, Fish Oil, Flax Seed Oil, Hemp Oil, Walnut Oil, Avocado Oil, Almond Butter, Brazil Nut Butter, Butter (unsalted), Extra Virgin Olive Oil

FRUITS
Apples, Avocado, Banana, Blackberries, Blueberries, Boysenberries, Cantaloupe, Casaba Melon, Cherries, Coconut, Cranberries, Currants, Dates, Elderberries, Gooseberries, Grapefruit, Grapes, Guava, Figs, Honeydew Melon, Kiwifruit, Kumquat, Lemons, Limes, Loganberries, Mango, Nectarines, Oranges, Papaya, Pears, Persimmon, Pineapple, Plums, Pomegranate, Prunes, Raisins, Raspberries, Rhubarb, Strawberries, Tangerines, Tomatoes, Watermelon

HERBS, SPICES & SEASONINGS
Anise, Celtic Sea Salt, Basil, Bay Leaf, Caraway, Cardamom, Carob, Cayenne, Chervil, Chili Powder, Chive, Cinnamon, Coriander, Cumin, Curry Powder, Dill Weed, Fennel Seed, Fenugreek, Ginger, Honey, Horseradish, Himalayan Salt, 90% Org Choc, Marjoram, Molasses, Mustard, Mustard Seed, Nutmeg, Oregano, Paprika, Parsley, Pepper (ground black), Peppermint, Rosemary, Saffron, Sage, Salt (sea, unrefined), Savory, Ketchup Organic, Spearmint, Tarragon, Thyme, Tumeric, Wasabi

BEVERAGES
Greens Drinks, Alkalising Salts, Goats Milk, Tea (Herbal), Vegetable Juices, Water, Coconut Milk, Rice Milk, Almond Milk, Wine (Red), Organic Coffee (caffeinated), Organic Green Tea

Tip!
- Always use safe cookware.
- Eat foods in their natural state as often as possible
- Drink reverse osmosis water when possible
- Always have gratitude towards your food
- Eat in a relaxed environment

Please use this food table to help you to plan your meals with more variety. For example, when you see on the following nutrition plans, "Fish Choice", simply look at the food table and you will see that there are multiple choices of fish. You simply select one and then, next time, when you see "Fish Choice" again, chose another one.

This plan gives you so much flexibility in preparing nutritious meals and allows you to have a wide variety of food in you nutrition plan

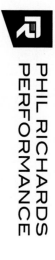

PHIL RICHARDS PERFORMANCE

NUTRITION PLAN
FOR FAT LOSS

	DAY 1	DAY 2	DAY 3	DAY 4	DAY 5	DAY 6	DAY 7
BREAKFAST	Stir Fry Vegetables 1 TBSP Coconut Oil Fish Choice 1 Avocado Bowl of Blueberries	Greens/Veggie Choice Dairy Choice Brown Rice 1 TBSP Extra Virgin Oil Bowl of Strawberries	Greens/Veggie Choice Meat Choice 1 TBSP Full Fat Organic Butter on vegetables Nuts & Seeds Bowl of Pineapples	Greens/Veggie Choice Poultry Choice 1 TBSP Coconut Oil or Extra Virgin Olive Oil Organic Apple	Stir Fry Vegetables Fish Choice Gluten free grain choice 1 TBSP Coconut Oil	Greens/Veggie Choice Meat Choice 1 Avocado 1 TBSP Extra Virgin Olive Oil Fruit Choice	CHEAT MEAL
SUPPLEMENTS	SUPPLEMENTS	SUPPLEMENTS	SUPPLEMENTS	SUPPLEMENTS	SUPPLEMENTS	SUPPLEMENTS	
LUNCH	Greens / Veg Choice Poultry Choice 2 TBSP Extra Virgin Olive Oil	Greens / Veg Choice Fish Choice 2 TBSP Extra Virgin Olive Oil	Greens / Veg Choice Dairy Choice 2 TBSP Extra Virgin Olive Oil	Greens / Veg Choice Meat Choice 2 TBSP Extra Virgin Olive Oil	Greens / Veg Choice Nuts & Seeds Fish Choice 2 TBSP Extra Virgin Olive Oil	Greens / Veg Choice Fish Choice Meat Choice 2 TBSP Extra Virgin Olive Oil Fruit Choice	Grain Choice Veggie Choice Meat Choice Fruit Choice
SUPPLEMENTS	SUPPLEMENTS	SUPPLEMENTS	SUPPLEMENTS	SUPPLEMENTS	SUPPLEMENTS	SUPPLEMENTS	SUPPLEMENTS
DINNER	Greens / Veg Choice Meat Choice Gluten Free Grain 1 TBSP Avocado Oil	Greens / Veg Choice Poultry Choice Small Jacket Potato 1 TBSP Walnut Oil	Greens/Veggie Choice Fish Choice 1 TBSP Full Fat Butter on Vegetables & 1 TBSP Extra Virgin Olive Oil Legumes	Greens/Veggie Choice Meat Choice 2 TBSP Extra Virgin Olive Oil Fruit Salad	Greens / Veg Choice Poultry Choice 1 TBSP Full Fat Butter on Vegetables Legumes or fruit	CHEAT MEAL (NO ALCOHOL)	Greens / Veg Choice Meat Choice Gluten free grains 1 TBSP Extra Virgin Olive Oil Legumes
SUPPLEMENTS	SUPPLEMENTS	SUPPLEMENTS	SUPPLEMENTS	SUPPLEMENTS	SUPPLEMENTS	SUPPLEMENTS	SUPPLEMENTS

Tip! Drink 1 litre of reverse osmosis water per 25kg of body weight daily!

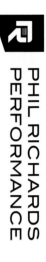

PHIL RICHARDS PERFORMANCE

SUPPLEMENT PLAN
FAT LOSS

20 MINUTES BEFORE BREAKFAST	BREAKFAST	LUNCH	DINNER	1 HOUR BEFORE BED ON AN EMPTY STOMACH
1 Teaspoon of Alkalising Salts	4 x Blood Builder Capsules	4 x Blood Builder Capsules	4 x Blood Builder Capsules	2 Scoops of Nitric Oxide Generator
1 Desert spoom of Collagen Formula	1 Teaspoon of Heart & Brain Oil	1 Teaspoon of Heart & Brain Oil	1 Teaspoon of Heart & Brain Oil	
In 500ml of water	3 x Iodine Forte Capsules 1 Heaped scoop of Heart Fuel	1 Desert spoom of Collagen Formula 1 Heaped teaspoon of Heart Fuel	1 Teaspoon of Brain Talk 1 Desert spoon of Collagen Formula	3 x Magnesium Relax
2 x Super Digestive Enzymes Capsules	2 x Super Digestive Enzymes Capsules	2 x Super Digestive Enzymes Capsules	2 x Super Digestive Enzymes Capsules	2 x Super Digestive Enzymes Capsules

45 MINUTES BEFORE TRAINING	DURING TRAINING SESSION	POST TRAINING SESSION
2 Scoops of Amino Work Capacity 1 Heaped Scoop of Heart Fuel	1 Scoop of Amino Work Capacity	1 Scoop of Anabolic Drive 1 Scoop of Brain Talk
In 750ml of water	In 750ml of water	In 750ml of water

BETWEEN MEAL TIMES:

In between breakfast, lunch & evening meals drink 1 litre of still mineral water with ONE heaped TABLESPOON of Goodness Greens mixed with ONE heaped TABLESPOON of Heavy Metal Chelator.

PHIL RICHARDS PERFORMANCE

NUTRITION PLAN FOR DETOXIFICATION & FAT LOSS

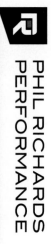

	DAY 1	DAY 2	DAY 3	DAY 4	DAY 5	DAY 6	DAY 7
BREAKFAST	Stir Fry Vegetables Fish Choice 1-2 TBSP Coconut Oil Nuts & Seeds	Greens/Veggie Choice Dairy Choice 1 TBSP Extra Virgin Olive Oil	Greens/Veggie Choice Poultry Choice 1 TBSP Extra Virgin Olive Oil	Greens/Veggie Choice Fish Choice 1 TBSP Extra Virgin Olive Oil	Stir Fry Vegetables Fish Choice 1 TBSP Coconut Oil Olive Oil	Greens/Veggie Choice Meat Choice 1 TBSP Extra Virgin Olive Oil	CHEAT BREAKFAST
Fruit Choice	Fruit Choice	Fruit Choice	Fruit Choice	Fruit Choice	Fruit Choice	Fruit Choice	
SUPPLEMENTS	SUPPLEMENTS	SUPPLEMENTS	SUPPLEMENTS	SUPPLEMENTS	SUPPLEMENTS	SUPPLEMENTS	SUPPLEMENTS
LUNCH	Greens / Veg Choice Poultry Choice 1 TBSP Extra Virgin Olive Oil Grain Choice (optional)	Greens / Veg Choice Fish Choice 1 TBSP Avacado Oil Nuts & Seeds Grain Choice (optional)	Greens / Veg Choice Dairy Choice 1 TBSP Extra Virgin Olive Oil Nuts & Seeds Grain Choice (optional)	Greens / Veg Choice Poultry Choice 1 TBSP Organic Butter Grain Choice (optional)	Greens / Veg Choice Fish Choice 1 TBSP Organic Butter Nuts & Seeds Grain Choice (optional)	Greens / Veg Choice Fish Choice 1 TBSP Extra Virgin Olive Oil Nuts & Seeds Grain Choice (optional)	Greens / Veg Choice Fish Choice 1 TBSP Extra Virgin Olive Oil Grain Choice (optional)
SUPPLEMENTS	SUPPLEMENTS	SUPPLEMENTS	SUPPLEMENTS	SUPPLEMENTS	SUPPLEMENTS	SUPPLEMENTS	SUPPLEMENTS
DINNER	Greens / Veg Choice Meat Choice 1 TBSP Organic Butter Herb choice	Greens / Veg Choice Poultry Choice 1-2 TBSP Extra Virgin Olive Oil Herb choice	Greens / Veg Choice Meat Choice 1 TBSP Organic Butter Nuts & Seeds	Greens / Veg Choice Meat Choice 1 TBSP Avacado Oil Herb choice	Greens / Veg Choice Meat Choice 1 TBSP Avacado Oil Herb choice	CHEAT MEAL	Greens / Veg Choice Poultry Choice 1 TBSP Organic Butter Herb choice
SUPPLEMENTS	SUPPLEMENTS	SUPPLEMENTS	SUPPLEMENTS	SUPPLEMENTS	SUPPLEMENTS	SUPPLEMENTS	SUPPLEMENTS

IMPORTANT POINTS:

- Always consult a health care professional before starting any nutrition or supplement program
- Use the food Table provided to get all the choices you need and ROTATE foods regularly to prevent food intolerances.
- The Grains we've provided in the food table are Gluten Free.
- Follow the supplement plan provided
- For your fluid intake, drink in between meals.

- Chew your food properly and I advise you always use super digestive enzymes with each meal.
- Please note Carbohydrate intake depends on exercise intensity & duration. Little exercise = Little Carbs – More Exercise = More Carbs.
- Cheat meal is your choice but try not to go over board
- Portion size - as much vegetables as you want but limit root vegetables. Fruit - small bowl e.g. berries or 1 piece of fruit (ALWAYS ORGANIC). Meat - size of the palm of your hand

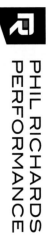

PHIL RICHARDS PERFORMANCE

SUPPLEMENT PLAN
FAT LOSS & DETOXIFICATION

30 MINUTES BEFORE EVERY MEAL	BREAKFAST	LUNCH	DINNER	1 HOUR BEFORE BED ON AN EMPTY STOMACH
½ Teaspoon of Alkalising Salts	1 Heaped Teaspoon of Super Brain Talk	1 Heaped Teaspoon of Super Brain Talk	1 Heaped Teaspoon of Super Brain Talk	2 Scoops of Nitric Oxide Generator
	1 Teaspoon of Ultimate Fish Oil Liquid	1 Teaspoon of Ultimate Fish Oil Liquid	1 Teaspoon of Ultimate Fish Oil Liquid	
In 500ml of water	2x Natures Multivitamins	2x Natures Multivitamins	2x Natures Multivitamins	
	2 Teaspoons of Collagen Formula	2x Teaspoons of Collagen Formula	2x Teaspoons of Collagen Formula	
	3x Iodine Forte Capsules			
	1 Scoop of Cardio Fuel	1 Scoop of Cardio Fuel	1 Scoop of Cardio Fuel	
	3x Probiotic Gut Heath	2x Super Digestive Enzymes	2x Super Digestive Enzymes	
	2x Super Digestive Enzymes			

45 MINUTES BEFORE TRAINING (ON AN EMPTY STOMACH)	DURING TRAINING SESSION	POST TRAINING SESSION
2 Scoops of Amino Work Capacity	1 Scoop of Amino Work Capacity	1 Scoop of Anabolic Drive
In 750ml of water	In 750ml of water	In 750ml of water

All of these supplements can be found on our website at www.philricardsperformance.co.uk

BETWEEN MEAL TIMES:
In between breakfast, lunch & evening meals drink 1 litre of still mineral water with ONE heaped TABLESPOON of Goodness Greens mixed with ONE heaped TABLESPOON of Heavy Metal Chelator.

NUTRITION PLAN

FOR FEMALE BODY BUILDER WHO NEEDED HIGH CARBS TO ACHIEVE LOW BODY FAT

	DAY 1	DAY 2	DAY 3	DAY 4	DAY 5	DAY 6	DAY 7
WORKOUT	SUPPLEMENTS	SUPPLEMENTS	SUPPLEMENTS	SUPPLEMENTS	SUPPLEMENTS	SUPPLEMENTS	SUPPLEMENTS
BREAKFAST	Porridge Coconut Milk 1 Tbsp Cocnut Oil	Porridge Coconut Milk 1 Tbsp Cocnut Oil	Porridge Coconut Milk 1 Tbsp Cocnut Oil	Porridge Coconut Milk 1 Tbsp Cocnut Oil	Porridge Coconut Milk 1 Tbsp Cocnut Oil	Porridge Coconut Milk 1 Tbsp Cocnut Oil	Porridge Coconut Milk 1 Tbsp Cocnut Oil
SUPPLEMENTS	Nuts & Seeds	Fruit Choice	Fruit Choice	Nuts & Seeds	Fruit Choice	Fruit Choice	Nuts & Seeds
LUNCH	Greens / Veg Choice Poultry Choice 1 TBSP Extra Virgin Olive Oil Fruit Choice	Greens / Veg Choice Fish Choice 1 TBSP Extra Virgin Olive Oil Fruit Choice	Greens / Veg Choice Meat Choice 1 Tbsp Coconut Oil Fruit Choice	Greens / Veg Choice Poultry Choice 1 TBSP Avacado Oil Nuts & Seeds Grain Choice Fruit Choice	Greens / Veg Choice Meat Choice 1 TBSP Avacado Oil Fruit Choice	Greens / Veg Choice Fish Choice 1 TBSP Extra Virgin Olive Oil Grain Choice	Greens / Veg Choice Poultry Choice 1 TBSP Extra Virgin Olive Oil Fruit Choice
SUPPLEMENTS							
DINNER	Greens / Veg Choice Meat Choice 1 TBSP Coconut Oil Grain Choice	Greens / Veg Choice Poultry Choice 1 TBSP Avacado Oil Grain Choice	Greens / Veg Choice Meat Choice 1 TBSP Avacado Oil Grain Choice	Greens / Veg Choice Meat Choice 1 TBSP Avacado Oil Grain Choice	Greens / Veg Choice Meat Choice 1 TBSP Avacado Oil Herb Choice Grain Choice	Greens / Veg Choice Fish Choice 1 TBSP Avacado Oil Grain Choice	Greens / Veg Choice Poultry Choice 1 TBSP Cocnut Oil Grain Choice
SUPPLEMENTS							

Tip! THIS PLAN HIGHLIGHTS NUTRITIONAL INDIVIDUALITY. YOU CAN SEE THAT THIS ATHLETE NEEDED HIGH AMOUNTS OF CARBOHYDRATES TO ACHIEVE LOWER BODY FAT. FOR THIS, SHE CONSUMED THE SAME BREAKFAST EVERYDAY AS SHE FOUND THAT THIS IS WHAT SHE NEEDED.

- Always consult a health care professional before starting any nutrition or supplement program
- Use the food Table provided to get all the choices you need and
- ROTATE foods regularly to prevent food intolerances.
- The Grains we've provided in the food table are Gluten Free.
- Follow the supplement plan provided
- For your fluid intake, drink in between meals.

- Chew your food properly and I advise you always use super digestive enzymes with each meal.
- Please note Carbohydrate intake depends on exercise intensity & duration.
- Little exercise = Little Carbs – More Exercise = More Carbs.
- Cheat meal is your choice but try not to go over board
- Portion size - as much vegetables as you want but limit root vegetables. Fruit - small bowl
  e.g. berries or 1 piece of fruit (ALWAYS ORGANIC), Meat - size of the palm of your hand

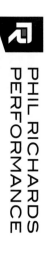

PHIL RICHARDS PERFORMANCE

SUPPLEMENT PLAN
FEMALE BODY BUILDER

20-30 MINUTES BEFORE BREAKFAST (UNLESS TRAINING)
1 Teaspoon of Alkalising Salts In 500ml of water

BREAKFAST	LUNCH	DINNER	1 HOUR BEFORE BED ON AN EMPTY STOMACH
6 x Nature's Multivitamin	6 x Nature's Multivitamin	6 x Nature's Multivitamin	2 Scoops of Nitric Oxide Generator
1 Heaped Teaspoon of Super Brain Talk	1 Heaped teaspoon of Super Brain Talk		3 x Magnesium Relax
1 Teaspoon of Ultimate Fish Oil Liquid	1 Teaspoon of Ultimate Fish Oil Liquid	1 Teaspoon of Ultimate Fish Oil Liquid	
3 x Iodine Forte Capsules	1 Tablespoon of Collagen Formula	1 Tablespoon of Collagen Formula	
3 x Probiotic Gut Health			
2 x Super Digestive Enzymes Capsules	2 x Super Digestive Enzymes Capsules	2 x Super Digestive Enzymes Capsules	2 x Super Digestive Enzymes Capsules

45-60 MINUTES BEFORE TRAINING ON AN EMPTY STOMACH	DURING TRAINING SESSION	POST TRAINING SESSION
1 1/2 Scoops of Amino Work Capacity 2 Scoops of Cardio Fuel	1 Scoop of Amino Work Capacity	1 Scoop of Anabolic Drive 4 weeks from competition we would use ; 1 scoop Amino work capacity instead of Anabolic Drive
In 750ml of water	In 750ml of water	In 750ml of water

BETWEEN MEAL TIMES:
In between breakfast, lunch & evening meals drink 1 pint of still mineral water with TWO heaped TABLESPOONS of Goodness Greens mixed with ONE heaped TABLESPOON of Heavy Metal Chelator.

NUTRITION PLAN FOR ENDURANCE

	DAY 1	DAY 2	DAY 3	DAY 4	DAY 5	DAY 6	DAY 7
WORKOUT SUPPLEMENTS	WORKOUT SUPPLEMENTS	WORKOUT SUPPLEMENTS	WORKOUT SUPPLEMENTS	WORKOUT SUPPLEMENTS	WORKOUT SUPPLEMENTS	WORKOUT SUPPLEMENTS	WORKOUT SUPPLEMENTS
BREAKFAST	Stir Fry Vegetables Fish Choice 1-2 TBSP Coconut Oil Nuts & Seeds	Greens/Veggie Choice Dairy Choice 1 TBSP Extra Virgin Olive Oil	Greens/Veggie Choice Meat Choice 1 TBSP Extra Virgin Olive Oil	Greens/Veggie Choice Poultry Choice 1 TBSP Extra Virgin Olive Oil	Stir Fry Vegetables Meat Choice 1 TBSP Coconut Oil Nuts & Seeds	Greens/Veggie Choice Meat Choice 1 TBSP Extra Virgin Olive Oil	CHEAT BREAKFAST
SUPPLEMENTS							
Fruit Choice	Fruit Choice	Fruit Choice	Fruit Choice	Fruit Choice	Fruit Choice	Fruit Choice	
SUPPLEMENTS							
LUNCH	Greens / Veg Choice Poultry Choice 1 TBSP Extra Virgin Olive Oil Nuts & Seeds Grain Choice	Greens / Veg Choice Fish Choice 1 TBSP Avacado Oil Olive Oil Nuts & Seeds Grain Choice	Greens / Veg Choice Poultry Choice 1 TBSP Extra Virgin Olive Oil Nuts & Seeds Grain Choice	Greens / Veg Choice Poultry Choice 1 TBSP Avacado Oil Olive Oil Nuts & Seeds Grain Choice	Greens / Veg Choice Fish Choice 1 TBSP Avacado Oil Olive Oil Nuts & Seeds Grain Choice	Greens / Veg Choice Fish Choice 1 TBSP Extra Virgin Olive Oil Nuts & Seeds Grain Choice	Greens / Veg Choice Fish Choice Olive Oil 1 TBSP Extra Virgin Nuts & Seeds Grain Choice
SUPPLEMENTS							
DINNER	Greens / Veg Choice Meat Choice 1 TBSP Organic Butter Herb Choice Fruit Choice	Greens / Veg Choice Poultry Choice 1 - 2 TBSP Extra Virgin Olive Oil Herb Choice Fruit Choice	CHEAT MEAL (NO ALCOHOL)	Greens / Veg Choice Fish Choice 1 TBSP Organic Butter Herb Choice Fruit Choice	CHEAT MEAL (NO ALCOHOL)	Greens / Veg Choice Poultry Choice 1 TBSP Organic Butter Herb Choice Fruit Choice	Greens / Veg Choice Poultry Choice 1 TBSP Organic Butter Herb Choice Fruit Choice
SUPPLEMENTS							

- Always consult a health care professional before starting any nutrition or supplement program
- Use the food Table provided to get all the choices you need and
- ROTATE foods regularly to prevent food intolerances.
- The Grains we've provided in the food table are Gluten Free.
- Follow the supplement plan provided
- For your fluid intake, drink in between meals.

- Chew your food properly and I advise you always use super digestive enzymes with each meal.
- Please note Carbohydrate intake depends on exercise intensity & duration.
- Little exercise = Little Carbs – More Exercise = More Carbs.
- Cheat meal is your choice but try not to go over board
- Portion size - as much vegetables as you want but limit root vegetables. Fruit - small bowl e.g. berries or 1 piece of fruit (ALWAYS ORGANIC). Meat - size of the palm of your hand

PHIL RICHARDS PERFORMANCE

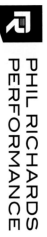

GAME DAY
FOR TEAM ATHLETE (Rugby/Football)
KICK OFF - 3pm

07:30am	08:00am	11:30am	14:10pm	14:25pm
1 Teaspoon of Alkalising Salts in 750ml of water	MEAT CHOICE, Steamed Vegetables & Boiled Rice (with 1 tablespoon of coconut oil) SUPPLEMENTS (as per indv. program)	FISH CHOICE, Steamed Vegetables & Boiled Rice Bowl of Berries SUPPLEMENTS: (as per indv. program)	2 x Scoops Amino Work Capacity 2 x Scoops Cardio Fuel In 1 litre of water	WARM UP

15:00pm	15:45pm	16:45pm	18:00pm
KICK OFF	HALF TIME 1-2 x Scoops Amino Work Capacity in 750ml of water	GAME OVER ROVER! 1-2 x Scoops Anabolic Drive	CLUB MEAL

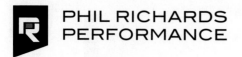

PHIL RICHARDS
PERFORMANCE

NUTRITIONAL STRATEGY AFTER FIGHT WEIGH IN

14.00 Weigh In
14.10 1 litre Water – 2 Scoops Anabolic Drive
15.15 Meal 1 – Fish Choice – Veggie Choices – Potatoes (Boiled) – Butter – Extra Virgin Oil – Rice Pudding
(Supplements)
17.00 1 litre Water – 2 Scoops Anabolic Drive
18.00 Meal 2 – Steak – Veggie Choices – Rice (Boiled) – Butter – Extra Virgin Oil – Ice Cream (Supplements)
21.00 2 Scoops Nitric Oxide Generator – 750 ml Water

Fight Day – Fight at 20.00
07.30 1 Teaspoon Of Alkalising Salts in 1 litre Water
08.00 Meal 3 - Fish Choice – Veggie Choices – Potatoes (Boiled) – Butter – Extra Virgin Oil – Bowl Of Fruit Salad
(Supplements)
10.30 1 litre Water – 2 Scoops Anabolic Drive
12.30 Meal 4 – Lamb – Veggie Choices – Rice (Boiled) – Butter – Extra Virgin Oil – Piece of Fruit (Supplements)
15.00 1 litre Water – 2 Scoops Anabolic Drive
16.00 Meal 5 – Fish Choice – Veggie Choices – Potatoes (Boiled) - Piece of Fruit
19.00 2 Scoops of Amino Work Capacity – 2 Scoops of Heart Fuel - 1 litre Water (finish drinking by 19.15).
20.00 Do The Business!

Food diary template and monitoring information

What did you have for breakfast?

FOOD	FLUIDS	SUPPLEMENTS / MEDICATION

Snack

FOOD	FLUIDS	SUPPLEMENTS / MEDICATION

What did you have for lunch?

FOOD	FLUIDS	SUPPLEMENTS / MEDICATION

Snack

FOOD	FLUIDS	SUPPLEMENTS / MEDICATION

What did you have for dinner?

FOOD	FLUIDS	SUPPLEMENTS / MEDICATION

Snack

FOOD	FLUIDS	SUPPLEMENTS / MEDICATION

How were your stress levels today?

How were your energy levels today?

AM Training _____

Hydration score _____

AM Training _____

Comments:

238

HABIT 10

GETTING THE MOST OUT OF YOUR EXERCISE PROGRAMME

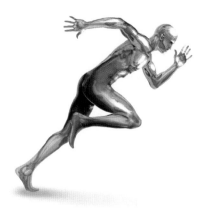

Those who experienced the environment created at Worcester Warriors (Professional Rugby) for any length of time know that it was brutal but time proved its effectiveness. It was based on the premise that if you subjected the body to a constant load of heavy stress it would adjust to this load and adapt to handle the increased stress. The first thing to understand is that the program was designed for hard men to become hard athletic, robust men, cream of the crop. Those of average mentality and a lack of willingness to succeed were not able to adapt to the demands of the program and fell by the way. Those who stuck around went on to be one of the most physically feared sides ever to grace the premiership. Men who went into battle ready for any onslaught that came their way and dealing with it relentlessly to the very bitter end.

Neil Taylor 3 X Commonwealth Weightlifter & Medalist and England Rugby Union Weightlifting Coach

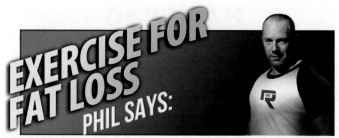

EXERCISE FOR FAT LOSS
PHIL SAYS:

The reason why exercise has been left until habit 10 is because, if you want to get outstanding results from your exercise/gym program, then you must ensure that everything in your life is also excellent. Most overweight people who attend the gym hate thier bodies and go on a mission to try and destroy their body to burn the fat. It would be more beneficial, from a weight loss perspective, to learn to love yourself, your body and realise that the mind and body work together and this, I beleive, will help any one who is overweight lose body fat far more efficiently.

For example, I remember training a middle aged man, who was exceptionally over weight. He trained 6 days a week, was an ex-boxer and was trying with 100% effort to lose the fat through exercise. In reality, he had so many anger management issues that I repeatedly told him that until he resolved those issues, the training he did was simply making him fatter. I witnessed him, after 6 monthsof beasting himself in the gym, gain 9lbs in weight. As I have said repeatedly, make sure that you are physically, mentally and emotionally healthy if you want to see the benefits of exercise for fat loss.

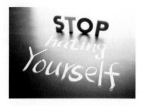

If you want a more in-depth view of strength and conditioning, then you can get a copy of my Strength Training for Athletic Development (STAD) manual which you can purchase from my website, www.philrichardsperformance.co.uk

- I have pushed athletes/teams to their absolute limits both physically and mentally and to do this I knew I had been in their shoes. From a very young age I used to cycle competitively doing time trials every week throughout the summer where pain become my friend. On joining an infantry regiment in the British Army at the age of 16, I learnt very quickly the fitter you were the less shit you were given and I thrived on the brutality that we were subjected too. In fact I remember that on one of my many visits to the regimental prison for being a naughty boy they give up trying to break me physically which was the usual for those who didn't have my level of fitness as the more physical punishment they threw at me the more I thrived. I have run a 12 hour mountain marathon and have also cycled 12 hours non - stop around a running track from 9 P.M. to 9 A.M. which left me with no skin left on my testicles at the end. In the gym I have squatted 260 kgs, dead lifted 270 kgs and benched pressed 170 kgs drug free. So I say this not to blow smoke up my ass but to become an expert in strength & conditioning it is wise to have worn the shoes of those who you are training

- The reasons why most exercise programmes fail is quite simple: most people exercise whilst they are in an unhealthy condition. I cannot emphasize enough how important it is to have the right lifestyle, nutrtional habits, the right thoughts and having people around you who love and care for you. These are essential for any fitness plan to work.

- The amount of people that I have personally observed over the last 30 years who think they can exericse their fat away and end up failing is astonishing. The reason was always because they did not have the factors listed above in place.

- Let's use 2 examples: 2 identical twin sisters (they have identical genes). They are both 45 years of age. Twin A is Lorna. Twin B is Sarah.

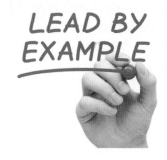

LEAD BY EXAMPLE

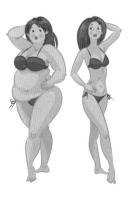

Sarah & Lorna

- The three questions I ask all of my athletes to answer when I meet them for the first time are:

1. What are the 5 most stressful things that have happened in your life?

2. How much love and happiness are in your life?
3. What's in your mouth?

- Lorna has had a wonderful life; she has 2 children, a loving husband, a beautiful home, no financial worries, has eaten healthily all of her life, has good dental health and has healthy body fat levels.

- Sarah also has 2 children, unruley teenagers, a husband who has had numerous affairs. She lives in rented accomodation, her husband is in and out of work and so she has the constant threat of eviction. She has 5 amalgam fillings and a couple of root canals. She is 45lbs overweight.

- Lorna can go straight into an exercise programme and, from my experience, can expect to see gains in fitness, sense of well-being and

Cliff Young's Story

- Every year, Australia hosts 543.7-mile (875-kilometer) endurance racing from Sydney to Melbourne. It is considered among the world's most gruelling ultra-marathons. The race takes five days to complete and is normally only attempted by world-class athletes who train specially for the event. These athletes are typically less than 30 years old and backed by large companies such as Nike.

- In 1983, a man named Cliff Young showed up at the start of this race. Cliff was 61 years old and wore overalls and work boots. To everyone's shock, Cliff wasn't a spectator. He picked up his race number and joined the other runners.

- The press and other athletes became curious and questioned Cliff. They told him, "You're crazy, there's no way you can finish this race". To which he replied, "Yes I can. See, I grew up on a farm where we couldn't afford horses or tractors, and the whole time I was growing up, whenever the storms would roll in, I'd have to go out and round up the sheep.

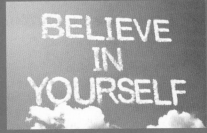

- We had 2,000 sheep on 2,000 acres. Sometimes I would have to run those sheep for two or three days. It took a long time, but I'd always catch them. I believe I can run this race."

- All of the professional athletes knew that it took about 5 days to finish the race. In order to compete, one had to run about 18 hours a day and sleep the remaining 6 hours. The thing is, Cliff Young didn't know that!

- When the morning of the second day came, everyone was in for another surprise. Not only was Cliff still in the race, he had continued jogging all night. Eventually Cliff was asked about his tactics for the rest of the race. To everyone's disbelief, he claimed he would run straight through to the finish without sleeping. Cliff kept running. Each night he came a little closer to the leading pack. By the final night, he had surpassed all of the young, world-class athletes. He was the first competitor to cross the finish line and he set a new course record!

reducing her body fat levels (if that was her goal). She could easily exercise 4/5 mornings a week and benefit from each session.

- If Sarah was to try to do this same exercise programme, there would be a strong likelyhood that, by the time she gets halfway through week 2, she is realising that she simply cannot keep up with dynamo Lorna. The exercise is making her feel sick, tired and fat, the opposite effect that it is having on Sarah.

- I come to the rescue of Sarah. I would advise Lorna to continue what she is doing as she is getting results. My plan with someone like Sarah would be quite simple, from an exercise perspective, I would meet her 3 times a week and take her for a 3-4 mile brisk walk in nature. Whilst walking with her, I would get her to unload all of her emotional worries and find out what makes her tick. I would also explain the importance of being happy because, without that, every programme is doomed to fail.

- I would explain to Sarah that we need to chase one rabbit at a time. We first need to tackle all of her emotional worries to help her reclaim her life.

- The most important point with Sarah would be to get her to understand that she is in charge of her thoughts, her thoughts are not in control of her. we become what we think about most. This point is invaluable because if you think you are fat and worthless, you become fat and worthless. You must think, "I am lean, happy and healthy. I deserve to be happy". If you keep thinking and believing in these thoughts then they will become a reality.

- Once Sarah has managed to get on top of her thoughts, my next step would be to go on the detoxification programme discussed in habit 2. My priority would be removing the amalgam fillings and root canals over a 6 month period with a competent dentist and a very comprehensive nutritional and supplement plan.

- As the process of the detox protocol was taking place, I would have Sarah using infrared sauna 3 times a week after a 30 minute walk-jog-sweat-talk programme. I personally would not bring in resistance training with someone like her for around 8-12 weeks. Not until we have gone through emotional and chemical detoxification and nutritional and lifestyle education. I would also begin to educate her on creating the right home environment.

- When I know all of these factors are in place, it is time to enter the gym. You must rememeber; exercise is stress. It is pointless putting stress on top of more stress. The exercise will cause more problems then benefits.

- If Sarah was not prepared to make the changes that I recommeneded, then I would sack her!

The the reason why so many people drop out of their fitness programmes over time - a lack of results.

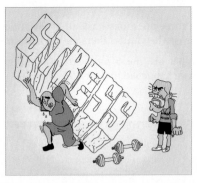

Don't train, unless you can gain

- The reason why I was so successful as an S&C coach was my ability to prescirbe exercise (stress) to players based on how they could cope and improve from a given exercise (stressor). I could recognise that, when a player was, for example, scheduled in to do a heavy weights sesison, if his body language was not right, he would benefit more from 1 hour of full body massage than lifting heavy weights.

- Always remember this quote from my great friend, the late, great Charlie Francis;

Don't train unless you can gain

Creating the ideal training environment for optimum results

- The reason why I had such outstanding results in professional sports was, not only I had acquired exceptional knowledge in my field of strength and conditioning and nutrition, I had also observed, from an early age as a soldier in the army, that the Sergeants that spoke to their soliders with the most respect, got the most

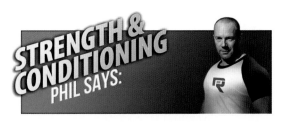

STRENGTH & CONDITIONING
PHIL SAYS:

I have had over 30 years of experience in writing and prescribing strength and conditioning programs for a wide range of requirements. These include preparing soliders for selection to Special Forces, working with members of the general public with an array of medical issues, preparing athletes for Olympic games, preparing teams for league games and cup finals and preparing boxers for title fights etc. This, I believe, has given me an incredible opportunity to share what I have learnt over my career as a world class strength and conditioning coach which I have done in this habit. Let me spell it out quite simply, there are no shortcuts to a lean and healthy body, as you are about to find out.

respect back and those soliders would literally die for their Sergeant if the situation arose.

- This was opposite to the Sergeants who disrespected their men, created an environment of unrest and uncomfortableness. For those Sergeants, the men would not go that extra yard for them.

- I had learnt that communication was very important from an early age and that, in my first coaching job in professional rugby, I realised very quickly that creating the right environment was very important and could be the difference between success and failure.

- For example, with my first team, I got the players to listen to audio tapes from coaches who had been exceptionally successful in the NFL. The subjects covered such things as; how to create a winning attitude, overcoming adversity, what it takes to create a winning team. Over a period of a couple of months, I had integrated severe physical training with psychological input on how to create a winning team.

- My first team in professional rugby won 3 league titles in 5 seasons and went to 2 cup finals. I feel that I had achieved my goal.

- This biggest challenge after that was leaving this team which was full of worldclass rugby players form all over the world and dropping down a division and working with a team with no international players. To be quite frank, they were an ordinary bunch of players. This team had a lot of money and had tried to get promoted to the premiership for the last 4 years before I arrived, and failed each time. When I arrived at this club, they had pretty much the same players and coaches as they had the last 2 seasons. I observed immediately that, if I

changed the environment, this team would get promoted. I had no doubt what so ever. I will never forget my first meeting with the players at this new team, when I told them in no uncertain terms that I would take no prisoners in anything that I did with them from field conditioning, nutritional plans, weight sessions that they followed. I had an 8 week training block where my aim was to educate these players on their nutrition and lifestyle. They did not have to worry about anything else as I had that covered. I knew, from my previous 5 years of working at the highest level, when a player becomes healthy, he can not only withstand any training plan, more importantly, he can also gain from the training plan.

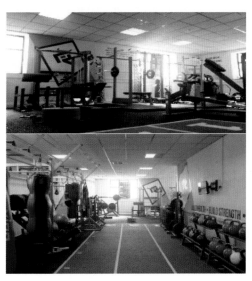

Phil Richards Performance Centre. Creating the right environment.

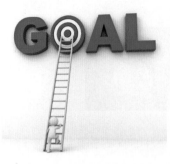

You must set yourself goals which are realistic, yet challenging. This will force you to constantly strive towards achieving outstanding results.

When you have a squad of extremely healthy players, anything is possible.

I cannot emphasise the importance of building health, then strength, and performance will always follow.

- I gave the players full responsibility of their nutirition, lifestyle and supplement plans. I monitored that through hydration testing, pH testing, body fat analysis and food diaries. Eventually, the whole squad bought into my philosiphy of health coming first. As I got the players healthy, the training could then only be described with one word, BRUTAL. I had pushed them harder then I had ever pushed any I had any other team previously. The results were spectacular. I witnessed ordinary rugby players becoming, extraordinary players. That season, we won 26 games out of 26. This had never occured before or since. This was in the 2003/2004 season. What was even more remarkable was that, on gaining promotion, every team had been relegated the following season. Thankfully this did not happen to us and we became known for our exceptional physicality in premiership rugby.

- The point I want to emphasize is that;

If you want outstanding results, you have to create an outstanding environment. After this, everything else will take care of itself.

- I also want to share with you my observation with working with one team. When we had a player that did not contribute to the environment in a positive way, he was simply removed from the environment.

- Remember from earlier in the book when we spoke about cells becoming their environment? Remember, we are also just a mass of trillions of cells - we also become our environment. I witnessed one coach who bullied 48 grown men in one club. The effect that he had on this group of people can only be described as devastating. Thankfully, he was removed from the environment and, as if by magic, everyone started to thrive again. Just like removing a cancer cell.

You must create the right training environment for the athlete to flourish! Remember, you become your environment.

- You must mentally prepare yourself for any training that you do. You cannot simply turn up to a training session. All of the athletes that I have worked with would mentally prepare themselves for the sessions and go through what they wanted to accomplish from that session.

Whether you think you can, or you think you can't, you're right

Henry Ford

Conclusion

- What I personally make sure of when I'm working with someone who has to be very lean and muscular is to use the STAD (Strength Training for Athletic Developmet) method to the full. Not only rotating exercises frequently but also sets, reps, rest periods, tempo, training days and even locations. This ensures not only variety, so we don't accommodate, but also mental stimulation. How many athletes/people do you know that train at the same time, same place, do the same exercises and guess what get the same results? This is the defintion of insanity.

- I now want to show you some example programs. I will show you programs that I prescirbe for someone who is severely overweight, for a champion boxer, a rugby team and a few more.

- Remember, these sessions are just examples. If they are not relevant for you, your training and your needs then simply use them as a template and find what works for you.

- If there are any exercises that you do not know how to do in these programs, or are unsure of the techniques, then speak to a qualified trainer or use the internet, which is an amazing tool to use.

- Remember, before undertaking any exercise program that you check with a medical professional to ensure that you have no underlying health problems.

- I realise that, for some people, this may be the first time they have done a weights session in the gym or have seen a program written down. The table below shows you how I set out the programs and what each column means and how to implement it. If you are unsure of anything then speak to a qualified personal trainer who can help.

EXERCISE	SETS	REPS	REST	TEMPO
This is the order in which to perform the exercises; A, B, C etc. If you see, for example A1 and A2, then this means that you should perform these as a super set. Rather than performing all of the sets for A1, perform one set of A1, then one set of A2. Then repeat for the necessary amount of sets.	The numer of times you will perform each exercise. For example, 6 sets of 6 squats	How many times you will lift a weight in a sinlge set.	How long you should rest between each set	The tempo of the lift may look like; 3 - 1 - X - 1 The 1st number refers to the eccentric part of the exercise (lowering the bar to your chest on a bench press), the 2nd number refers to the isometric pause in the stretched position (bar is touching your chest), the 3rd number refers to the concentric contraction (pressing the bar up), and the 4th number refers to the isometric pause in the shortened position (bar is locked out over your chest).

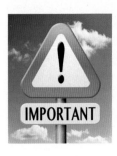

The less functional your job is (e.g. sitting down all day looking at a computer), the more functional your training needs to be. For example, cable wood chops, swiss ball work, chin ups, lunges etc.are some of the exercises that you could do.

On the flip side, the more functional your job (e.g. a builder), the less functional your training needs to be. This obviously does not apply to professional athletes whose training must be specific to their sport.

246

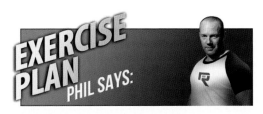

This is a program that I have designed for an extremely overweight, 45 year old female, who has done very little exercise in the last 25 years. The key to the program is to combine both aerobic and anaerobic exercises in a way that is very achievable. I am trying to enhance the functioning of her mitochondria with the brisk walking and then, with the weight training, my aim is to increase her lean muscle mass, which will raise her metabolic rate.

Each week, I will increase the intensity, if I feel that they can cope with the intensity so far. You must remember, with exercise, some days you feel great, some days you don't. On the days that you feel great, ramp it up. On the days you don't, you may have to take your foot off the pedal.

WEEK 1

MONDAY	TUESDAY	WEDNESDAY	THURSDAY	FRIDAY	SATURDAY	SUNDAY
A.M. 20 MINUTE BRISK EACH MORNING WALK IN A FASTED STATE (1 SCOOP AMINO WORK CAPACITY)						
	P.M. ALL OVER WEIGHTS 1		P.M. ALL OVER WEIGHTS 2			P.M. ALL OVER WEIGHTS 3

WEEK 2

MONDAY	TUESDAY	WEDNESDAY	THURSDAY	FRIDAY	SATURDAY	SUNDAY
A.M. 25 MINUTE BRISK EACH MORNING WALK IN A FASTED STATE (1 SCOOP AMINO WORK CAPACITY)						
	P.M. ALL OVER WEIGHTS 1		P.M. ALL OVER WEIGHTS 2			P.M. ALL OVER WEIGHTS 3

WEEK 3

MONDAY	TUESDAY	WEDNESDAY	THURSDAY	FRIDAY	SATURDAY	SUNDAY
A.M. 30 MINUTE BRISK EACH MORNING WALK IN A FASTED STATE (1 SCOOP AMINO WORK CAPACITY)						
	P.M. ALL OVER WEIGHTS 1		P.M. ALL OVER WEIGHTS 2			P.M. ALL OVER WEIGHTS 3

WEEK 4

MONDAY	TUESDAY	WEDNESDAY	THURSDAY	FRIDAY	SATURDAY	SUNDAY
A.M. 40 MIN WALK/JOG		A.M. 40 MIN WALK/JOG		A.M. 40 MIN WALK/JOG		
	P.M. ALL OVER WEIGHTS 1		P.M. ALL OVER WEIGHTS 2			P.M. ALL OVER WEIGHTS 3

ALL OVER 1

EXERCISE	SETS	REPS	REST
A BIKE	1	10 MINUTES	
B1 HORIZONTAL SINGLE ARM PULLY ROWS	3	12	75 SECS
B2 LEG EXTENSION	3	12	75 SECS
C1 SEATED CHEST PRESS	3	12	75 SECS
C2 HIP ABDUCTOR	3	12	75 SECS
D1 HIP ADDUCTOR	3	10	75 SECS
D2 STANDING DUMBELL CURLS	3	10	75 SECS

ALL OVER 2

EXERCISE	SETS	REPS	REST
A ROWING	1	10 MINUTES	
B1 SMITH MACHINE SQUAT (PARALLEL)	3	12	75 SECS
B2 SEATED ROW	3	12	75 SECS
C1 PEC DEC	3	12	75 SECS
C2 LEG CURL	3	12	75 SECS
D1 SEATED LOWER BACK EXTENSION	3	10	75 SECS
D2 TRICEP EXTENSION	3	10	75 SECS

ALL OVER 3

EXERCISE	SETS	REPS	REST
A INCLINE TREADMILL	1	10 MINUTES	
B1 LEG PRESS	3	12	75 SECS
B2 SEATED SHOULDER PRESS	3	12	75 SECS
C1 DUMBELL STEP-UPS	3	12	75 SECS
C2 LATERAL RAISE	3	12	75 SECS
D1 SEATED LEG CURL	3	10	75 SECS
D2 PREACHER CURLS	3	10	75 SECS

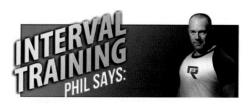

INTERVAL TRAINING PHIL SAYS:

There seems to be a lot of fitness experts who advocate high-intensity interval training (HIIT) and sprint training for fat loss. The science for this type of training looks very convinving, however, after 30 years of training athletes, I found that this method worked only with mainly fast twitch fibre athletes (e.g. sprinter, weight lifter, winger in rugby etc.)

For example, if you were an uneducated trainer and you read an article on the benfits of HIIT and sprint training, and their first client happened to be a 45 year old female who was exceptionally overweight, has not exercised in over 25 years, has 3 children in an unhappy marriage, 5 amalgam fillings in her mouth. In their enthusiasm, they believe that the quickest way for this ladie to drop body fat is to adopt the HIIT and sprint training method. They give this ladie a 5 minute gentle warm-up, which she struggles with. They then pull out a stop watch and say "GO", 30 seconds flat out. After 1 sprint, she is panting like a rhino, who has just been doing hill sprints with an elephant on its back. She looks you in the eye and says "what the f**k are you doing?"

The point each person should do what is relevant at the present moment to ensure that you can cope with the exercise and see improvements long term. You should also exercise according to your body. If you are a fast twith fibre person then you probably will thrive off HIIT, so long as other things in your life are right and you have a certain level of fitness. Mixed or slow twitch fibre type people will benefit less from HIIT and more from the aerobic training.

Let me repeat, I am an advocate of HIIT and sprint training but only when it is relevant to that person and when I know results will follow. I use this type of training myself for a very long time and it had a minimum effect on my body composition. It was only when I started doing long runs and higher rep weight training that my body fat percentage come back to a healthy range.

There is one more twist to the story though. If you have someone who is struggling with depression, from my research, the aerobic training will increase seratonin levels, which will give you a much better sense of well being. HIIT will increase your noradrenaline, adrenaline and dopamine levels which can make you feel edgy.

Rugby Training

Next I have added an 8 week preseaon plan that I have used with some of the teams I have worked with. This preseason plan helped teams win League and Cup Titles and take players from ordinary to extraordinary. But first, I want to share a story with you about how you have to fight for results, sometimes literally. So I have put this in to show you how the big boys train.

Sometimes you simply have to fight for everything if you want RESULTS:

My first year with Worcester Warriors is probably one of the most satisfying that I had in my professional career as a strength & conditioning coach in professional sport. From applying my philosophy on strength & conditioning (simple, direct & brutal), we won 26 games out of 26 games and were then promoted to the premiership of English Rugby, which is one of the most physical in the world. Every team before us that had been promoted had been relegated the following season. I was determined not to continue that tradition that, was for sure. I had been in rugby at this stage long enough to know that if you could get fifteen hard f...ckers on the field who can play rugby, the law of averages was quite simple, you had to win some games, even if you have a very basic core of players. I set about the Summer of 2004 plotting on creating that physical monster that I knew would shock the hardened teams of the English Premiership that would look upon us as a soft touch and an easy win.

That first week of an 8 week pre season in preparation of the new season ahead saw me take the team to an army camp where the focus on the day was the boxing competition that I had set up for them in the afternoon, after a morning of getting beasted on the assault course. I had carefully paired players off against each other and had an army physical training sergeant major referee each fight, which in the army is called milling. It is a one minute round where you simply beat the shit out of each other and it is about as tactical as firing a large nuclear bomb at a small island. Well, I can honestly say that afternoon was probably the best bonding session that I had put together, to get a group of players to find a new found respect for each other and I remember giving a speech at the end of that monumental afternoon and telling the players, in a no nonsense way, "what we will endure over the next nine 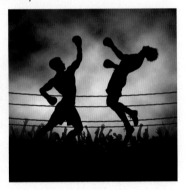 months when the season starts is what we endured this afternoon". We would have to fight for every second, of every minute, of every game if we are going to survive the season ahead and I'm very proud to say we did we become the first team to be promoted and not to be relegated the following season.

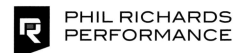

WEEK 1

MONDAY	TUESDAY	WEDNESDAY	THURSDAY	FRIDAY	SATURDAY	SUNDAY
A.M Upper Body Weights 1	A.M Swim Recovery & Massage	A.M Lower Body Weights 1	A.M Swim Recovery & Massage	A.M All Over Body Weights 1	DAY OFF	DAY OFF
P.M Boxing & Med Ball Cicuit	-	P.M Strongman Conditioning	-	P.M 5 Mile Stretcher Race & Night out (Team Bond- ing)	DAY OFF	DAY OFF

WEEK 2

MONDAY	TUESDAY	WEDNESDAY	THURSDAY	FRIDAY	SATURDAY	SUNDAY
A.M Upper Body Weights 1	A.M Swim Recovery & Massage	A.M Lower Body Weights 1	A.M Swim Recovery & Massage	A.M All Over Body Weights 1	DAY OFF	45 min run
P.M Shield & Bag Conditioning Drills	P.M -	P.M Strongman Conditioning	-	P.M Bike, Boxing & Med Ball Circuit	DAY OFF	

WEEK 3

MONDAY	TUESDAY	WEDNESDAY	THURSDAY	FRIDAY	SATURDAY	SUNDAY
A.M Upper Body Weights 1	A.M Rugby Session	A.M Lower Body Weights 1	A.M Swim Recovery & Massage	A.M All Over Body Weights 1	A.M Milling (Boxing)	DAY OFF
P.M Ball, Sheild & Bag Conditioning Drills	P.M -	P.M Phosphates - Tyres & Rugby Drills	-	P.M Bike, Rugby Session	P.M Night Out (Team Bonding)	

Stretcher Please!

In my last pre season with the Worcester Warriors I started it with an 8 mile stretcher race, hoping I would break someone. This wasn't a normal stretcher run - there were 6 players per stretcher. This meant one player on each corner carrying the stretcher, one player on the stretcher and the spare player had to carry two 25 kg plates - so in reality everyone was fucked. Even the player on the stretcher couldn't rest because he could have one player on a corner who is six foot eight and another on the opposite corner who his five foot seven and he literally is hanging on for dear life. I made the course exceptionally difficult; even though we were following a canal for four miles up four miles back, I made them continually go up the canal banks where underfoot was

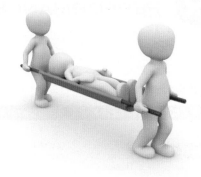

extremely difficult. There were six groups of six players ready to race each other literally to the death because the losing team would be punished with a mile car push, which is about as pleasurable as an afternoon bungee jumping without a bungee off a tall bridge

When I blew my whistle to signal the start of the race I was like a kid at Christmas, so excited, knowing someone was going to break and the rest would become stronger. There was a coach allocated to each group of players to make sure the player on the stretcher was rotated literally every minute to make sure everyone got a turn on the stretcher and that the lightest player didn't get threatened with his life if he got off the stretcher in place of some 23 stone hairy assed prop.

I put the players under so much pressure not to be last, I was literally screaming constantly at them to raise their standards, to push as hard as they could and to sort out any if there were any weak members of their team. Twenty minutes in to the race it was getting heated, a few arguments breaking out. One player dropped a 25 kg plate into the canal so he had to swim around in there for a bit whilst his stretcher team mates screamed some rather unpleasant names at him because it was costing them some invaluable time. It was absolute carnage, the exact thing I wanted- everyone working together under pressure, just like a game situation.

My team were at the front fighting for every yard, I'm running back and fourth checking the progress of the other teams and shouting encouragement and abuse. Then I get news the team at the back is missing a player, he's gone missing in action. I'm fucking stunned. How could you let your team mates down? Take your work load on? If you do that in a stretcher race then you are sure to do it in a game. This player had only just joined the team as well so he needed an excellent excuse, which in my book was either he was dead or lost a fucking limb.

Anyway we are now in full swing of the stretcher race, there were fights breaking out amongst the players who were so eager to win - if you weren't putting in you were getting punched. The effort that I witnessed during the stretcher race pleased me immensely. I knew hand-on-heart I had a group of players who would not take a backward step on the battlefield. I didn't even punish the losing team with the car push because how can you punish a group who have given 100% effort even I've got a heart.

So, where the fuck was our missing player? I make all the players hold a pressup position whilst I located him. I'm running around the ground frantically trying to locate him. On passing the physio room I thought I saw a player in there with an ice pack on his head but thought, "no, it can't be!". I back pedaled to take a second look and it was our missing player. I won't mention his nationality to spare his countries blushes but as he his explaining to me in his broken English that it was too hot for him, I explained back in my broken English that I thought he was a spineless twat. He was removed from the team shortly after.

Conclusion - if you want results you have to go through uncomfortable times. Make sure you have the right people on your team to get the job done properly. It only takes one person to collapse a team/ organisation.

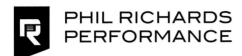

WEEK 4

MONDAY	TUESDAY	WEDNESDAY	THURSDAY	FRIDAY	SATURDAY	SUNDAY
A.M Upper Body Weights 2	A.M Rugby Session	A.M Lower Body Weights 2	A.M Swim Recovery & Massage	A.M All Over Body Weights 2	DAY OFF	DAY OFF
P.M Speed Session for relevant positions or work capacity	P.M Rugby Session	P.M Rugby Session	-	P.M Rugby Session (BRUTAL)	-	-

WEEK 5

MONDAY	TUESDAY	WEDNESDAY	THURSDAY	FRIDAY	SATURDAY	SUNDAY
A.M Upper Body Weights 2	A.M Rugby Session	A.M Lower Body Weights 2	A.M Swim Recovery & Massage	A.M All Over Body Weights 2	A.M Rugby Session	DAY OFF
P.M Speed Session for relevant positions or work capacity	P.M Rugby Session	P.M Rugby Session	-	P.M Bike - Rugby Session	-	

WEEK 6

MONDAY	TUESDAY	WEDNESDAY	THURSDAY	FRIDAY	SATURDAY	SUNDAY
A.M All Over Body Weights 3	A.M Rugby Session	A.M All Over Body Weights 4	A.M Swim Recovery & Massage	A.M Team Run (VERY INTENSE)	A.M Pre-Season Friendly (Go as hard as possible)	DAY OFF
P.M Speed Session for relevant positions or work capacity	P.M Rugby Session	P.M Rugby Session	-	-	P.M Night Out (Team Bonding)	-

Gentlemen, please start crawling!

My first training session with London Harlequins (a giant of English Rugby) was undoubtedly one of the most satisfying of my career as I genuinely disliked everything I had previously seen from my experience with other teams playing against them. I can honestly say they were the softest least physical team I had seen at the professional level. So when I got the chance to work with this team, I was more excited than a dog with three dicks.

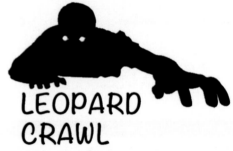

LEOPARD CRAWL

I remember the session quite vividly, standing on this beautiful rugby field, nice hot summer's day in London. All the players eagerly awaiting the upcoming training session and had been pre-warned by former rugby players that I had some mental health issues when it came to physical training. Anyway, I get the players to line up on the dead ball line and give the instruction to get on their bellies and start doing some lower back stretches. I observed their relief - but they did not know that they were just about to get a fucking beasting from hell.

After about the fourth stretch I instructed the players "Whilst you are still on your bellies, start leopard crawling you bunch of f***ers". I made them leopard crawl for a good thirty minutes. They were absolutely busted and I remember one of the players saying to me that it was the most pointless things he has ever done in his life, to which I replied "I totally agree but it give me huge fucking satisfaction, putting you through that pain".

And, boom our pre season was under way. I was only with this team for just over 4 months as I didn't like the constant noise of London but I can honestly say they become one of the most successful teams in the English premiership and I like to think I played a small part in teaching them to push themselves to their absolute limits and creating an environment that demanded results.

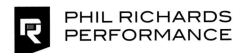

PHIL RICHARDS
PERFORMANCE

8 WEEK PREPARATION
PRE-SEASON RUGBY

WEEK 7

MONDAY	TUESDAY	WEDNESDAY	THURSDAY	FRIDAY	SATURDAY	SUNDAY
A.M All Over Body Weights 3	A.M Rugby Session (SKILLS)	A.M All over body weights 4	A.M Swim Recovery & Massage	A.M Team Run (VERY INTENSE)	A.M Pre-Season	DAY OFF
P.M Video & Massage	P.M Rugby Session (TEAM)	P.M Rugby Session	-	-	-	

WEEK 8

MONDAY	TUESDAY	WEDNESDAY	THURSDAY	FRIDAY	SATURDAY	SUNDAY
A.M All over body weights 3	A.M Rugby Session (SKILLS)	A.M All over body weights 4	A.M Swim Recovery & Massage	A.M Team Run (VERY INTENSE)	A.M First game of season!!	DAY OFF
P.M Video & Massage	P.M Rugby Session (TEAM)	P.M Rugby Session	-	-	-	

"PHIL WAS AN IMPORTANT PART OF A VERY SUCCESSFUL SWANSEA RUGBY SQUAD THAT DOMINATED WELSH RUGBY FOR A 4 YEAR PERIOD, HIS CONTRIBUTION WAS ENORMOUS, HE INSURED THAT WE COULD COMPETE PHYSICALLY WITH ANY OTHER TEAM IN EUROPE.

PLAYERS HAVE HUGE RESPECT FOR PHIL BECAUSE OF HIS DESIRE AND ENTHUSIASM TO HELP THEM BE THE BEST THEY CAN BE. THIS ABILITY WAS SO IMPORTANT TO THE COLLECTIVE TEAM EFFORT IN GETTING THE BEST OUT OF EVERY INDIVIDUAL"

JOHN PLUMTREE
SWANSEA RUGBY COACH 1997-2001, NOW NATAL SHARKS

255

Golf Episode Do not become complacent when things are going well.

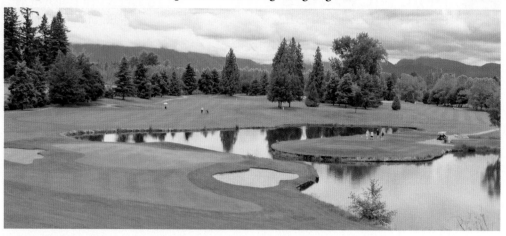

Sometimes you have to do what you have got to do to make sure you get what you want. With me, that was always RESULTS, no matter what method I used. I remember one preseason trip with Swansea Rugby Club (Now part of the Ospreys Rugby Team) in particular where I felt that the players were becoming complacent due to the fact that we had been very successful for a few seasons previously. Well for those of you reading this who are not familiar with preseason it is a period of very intense training in preparation for the upcoming season.

The team had decided to go away for a few days, play a pre season friendly and get some intense training in as well. On one particular evening I actually encouraged the players to go out have a few beers knowing full well a few beers to a rugby player is an excuse to get absolutely shit faced. Unbeknown to the players, I had planned an early morning meeting with hell for them, I had an early morning call at 4 A.M. arranged for every room and the players had been given a curfew that they must be back from the pub by 3 A.M or they would be fined. I was like a kid at Christmas waiting in reception at 3.55 A.M. knowing that very shortly that I was going to find out if this group of players were going to be able to cope with what I was about to throw at them.

As if by magic, they started wandering into reception as if they had been abducted by the mysterious beer monster who had forced them to drink on average 30 pints - they were, as predicted, shit faced. Trying to address 36 plus pissed up rugby players at 4 A.M. is no easy task, especially as they had only just fallen asleep, but I had a knack of being a total bastard when needed to be in these situations - one thing my early army days taught me. To get the players attention I blew my whistle in reception as loud as I could and explain, in a no - nonsense way, that we were just about to go through hell and the objective was to do forward rolls, crawl, wheel barrow, piggy back or run depending on my command around this beautiful 18 hole golf course. And there was one more twist, if there was any noise, e.g. talking, laughing crying, and we would go back to hole 1 (the start) and start again. We all got outside and the players were now in a state of panic because, from previous encounters with me on these types of situations, they knew they were just about to go through a very fucking painful couple of hours.

The start of the course was slightly down hill for approximately 60 meters so I made the players do forward rolls down as fast as they could knowing full well they were intoxicated and I was hoping to get my first spewer early as this is always entertaining for everyone else. Well I didn't get a spewer - I got a disappearance. One of the players had got disorientated and, unbeknown to me because I couldn't because it was still very dark, went off the side of the golf course, fell off a cliff and landed in a shit load of stingy nettles. He was screaming, "it doesn't hurt". After about 10 minutes of pulling the player to freedom we started again, remember I said no noise or we go back to hole one. I blew my whistle again and they were off, myself and head coach screaming at the players deliberately putting massive pressure on them to talk, laugh anything to make a noise so we could get them to start again.

20 minutes into our nature ramble around the golf course I spotted a massive lake - my prayers had been answered. I got all the players into the lake chest deep and gave the command that when they hear

the first whistle they must dunk their heads under water. When they hear the second whistle, they can come up and breathe. I kept this going for a good 5 minutes, the players were extremely cold but I wanted one of them to crack - just fucking one, so we could break them on the golf course! No not one cracked in the lake so we resumed our fun of crawling, carrying each other, wheel barrowing and everything else which you can make exceptionally difficult for someone on a golf course at the crack of the arse time of the morning.

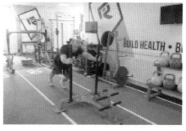

Prowler work

Anyway cut a long story short, after four grueling hours we finished the training/mental session and I got the players in a huddle and told them that was an exceptional effort and they must remember that if we were going to win the league that season, then that was the effort that would be required every time. We had our most sucessful season ever that year.

There is a final twist to this little story. As it had been a long morning on the golf course, I was having a shower and my phone went off in my hotel room. It was the hotel receptionist informing me that the grounds man of the golf course was very eager to speak to me. On meeting the grounds man in the hotel reception he was shaking like a shitting dog and I thought he had a speech impediment but I realised that it was just rage. He eagerly wanted to show me his golf course, I'm just thinking "mate I've been on it for the last 4 hours so hurry up". What I hadn't realised that a golf course is not supposed to have 36 plus hairy assed players wearing rugby boots and with the average weight being around 17 stone on it due to the possibility of ripping the course to pieces. He showed me some damage on the second hole and, in all fairness, it looked like a bunch of rhinoceroses had been playing murder ball there all night the ground was cut up so much. On explaining to the rather excitable grounds man on the possibility that it could have been local rabbits that did it, he exploded into an uncontrollable outburst, with some of the most abusive language that my delicate ears had ever heard and we parted company on that note. I walked away knowing - job done!

Boxing Training

The session doesn't have to be long to be effective no matter how fit you are!

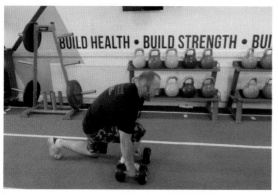

In preparation for another fight, I was getting ready to take Amir Khan through another training session. It was very early in our preparation, I think it might have been the first day of an 8 week plan that we did when I was training him. I had a professional strength & conditioning coach interning with that day (Paul Hatton) who himself is know a very accomplished strength coach and I rate him in my top 3 strength coaches in UK sport, along with Craig White & Neil Taylor.

The session was quite simple - I had a prowler loaded with 60 kgs, plus obviously the weight of the prowler (the one I used then was about 40 kgs), bearing in mind Amir was only about 63kgs at this time. I explained to Amir that all I wanted him to do was to push the prowler the full length of the track which was 60 meters using real big steps to get nice and warm and make sure he didn't stop. Now when you tell Amir not to stop let me tell you he will not stop. Out of all the athletes I've trained over the years he was one of the toughest.

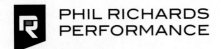

WEEK 1

MONDAY	TUESDAY	WEDNESDAY	THURSDAY	FRIDAY	SATURDAY	SUNDAY
A.M Upper Body Weights 1	A.M Swim Recovery & Massage	A.M Lower Body Weights 1	A.M Swim Recovery & Massage	A.M All Over Body Weights 1	DAY OFF	45 min run
P.M Bike & Bag Intervals	-	P.M Prowler & Tyre Work	-	P.M Bike, Bag & KB Intervals	DAY OFF	

WEEK 2

MONDAY	TUESDAY	WEDNESDAY	THURSDAY	FRIDAY	SATURDAY	SUNDAY
A.M Upper Body Weights 1	A.M 6 x 400m Track	A.M Lower Body Weights 1	A.M Swim Recovery & Massage	A.M All Over Body Weights 1	DAY OFF	45 min run
P.M Bike & Bag Intervals	P.M Swim Recovery & Massage	P.M Prowler & Tyre Work	-	P.M Bike, Bag & KB Intervals	DAY OFF	

WEEK 3

MONDAY	TUESDAY	WEDNESDAY	THURSDAY	FRIDAY	SATURDAY	SUNDAY
A.M Upper Body Weights 1	A.M 8 x 400m Track	A.M Lower Body Weights 1	A.M Swim Recovery & Massage	A.M All Over Body Weights 1	A.M Field Conditioning	45 min run
P.M Bike & Bag Intervals	P.M Swim Recovery & Massage	P.M Prowler & Tyre Work	-	P.M Bike, Bag & KB Intervals	-	

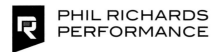

WEEK 4

MONDAY	TUESDAY	WEDNESDAY	THURSDAY	FRIDAY	SATURDAY	SUNDAY
A.M Boxing Training	A.M Swim Recovery & Massage	A.M Boxing Training	A.M Swim Recovery & Massage	A.M All Over Body Weights 1	A.M Rest	45 min run
P.M Upper Body Weights 2	-	P.M Lower Body Weights 2	-	P.M All Over Body Weights 2	-	

WEEK 5

MONDAY	TUESDAY	WEDNESDAY	THURSDAY	FRIDAY	SATURDAY	SUNDAY
A.M Boxing Training & Sparring	A.M 8 x 400m Track	A.M Boxing Training & Sparring	A.M Swim Recovery & Massage	A.M Boxing Training & Sparring	A.M Rest	45 min run
P.M Upper Body Weights 2	P.M Swim Recovery & Massage	P.M Lower Body Weights 2	-	P.M All Over Body Weights 2	-	

WEEK 6

MONDAY	TUESDAY	WEDNESDAY	THURSDAY	FRIDAY	SATURDAY	SUNDAY
A.M Boxing Training & Sparring	A.M 10 x 400m Track	A.M Boxing Training & Sparring	A.M Swim Recovery & Massage	A.M Boxing Training & Sparring	A.M Field Conditioning	A.M Rest
P.M Upper Body Weights 2	P.M Swim Recovery & Massage	P.M Lower Body Weights 2	-	P.M All Over Body Weights 2	-	-

259

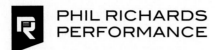
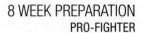

WEEK 7

MONDAY	TUESDAY	WEDNESDAY	THURSDAY	FRIDAY	SATURDAY	SUNDAY
A.M Boxing Training & Sparring	A.M Swim Recovery & Massage	A.M Boxing Training & Sparring	A.M Swim Recovery & Massage	A.M Boxing Training & Sparring	A.M Swim Recovery & Massage	45 min run if needed to for weight. If not rest.
P.M Upper Body Weights 2	-	P.M Lower Body Weights 2	-	P.M All Over Body Weights 2	-	

WEEK 8

MONDAY	TUESDAY	WEDNESDAY	THURSDAY	FRIDAY	SATURDAY	SUNDAY
A.M Swim Recovery & Massage	A.M Swim Recovery & Massage	A.M Boxing Training Technical Skills (light)	A.M Day Off	A.M Weigh In	-	
P.M All Over Body Weights 3	-	P.M Lower Body Weights 2	-	P.M Light Pad Work	A.M Fight Night	

Anyway, Amir went off like a grayhound out of the traps. I turned to Paul my internee and said "That's it. The session will be finished in approximately 90 seconds". Paul looked at me in astonishment bearing in mind he had come to see a full on training session, after traveeling 2 hours to get to it, and said, "You are having a laugh", to which I replied, "When the prowler hits the blue mat at the end of the track, watch whats happens".

As predicted Amir fought with that prowler every inch of the way and did not stop. Approximately 90 seconds later, the prowler hits the blue mat and Amir got up from the pushing position and started walking towards us. At first he looked to be ok but I knew what was going to happen, as I had seen it multiple times with elite rugby players I had trained. The steady walked turned into bambi on ice, to us carrying Amir to the changing room and it took a good two hours for Amir's head to come back to normality. Intensity is the key when you are looking to get results and as the old saying goes, "you can either train long or hard but you can't do the both in the same session".

"PHIL HAS MADE ME DO SESSIONS AND WHEN I HAVE FINISHED THEM I DON'T KNOW WHERE MY HEAD IS. BUT IT IS GOOD TO FEEL LIKE THAT BECAUSE IN A FIGHT I KNOW I WILL FEEL LIKE THAT AT SOME STAGE. I HAVE NEVER FELT THE PAIN OR EXHAUSTION THAT I FEEL WITH PHIL.

"THERE HAVE BEEN SOME SESSIONS THAT HAVE BEEN SO TOUGH, I WANTED TO HIDE IN A CORNER BECAUSE THERE WERE ANOTHER FIVE SESSIONS TO DO.
"HE TAKES YOU TO AN UNCOMFORTABLE ZONE BUT I NEED TO KNOW HOW I FEEL WHEN I AM IN IT. I FEEL MORE FOCUSED THAN EVER, STRONGER THAN EVER, TOO."

AMIR KHAN
WORLD CHAMPION BOXER

UPPER BODY 1

EXERCISE	SETS	REPS	TEMPO	REST
A1 Viking Press	5	6 - 8	3 - 1 - X - 1	75 Seconds
A2 Cable Snatch	4	12	1 - 1 - 1 - 1	75 Seconds
ONCE ALL SETS HAVE BEEN COMPLETED REST FOR 5 MINUTES				
B1 Incline Bench Press	4	8 - 12	3 - 1 - X - 1	75 Seconds
B2 T-Bar Rows	4	8 - 12	Controlled	75 Seconds
ONCE ALL SETS HAVE BEEN COMPLETED REST FOR 5 MINUTES				
C Med Ball Throws	5	10	X - X - X - X	75 Seconds

LOWER BODY 1

EXERCISE	SETS	REPS	TEMPO	REST
A1 Box Squats	8	1 - 5	2 - 1 - X - 1	1 - 3 Minutes
ONCE ALL SETS HAVE BEEN COMPLETED REST FOR 5 MINUTES				
B1 Prowler Push	4	20 Meters	X - X - X - X	75 Seconds
B2 Lateral Step Overs	4	10 each side	X - X - X - X	75 Seconds
ONCE ALL SETS HAVE BEEN COMPLETED REST FOR 5 MINUTES				
C1 Cable Hyper Ext Rows	4	20	2 - 1 - X - 1	75 Seconds
C2 Standing Cable Crunches	4	20	3 - 1 - X - 1	75 Seconds

262

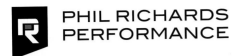

ALL OVER 1

EXERCISE	SETS	REPS	TEMPO	REST
A1 Log Clean & Press	8	3	X - X - X - X	60 Seconds
ONCE ALL SETS HAVE BEEN COMPLETED REST FOR 5 MINUTES				
B1 Lunge & Reach	4	6 - 8 each leg	2 - 1 - X - 1	75 Seconds
B2 Any Grip Chin	4	8 - 10	3 - 1 - X - 1	75 Seconds
ONCE ALL SETS HAVE BEEN COMPLETED REST FOR 5 MINUTES				
C1 Kettle Bell Rotations	3	20	2 - 1 - X - 1	75 Seconds
C2 Hanging Leg Raises	3	20	3 - 1 - X - 1	75 Seconds

UPPER BODY 2

EXERCISE	SETS	REPS	TEMPO	REST
A1 Dumb Bell Shoulder Press	5	6 - 8	3 - 1 - X - 1	75 Seconds
A2 Dumb Bell Shrug & External Rotation	5	12	1 - 1 - 1 - 1	75 Seconds
ONCE ALL SETS HAVE BEEN COMPLETED REST FOR 5 MINUTES				
B1 Incline Dumb Bell Chest Press	4	8 - 12	3 - 1 - X - 1	75 Seconds
B2 Single Arm Cable Rows	4	8 - 12	Controlled	75 Seconds
ONCE ALL SETS HAVE BEEN COMPLETED REST FOR 5 MINUTES				
C Hurdle Jumps	5	10	X - X - X - X	90 Seconds

263

LOWER BODY 2

EXERCISE	SETS	REPS	TEMPO	REST
A1 Dead Lifts	8	1 - 5	2 - 1 - X - 1	1 - 3 Minutes
ONCE ALL SETS HAVE BEEN COMPLETED REST FOR 5 MINUTES				
B1 Russian Step Ups	4	10 each leg	2 - 1 - X - 1	75 Seconds
B2 Back Attack	4	20	2 - 1 - X - 1	75 Seconds
ONCE ALL SETS HAVE BEEN COMPLETED REST FOR 5 MINUTES				
C1 Weighted Side Bends	4	12 each side	2 - 1 - X - 1	75 Seconds
C2 Swiss Ball Reverse Crunch	4	20	3 - 1 - X - 1	75 Seconds

ALL OVER 2

EXERCISE	SETS	REPS	TEMPO	REST
A1 Power Cleans	8	1 - 3	X - X - X - X	1 - 3 Minutes
A2 Super Yolk Walks	4	20 Meters	2 - 1 - X - 1	75 Seconds
ONCE ALL SETS HAVE BEEN COMPLETED REST FOR 5 MINUTES				
B1 Rack Bench Press	4	8 - 10	3 - 1 - X - 1	75 Seconds
B2 Lying Tricep Ext	3	8 - 12	2 - 1 - X - 1	75 Seconds
ONCE ALL SETS HAVE BEEN COMPLETED REST FOR 5 MINUTES				
C Pulley Curls	3	20	3 - 1 - X - 1	75 Seconds

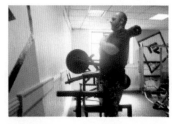

Back Attack

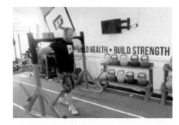

Super Yolk Walks

Sometimes it comes down to bare knuckles!

I believe my greatest attribute as a strength & conditioning coach was prescribing for the moment; it is only the naive coach who will rigidly stick to a plan. I could share many examples of this in my personal career but one that springs to mind is when a team I was working with had just lost to a rival team. There was an incredible amount of frustration amongst the players at this particular loss. So come two days after the game, the players had had some rest time and were then scheduled in to do a weights session.

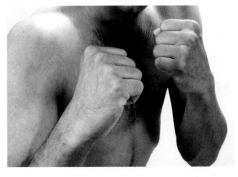

I observed the players entering the gym, their body language was telling me "I feel sorry for myself", and all the rest of the bull crap. Ok, change of plan! I set a room out with just boxing gloves, threw them in at full speed and I got them to start fighting each other. It was great! I saw an enormous amount of frustration being let out in that session. Every round I made sure they would fight a different partner. The last round was bare knuckle stuff, real-in-your-face shit. There was grappling on the floor, eye gouging, testicle squeezing and that was it session over. No weights, just fuck off and leave yesterday's game go and only focus on the next one.

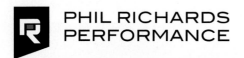
ALL OVER 3

EXERCISE	SETS	REPS	TEMPO	REST
A1 Bench Press	4	6 - 8	4 - 1 - X - 1	1 - 3 Minutes
ONCE ALL SETS HAVE BEEN COMPLETED REST FOR 5 MINUTES				
B1 Cable Snatch	4	12	2 - 1 - X - 1	75 Seconds
B2 Reverse Hypers	4	15	3 - 1 - X - 1	75 Seconds
ONCE ALL SETS HAVE BEEN COMPLETED REST FOR 5 MINUTES				
C1 T-Bar Rows	3	8 - 12	2 - 1 - X - 1	75 Seconds
C2 Pulley Curls	3	12	3 - 1 - X - 1	75 Seconds

Team Work: we can all learn an invaluable lesson on this from geese.

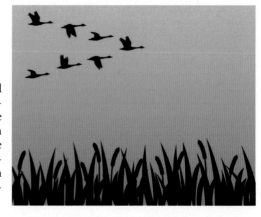

I remember reading this story about geese and how they work as a team when they fly and handing the message out to Swansea RFC, which at the time was stacked with international players from all over the world. We were headed for a game with Pontypool RFC, which were in a division below us and, in reality, should not have lived with us in terms of rugby ability and our superior fitness levels.

When you see geese flying along in "V" formation, you might consider what science has discovered as to why they fly that way. As each bird flaps its wings, it creates an uplift for the bird immediately following. By flying in "V" formation, the whole flock adds at least 71 percent greater flying range than if each bird flew on its own. People who share a common direction and sense of community can get where they are going more quickly and easily because they are traveling on the thrust of one another.

When a goose falls out of formation, it suddenly feels the drag and resistance of trying to go it alone — and quickly gets back into formation to take advantage of the lifting power of the bird in front. If we have as much sense as a goose, we will stay in formation with those people who are headed the same way we are.

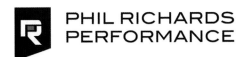

Week 1	Morning	Evening
Monday	All over weights 1	30 minute run (with fan)
Tuesday		
Wednesday	All over weights 2	30 minute bike (with fan)
Thursday		
Friday	All over weights 3	30 minute row (with fan)
Saturday	Swim – Sauna – Hot Tub	
Sunday		

Week 2	Morning	Evening
Monday	Upper Body 1	Swim – Sauna – Hot Tub
Tuesday		
Wednesday	Lower Body 1	Swim – Sauna – Hot Tub
Thursday		
Friday	Upper Body 2	Swim – Sauna – Hot Tub
Saturday	Lower Body 2	
Sunday		

Week 3	Morning	Evening
Monday	Chest & Back 1	35 minute run (with fan)
Tuesday		
Wednesday	Legs & Abs 1	35 minute bike (with fan)
Thursday		
Friday	Shoulders & Arms 1	35 minute row (with fan)
Saturday		
Sunday		

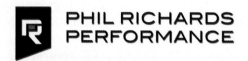 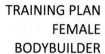

Week 4	Morning	Evening
Monday	All over weights 4	Swim – Sauna – Hot Tub
Tuesday		
Wednesday	All over weights 5	Swim – Sauna – Hot Tub
Thursday		
Friday	All over weights 6	Swim – Sauna – Hot Tub
Saturday		
Sunday		

Week 5	Morning	Evening
Monday	Upper Body 3	40 minute run (with fan)
Tuesday		
Wednesday	Lower Body 3	40 minute bike (with fan)
Thursday		
Friday	Upper Body 4	40 minute row (with fan)
Saturday	Lower Body 4	
Sunday		

Week 6	Morning	Evening
Monday	Chest & Back 2	Swim – Sauna – Hot Tub
Tuesday		
Wednesday	Legs & Abs 2	Swim – Sauna – Hot Tub
Thursday		
Friday	Shoulders & Arms 2	Swim – Sauna – Hot Tub
Saturday		
Sunday		

PHIL RICHARDS PERFORMANCE

WEIGHTS PLAN (EUROPEANS)
NATURAL BODY BUILDER

WEEK 1: ALLOVER BODY 1

EXERCISE	SETS	REPS	TEMPO	REST
A1 Snatch Grip Dead Lifts	10	3 - 5	2 - 1 - X - 1	1-3 minutes
ONCE ALL SETS HAVE BEEN COMPLETED REST FOR 3 MINUTES				
B1 Incline D/Bell Bench	4	8 - 12	4 - 1 - X - 1	60 Seconds
B2 Lat Pull Downs	4	8 - 12	3 - 1 - X - 1	60 Seconds
ONCE ALL SETS HAVE BEEN COMPLETED REST FOR 3 MINUTES				
C1 Standing Cable Crunches	3	20	Controlled	60 Seconds
C2 D/Bell Upright Row from floor	3	10 each side	3 - 1 - X - 1	60 Seconds

WEEK 1: ALLOVER BODY 2

EXERCISE	SETS	REPS	TEMPO	REST
A1 Ski Squats (Go Deep)	10	5	2 - 1 - X - 1	1 minute
ONCE ALL SETS HAVE BEEN COMPLETED REST FOR 3 MINUTES				
B1 Lying leg curls	4	8 - 10	4 - 1 - X - 1	60 Seconds
B2 Preacher Curl	4	8 - 12	4 - 1 - X - 1	60 Seconds
ONCE ALL SETS HAVE BEEN COMPLETED REST FOR 3 MINUTES				
C1 Leg Extension	4	15	4 - 1 - X - 2	60 Seconds
C2 Lying Tricep Extension	4	12	3 - 1 - X - 1	60 Seconds
D Incline Sit ups	3	30	3 - 1 - X - 1	90 Seconds

269

WEEK 1: ALLOVER BODY 3

EXERCISE	SETS	REPS	TEMPO	REST
A1 Rack Bench Press	5	6 - 8	2 - 1 - X - 1	60 Seconds
A2 Leg Press	5	20	2 - 1 - X - 1	60 Seconds
ONCE ALL SETS HAVE BEEN COMPLETED REST FOR 3 MINUTES				
B1 Cable Snatch (Horizontal)	4	15	2 - 1 - X - 1	60 Seconds
B2 Seated Bench Press	4	15	4 - 1 - X - 1	60 Seconds
ONCE ALL SETS HAVE BEEN COMPLETED REST FOR 3 MINUTES				
C1 Hip Abductor	4	20	3 - 1 - X - 1	60 Seconds
C2 Hip Abduction	4	20	3 - 1 - X - 1	60 Seconds

WEEK 2: UPPER BODY 1

EXERCISE	SETS	REPS	TEMPO	REST
A1 Standing Shoulder Press	5	6 - 8	2 - 1 - X - 1	75 Seconds
A2 Supinated Chins	5	6 - 8	4 - 1 - X - 2	75 Seconds
ONCE ALL SETS HAVE BEEN COMPLETED REST FOR 3 MINUTES				
B1 Incline Bench Press	4	8 - 12	3 - 1 - X - 1	75 Seconds
B2 Seated Rows	4	8 - 10	3 - 1 - X - 1	75 Seconds
ONCE ALL SETS HAVE BEEN COMPLETED REST FOR 3 MINUTES				
C1 Pulley Tricep Extensions	3	20	3 - 1 - X - 1	60 Seconds
C2 Pulley Bicep Curls	3	20	3 - 1 - X - 1	60 Seconds
D Sprints Treadmill	5	1 MInutes	X - X - X - X	60 Seconds

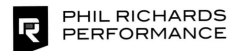

WEIGHTS PLAN (EUROPEANS)
NATURAL BODY BUILDER

WEEK 2: LOWER BODY 1

EXERCISE	SETS	REPS	TEMPO	REST
A1 Good Mornings	5	10	2 - 1 - X - 1	1 - 3 Minutes
A2 Backward Sled Drags	5	40 Meters	X - X - X - X	75 Seconds
ONCE ALL SETS HAVE BEEN COMPLETED REST FOR 3 MINUTES				
B1 Leg Press	4	12 -15	3 - 1 - X - 0	75 Seconds
B2 Cable Hyper Extensions	4	20	3 - 1 - X - 0	75 Seconds
B3 Swiss Ball Reverse Crunches	3	20	3 - 1 - X - 1	60 Seconds
ONCE ALL SETS HAVE BEEN COMPLETED REST FOR 3 MINUTES				
C Bike Sprints	6	1 Minute	FLAT OUT	60 Seconds

WEEK 2: UPPER BODY 2

EXERCISE	SETS	REPS	TEMPO	REST
A1 Flat D/B Press	5	8 - 10	4 - 1 - X - 1	75 Seconds
A2 B.O.L.R	5	8 - 10	1 - 1 - 1 - 1	75 Seconds
ONCE ALL SETS HAVE BEEN COMPLETED REST FOR 3 MINUTES				
B1 Seated Bench	4	12 - 15	4 - 1 - X - 1	75 Seconds
B2 Preacher Curls	4	12 - 15	3 - 1 - X - 1	75 Seconds
ONCE ALL SETS HAVE BEEN COMPLETED REST FOR 3 MINUTES				
C1 KBR	4	20	2 - 1 - X - 1	75 Seconds
C2 Over Cable Tricep Ext	4	12	4 - 1 - X - 1	75 Seconds
D Rowing	6	1 MInute	FLAT OUT	60 Seconds

WEEK 2: LOWER BODY 2

EXERCISE	SETS	REPS	TEMPO	REST
A1 Dead Lifts	8	1 - 3	2 - 1 - X - 1	No Rest
A2 Hurdle Jumps	8	5	X - X - X - X	90 Seconds
ONCE ALL SETS HAVE BEEN COMPLETED REST FOR 3 MINUTES				
B1 Leg Extensions	4	15	4 - 1 - X - 1	60 Seconds
B2 Leg Curls	4	15	4 - 1 - X - 1	60 Seconds
ONCE ALL SETS HAVE BEEN COMPLETED REST FOR 3 MINUTES				
C1 Prowler Push	4	50 Meters	FLAT OUT	3 Minutes

WEEK 3: CHEST & BACK 1

EXERCISE	SETS	REPS	TEMPO	REST
A1 Weighted Press Ups	5	8 - 12	3 - 1 - X - 1	60 Seconds
A2 T Bar Rows	5	12	4 - 1 - X - 1	60 Seconds
ONCE ALL SETS HAVE BEEN COMPLETED REST FOR 3 MINUTES				
B1 D/B Bench Press	4	8 - 12	3 - 1 - X - 1	75 Seconds
B2 Any Grip Chin	4	12	4 - 1 - X - 2	75 Seconds
ONCE ALL SETS HAVE BEEN COMPLETED REST FOR 3 MINUTES				
C1 Pulley Curls	4	15	4 - 1 - X - 2	75 Seconds
C2 Tricep Extensions	4	12	4 - 1 - X - 2	75 Seconds

WEIGHTS PLAN (EUROPEANS)
NATURAL BODY BUILDER

WEEK 3: LEGS & ABS 1

EXERCISE	SETS	REPS	TEMPO	REST
A1 Good Mornings	5	10	3 - 1 - X - 1	60 Seconds
A2 Leg Extensions	5	20	3 - 1 - X - 1	60 Seconds
ONCE ALL SETS HAVE BEEN COMPLETED REST FOR 3 MINUTES				
B1 Leg Press	4	8 - 12	4 - 1 - X - 1	60 Seconds
B2 Cable Crunch	4	20	2 - 1 - 1 - 1	60 Seconds
ONCE ALL SETS HAVE BEEN COMPLETED REST FOR 3 MINUTES				
C1 KBR	4	20	2 - 1 - 1 - 1	60 Seconds

WEEK 3: SHOULDERS & ARMS 1

EXERCISE	SETS	REPS	TEMPO	REST
A1 Standing Shoulder Press	5	10	3 - 1 - X - 1	60 Seconds
A2 Towel Chins	5	8	3 - 1 - X - 1	60 Seconds
ONCE ALL SETS HAVE BEEN COMPLETED REST FOR 3 MINUTES				
B1 Lateral Raises	4	20	3 - 1 - X - 1	60 Seconds
B2 Cable Crossovers	4	20	3 - 1 - X - 1	60 Seconds
ONCE ALL SETS HAVE BEEN COMPLETED REST FOR 3 MINUTES				
C1 Lying Tricep Ext	4	20	2 - 1 - 1 - 1	60 Seconds
C2 D/B Curls	4	15	4 - 1 - 1 - 1	60 Seconds

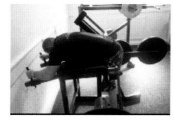 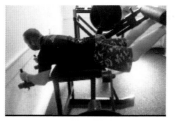

Reverse Hyper

WEEK 4: ALLOVER BODY 4

EXERCISE	SETS	REPS	TEMPO	REST
A1 Power Cleans	8	1 - 3	X - X - X - X	1-3 Minutes
ONCE ALL SETS HAVE BEEN COMPLETED REST FOR 3 MINUTES				
B1 Back Squats Deep	5	10	4 - 1 - X - 1	60 Seconds
B2 Any Grip Chin	4	8 - 12	3 - 1 - X - 1	60 Seconds
ONCE ALL SETS HAVE BEEN COMPLETED REST FOR 3 MINUTES				
C1 Standing Cable Crunches	4	20	Controlled	60 Seconds
C2 D/Bell Upright Row from floor	4	10 each side	3 - 1 - X - 1	60 Seconds
D Bike Sprint	8	1 Minute	FLAT OUT	60 Seconds

WEEK 4: ALLOVER BODY 5

EXERCISE	SETS	REPS	TEMPO	REST
A1 Barbell Lunge	5	5 Each Leg	2 - 1 - X - 1	60 Seconds
A2 Dips	5	8 - 10	4 - 1 - X - 1	60 Seconds
ONCE ALL SETS HAVE BEEN COMPLETED REST FOR 3 MINUTES				
B1 Leg Extensions	4	20	3 - 1 - X - 1	60 Seconds
B2 Preacher Curls	4	10 each arm	4 - 1 - X - 1	60 Seconds
ONCE ALL SETS HAVE BEEN COMPLETED REST FOR 3 MINUTES				
C1 Straight Leg Raises	4	20	3 - 1 - X - 1	60 Seconds
C2 Good Mornings	4	10	3 - 1 - X - 1	60 Seconds
D Treadmill	6	1 Minute	FLAT OUT	60 Seconds

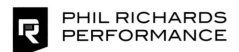

WEIGHTS PLAN (EUROPEANS)
NATURAL BODY BUILDER

WEEK 4: ALLOVER BODY 6

EXERCISE	SETS	REPS	TEMPO	REST
A1 Rack Bench Press	5	10	4 - 1 - X - 1	60 Seconds
A2 Lying Leg Curls	5	12	4 - 1 - X - 1	60 Seconds
ONCE ALL SETS HAVE BEEN COMPLETED REST FOR 3 MINUTES				
B1 Leg Press	4	20	4 - 1 - X - 1	60 Seconds
B2 Cable Tricep Ext	4	20	2 - 1 - X - 1	60 Seconds
B3 Supinated Chins	4	12	4 - 1 - X - 1	60 Seconds
ONCE ALL SETS HAVE BEEN COMPLETED REST FOR 3 MINUTES				
C1 Prowler Push	5	20 Meters	FLAT OUT	90 Seconds
C2 Rowing	5	1 Minute	FLAT OUT	90 Seconds

WEEK 5: UPPER BODY 3

EXERCISE	SETS	REPS	TEMPO	REST
A1 Incline Bench Press	5	6 - 8	4 - 1 - X - 1	1 - 3 minutes
A2 Lateral Raises	5	12 - 15	1 - 1 - X - 1	75 Seconds
A3 Press Up & Twist	5	6 each side	1 - 1 - 1 - 1	75 Seconds
A4 Cable Snatch	5	20	4 - 1 - X - 1	75 Seconds
ONCE ALL SETS HAVE BEEN COMPLETED REST FOR 3 MINUTES				
B Backward Sled Drags	5	50 Meters	FLAT OUT	120 Seconds

WEEK 5: LOWER BODY 3

EXERCISE	SETS	REPS	TEMPO	REST
A1 Ski Squats	5	5	2 - 1 - X - 1	60 Seconds
ONCE ALL SETS HAVE BEEN COMPLETED REST FOR 3 MINUTES				
B1 Russian Step Up	4	6 - 8 each leg	X - X - X - X	60 Seconds
B2 Lateral Step Overs	4	10 each side	3 - 1 - X - 1	60 Seconds
ONCE ALL SETS HAVE BEEN COMPLETED REST FOR 3 MINUTES				
C1 Swiss Ball leg Curls	4	12	2 - 1 - X - 1	60 Seconds
C2 Standing Cable Crunches	4	20	3 - 1 - X - 1	60 Seconds
C3 Cable Pull Throughs	4	20	3 - 1 - X - 1	60 Seconds

WEEK 5: UPPER BODY 4

EXERCISE	SETS	REPS	TEMPO	REST
A1 Cable Snatch	5	15	X - X - X - X	60 Seconds
A2 Incline Bench	5	6 - 8	4 - 1 - X - 1	60 Seconds
ONCE ALL SETS HAVE BEEN COMPLETED REST FOR 3 MINUTES				
B1 Seated Cable Rows	4	12 - 15	4 - 1 - X - 1	60 Seconds
B2 Seated Bench Press	4	12 - 15	3 - 1 - X - 1	60 Seconds
ONCE ALL SETS HAVE BEEN COMPLETED REST FOR 3 MINUTES				
C1 Single Arm Cable Curls	3	12	2 - 1 - X - 1	60 Seconds
C2 Single Arm Tricep Press	3	12	2 - 1 - X - 1	60 Seconds

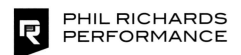

PHIL RICHARDS PERFORMANCE

WEIGHTS PLAN (EUROPEANS)
NATURAL BODY BUILDER

WEEK 5: LOWER BODY 4

EXERCISE	SETS	REPS	TEMPO	REST
A1 Backward Sled Drags	5	40 Meters	2 - 1 - X - 1	2 Minutes
A2 Lying Leg Curls	5	15	4 - 1 - X - 1	60 Seconds
ONCE ALL SETS HAVE BEEN COMPLETED REST FOR 3 MINUTES				
B1 Leg Extension	4	12	4 - 1 - X - 1	60 Seconds
B2 Lying Leg Press	4	20	4 - 1 - X - 1	60 Seconds
B3 Hip Abductor	4	20	4 - 1 - X - 1	60 Seconds
ONCE ALL SETS HAVE BEEN COMPLETED REST FOR 3 MINUTES				

WEEK 6: CHEST & BACK 2

EXERCISE	SETS	REPS	TEMPO	REST
A1 Thick Grip D/B Bench Press	5	8 - 12	3 - 1 - X - 1	60 Seconds
A2 Single Arms Rows	5	12	2 - 1 - X - 1	60 Seconds
ONCE ALL SETS HAVE BEEN COMPLETED REST FOR 3 MINUTES				
B1 Swiss Ball Press Up	4	10	3 - 1 - X - 1	60 Seconds
B2 Lat Pull Downs	4	12 - 15	2 - 1 - X - 1	60 Seconds
ONCE ALL SETS HAVE BEEN COMPLETED REST FOR 3 MINUTES				
C Rowing	8	1 Minute	FLAT OUT	60 Seconds

WEEK 6: LEGS & ABS 2

EXERCISE	SETS	REPS	TEMPO	REST
A1 Good Mornings	5	10	3 - 1 - X - 1	60 Seconds
A2 Leg Extensions	5	20	3 - 1 - X - 1	60 Seconds
ONCE ALL SETS HAVE BEEN COMPLETED REST FOR 3 MINUTES				
B1 Leg Press	4	20	3 - 1 - X - 1	60 Seconds
B2 Hanging Leg Raises Weighted	4	20	2 - 1 - 1 - 1	60 Seconds
ONCE ALL SETS HAVE BEEN COMPLETED REST FOR 3 MINUTES				
C1 KBR	4	20	2 - 1 - 1 - 1	60 Seconds
D Bike Sprint	6	1 Minute	FLAT OUT	60 Seconds

WEEK 6: SHOULDERS & ARMS 2

EXERCISE	SETS	REPS	TEMPO	REST
A1 Standing Shoulder Press	4	12	3 - 1 - X - 1	60 Seconds
A2 Any Grip Chins	4	12	3 - 1 - X - 1	60 Seconds
ONCE ALL SETS HAVE BEEN COMPLETED REST FOR 3 MINUTES				
B1 Lateral Raises	4	20	3 - 1 - X - 1	60 Seconds
B2 Preacher Curls	4	20	4 - 1 - X - 1	60 Seconds
ONCE ALL SETS HAVE BEEN COMPLETED REST FOR 3 MINUTES				
C1 Lying Tricep Ext	3	12 - 15	2 - 1 - 1 - 1	60 Seconds
C2 Cable Snatch	3	15	2 - 1 - 1 - 1	60 Seconds
ONCE ALL SETS HAVE BEEN COMPLETED REST FOR 3 MINUTES				
D Prowler	4	60 Meters	FLAT OUT	120 Seconds

When the head goose gets tired, it rotates back in the wing and another goose flies point. It is sensible to take turns doing demanding jobs, whether with people or with geese flying south. Geese honk from behind to encourage those up front to keep up their speed.

What messages do we give when we honk from behind? Finally — and this is important — when a goose gets sick or is wounded by gunshot, and falls out of formation, two other geese fall out with that goose and follow it down to lend help and protection. They stay with the fallen goose until it is able to fly or until it dies, and only then do they launch out on their own, or with another formation to catch up with their group.

If we have the sense of a goose, we will stand by each other like that

Well, the players had read the geese story and after a few minutes they started honking and laughing. I'm sitting down the front of the bus thinking "I now know you fuckers are thinking you are the dogs bollocks" and when a team is in this mental state there is usually a lesson in humility coming! I remember doing the warm up and the players didn't have that edge as they usually had before games, they thought they were above Pontypool and literally thought that they only had to go through the motions and we would win. I remember about five minutes into the game knowing we were going to lose, thinking about the post match analysis. I was going to open it up with Honk Fucking Honk. We went on and won the league that season, after that loss the players learnt very quickly to work as a team just like the geese and never became complacent.

Remember, we all make mistakes. It is only fools who keep repeating the same mistakes and expect a different outcome.

Next I've put a 6 week plan that I used with a female fitness model. This sport requires the athletes to have minimum body fat and have an athletic look. I worked closely with Nina Ross and came up with the following 6 week plan. The plan had to be planned around her job and her role as Mum, to her amazing little girl, Annabel.

Nina Ross British Champion Bodybuilder

When I first met Phil back in September 2011 I thought I was reasonably educated and quite well read in the field of health and nutrition however, i was soon blown away by the knowledge i gained from Phil both on a health and nutrition perspective which he also would deliver in such a digestible way that my understanding and my own performance progressed to another level.

Phil not only taught me some valuable lessons about health and nutrition but his expertise in the field of strength training quite simply took away all the complexity that is easy to get tangled in and showed me methods that not only made sense but also gained phenomenal results. I have gained 3 British titles since working with Phil and he has now given me the confidence and the knowledge to take ownership of not only my own progress but also to help others reach their goals. Phil is a great teacher and without him would never have made the necessary changes to reach international level.

Conclusion

Now you can see, for exercise to be effective in getting you results, it is imperative for you to first get healthy. Remember, exercise is a form of stress; you cannot keep loading stress on top of more stress. So, find ways in your life to reduce stress, and this will allow exercise to give you the results you need to become lean and healthy.

If you are new to exercise, find a good trainer who is well qualified both in nutrition and exercise. Look at their track record and their testimonials and make sure you are able to work with them.

Above all else, make sure you have a goal that allows you to train with a purpose during every single training session.

Final word

I hope that you have enjoyed reading the 10 Habits for Maximum Fat Loss, as much as I have in putting them together. May I wish you the very best for the future, and, remember, you deserve to be happy, healthy and lean - you have just got to apply the 10 habits and you will achieve.

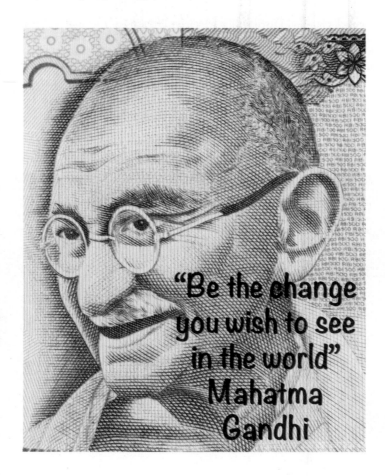

"Be the change you wish to see in the world"
Mahatma Gandhi